SWNHS

C20108929

D1142014

nt Decisions

ary

Library
Knowledge Spa
Royal Cornwall Hospital
Treliske
Truro. TR1 3HD

General Surgery Outpatient Decisions

SECOND EDITION

Edited by

MICHAEL GAUNT MD, FRCS

*Consultant Vascular Surgeon, Cambridge University Hospitals NHS
Foundation Trust, Cambridge, UK
Associate Lecturer, Cambridge University, UK*

TJUN TANG MRCS

*Specialist Registrar in General & Vascular Surgery, Eastern Deanery, UK
Clinical Research Associate, Cambridge Vascular Unit, Cambridge University
Hospitals NHS Foundation Trust, Cambridge, UK*

and

STEWART WALSH MSc, MRCS

*Specialist Registrar in General & Vascular Surgery, Eastern Deanery, UK
Clinical Research Associate, Cambridge Vascular Unit, Cambridge University
Hospitals NHS Foundation Trust, Cambridge, UK*

Foreword by

STEPHEN BREARLEY MChir, FRCS
*Consultant Surgeon
Director, The Whipps Cross Higher Surgery Course*

Radcliffe Publishing
Oxford • New York

Radcliffe Publishing Ltd
18 Marcham Road
Abingdon
Oxon OX14 1AA
United Kingdom

www.radcliffe-oxford.com
Electronic catalogue and worldwide online ordering facility.

© 2008 Michael Gaunt, Tjun Tang and Stewart Walsh

First Edition 2000 (published by Arnold)

Michael Gaunt, Tjun Tang and Stewart Walsh have asserted their right under the Copyright, Designs and Patents Act 1998 to be identified as the authors of this work.

All rights reserved. No part of this publication may be reproduced, stored in a retrieval system or transmitted, in any form or by any means, electronic, mechanical, photocopying, recording or otherwise, without the prior permission of the copyright owner.

British Library Cataloguing in Publication Data

A catalogue record for this book is available from the British Library.

ISBN-13: 978 184619 191 6

Typeset by Pindar NZ, Auckland, New Zealand
Printed and bound by TJI Digital, Padstow, Cornwall, UK

Contents

Foreword

Doctors in clinical practice spend most of their time making decisions, often without realising it. The decisions most often recognised as such are those concerning treatment – not simply what treatment to recommend but whether to recommend any treatment at all – but decision making starts whenever a doctor first meets a patient, not when the patient's work up has been completed. Doctors are constantly having to decide what questions to ask in the light of the patient's presenting complaint, what physical examination to undertake, whether to investigate further, what investigations to do, what explanation to give to the patient at each stage, whether the information gleaned is sufficient to make a sound diagnosis and develop a treatment plan, and so on.

In order to be soundly based, all these decisions need to be founded on an understanding of the pathology of surgical and other diseases, the symptoms to which they may give rise, the physical signs which they may produce and the investigations which may be used to detect them, including the reliability of those investigations. Much of this information is conveniently brought together in this book, which aims to lead the inexperienced surgical trainee systematically through the assessment and management of a wide range of conditions frequently seen in surgical outpatient clinics, pointing out some common pitfalls along the way.

That such a book is needed is beyond doubt. Just as well-informed and thoughtful decision making leads to optimal patient care, poor decision making, even over apparently trivial matters, may lead to patients being harmed and to litigation. Many more actions in medical negligence result from poor decisions than from poor surgical technique. Yet it is still not rare for young surgeons to be asked to see patients in clinics without direct supervision and without their having been given any specific training in how to meet the particular demands of outpatient work. The decisions these doctors make, whether to investigate, to treat, to follow-up or to discharge, may not be systematically checked. Surgical trainees who may be about to face the challenge of outpatient work for the first time, or in an unfamiliar speciality, are likely to find that the advice and wisdom contained in this volume gives them the framework they need to perform effectively from the outset.

The book may also be useful to those approaching surgical exams. Nowadays, surgical viva voce examinations tend to focus not on surgical topics but on clinical scenarios. The examiners want to find out whether candidates can analyse clinical information logically, draw appropriate conclusions and propose rational management strategies. These are precisely the intellectual processes which this book seeks to inculcate and to foster.

Sadly, there are still a few surgeons who see outpatient clinics as a regrettable necessity in order to recruit patients on whom they can operate. Often this point of view seems to go hand in hand with an unsophisticated and unthinking approach to decision making. The reflex response which equates one hernia with one operation or bleeding at stool with a flexible sigmoidoscopy is neither stimulating for the doctor nor good for the patient. Sophistication in diagnosis and decision making not only leads to optimal patient care but enormously increases the job satisfaction of the doctor. I hope that readers of this book will find that it increases their enjoyment of outpatient work, as well as helping them to perform to a high standard in the clinic.

Stephen Brearley MChir, FRCS
Consultant Surgeon
Director, The Whipps Cross Higher Surgery Course
August 2008

Preface to second edition

Welcome to the second edition of *General Surgery Outpatient Decisions*. I found publication of the first edition a very rewarding experience, especially when people who had read the book took time to contact me and tell me how much they enjoyed it. Occasions that stick in the memory include when a professor of surgery from Turkey who was visiting Cambridge tracked me down in Addenbrooke's Hospital to tell me that he had found my book in the library and had spent three hours sitting on the floor reading it. More recently a delegate approached me after a teaching session at another hospital to tell me how he used the book every day and recommended it to all his junior colleagues. The book was now dog-eared and full of his notes, written in the margin, which was exactly how I envisaged the book would be used.

Since the first edition was published, surgical outpatient services have undergone tremendous change. The traditional general surgical clinic has largely been replaced by specialist clinics where decisions on patient management are taken by multidisciplinary teams (MDTs). Breast clinics are the most striking example of this approach and there is no doubting the improvement in care and outcomes that has resulted. Therefore, this new edition is a multi-author edition to take account of the multidisciplinary approach. However, working in MDTs brings its own challenges, not least because surgeons are still expected to take overall responsibility for the patient, especially when things go wrong. Increasing sub-specialisation also brings challenges to the trainee surgeon experiencing that speciality for the first time. MDTs develop their own way of working and decision making, which can be difficult to understand for the newcomer. In order to reflect this new way of working, I have recruited two surgical registrars of the highest calibre: Tjun Tang and Stewart Walsh, whose experience of working in this environment is still current.

Once again, this book attempts to provide the necessary background information to enable rational decision making in a concise and economical style. I hope you find this book useful in your everyday practice and in preparation for your professional examinations, where the question, 'Yes the theory is all very well but what would you actually do?' can be the most difficult to answer; and may make the difference between success and failure.

When I wrote the first edition I had no idea how far across the world it would spread. A medical secretary from our hospital, on holiday in Vietnam, wandered into a bookshop, found my book for sale there and took a photograph to prove it! Although this book is written by surgeons working in the British National Health Service, I believe the medical problems described in this book are common to all healthcare systems. All surgeons have to be trained and go through the process of dealing with unfamiliar clinical conditions for the first time. Therefore, I hope surgeons from all countries will use this book as a useful foundation on which to build their own personal knowledge.

Finally, I would like to thank my fellow editors and the expert contributors to this book for their hard work and dedication to the cause.

Michael Gaunt
Cambridge, UK
August 2008

Introduction

A new batch of trainee surgeons attends their first outpatient clinic of a new speciality. They are anxious. They may have had some experience of this speciality as medical students and, like all good doctors, have read a textbook about the subject before starting in the post. However, they have yet to acquire a 'feel' for the speciality and to obtain the practical knowledge necessary to enable them to identify the crucial issues in each consultation and to function efficiently. The result of this uncertainty is that in outpatient clinics all over the world as the jobs rotate, trainee surgeons spend the first few weeks seeing patients who have been brought back for review by their predecessors. They in turn, unable to identify anything specifically wrong with the patients but not confident enough to discharge them, bring the patients back for their successors to do the same. The cycle continues at great inconvenience to the patients and at great cost to all healthcare systems. The clinics are crowded and time available to see those patients who are in real need is reduced, thus increasing the possibility of mistakes.

In general, few doctors receive any formal training in how to conduct an outpatient consultation or how to compose and dictate an outpatient letter. The result of poorly structured consultations and difficulties with communication is letters such as this one:

> Dear Dr. I reviewed Mrs Smith who is a delightful old lady in the outpatient clinic today her symptoms do not seem too bad at the moment although she is getting more pain now so I advised her just to increase the painkillers if and when she thought it was necessary and we will review the situation again at her next outpatient visit.

Despite the lack of punctuation, this doctor is trying to project the image of a bright and confident clinician who is constantly amused by the stream of old characters referred to him by the kind-hearted GP. However, any doctor who does not know the patient will have gained no useful information from this letter. The diagnosis is not mentioned or put into context with regard to other co-existing conditions or the patient's overall prognosis. The current dose of painkiller is not mentioned and no attempt has been made to explain why Mrs Smith is getting more pain. What is the overall treatment plan and what are the alternative therapeutic options if increasing the painkillers does not work? The only plan is to review the patient again, but when – next week, next month, next year? Unfortunately, these types of letters are often attached to very large sets of notes, which the next clinic doctor has to spend valuable time reading in order to ascertain the exact purpose of the consultation. Also, when the GP is called to see 'this delightful old lady' as an emergency because she has reached the maximum dose of painkiller and is still in pain, the GP may be more inclined to admit her to hospital, because the latest outpatient letter does not suggest any alternative course of action.

Mr Jones is 41 years old and is attending the surgical clinic to have his piles injected. He has been coming every three months for the past two years. On his first visit he saw the senior surgeon, who thought his small amount of rectal bleeding was probably due to haemorrhoids and would settle down with injection sclerotherapy. Injecting piles is an unpleasant task, which is often delegated to the most junior member of the team. Therefore, Mr Jones has seen several different trainee surgeons who have each injected the piles every three months. Each time, the bleeding improves for a few weeks after the injection but then returns. Unfortunately, as well as piles Mr Jones also has a rectal carcinoma at 10cm from the anal margin. At the time of his first consultation it was small and obscured by faeces and therefore not seen by the consultant. Now it is much bigger, but still not visible to the trainee surgeon injecting his piles. If the senior surgeon had known that the bleeding had not settled down he would have investigated further and the carcinoma would have been detected. Unfortunately, the senior surgeon is busy seeing the new referrals and the 'difficult' cases, and the clinic nurse automatically sends the 'piles' down to the trainee surgeon. By the time the cancer is diagnosed it will probably be inoperable.

These are just a few examples of the kinds of things that can go wrong in outpatient clinics of all specialities. They are problems caused by inexperience, unfamiliarity, the fear of making mistakes, the pressure of patient numbers and a lack of training.

Doctors tend to learn by experience, with all the pitfalls that entails. Most public healthcare systems are so busy that not every patient can be seen by the senior surgeon every time; and junior medical staff are integral to the running of the outpatient service. Inevitably the level of ability and experience of junior staff will vary, but for the patient only one level of care is acceptable – the best. Some may say this is well known and junior staff are expected to deal only with straightforward new cases or routine follow-ups. But straightforward cases are only straightforward up to the point where the patient reports a new symptom or complication. Follow-ups are considered easy, but is this true? In standard textbooks the new doctor will find little help on how to follow up patients. The new doctor may be faced with the choice of either walking down to the senior doctor's room, past the crowded waiting area full of disgruntled patients and exasperated clinic nurses, to ask the advice of the busy consultant for the fifth time this clinic; or ignoring the new symptom; or bringing the patient back to clinic after a time to see someone else; or perhaps ordering an investigation to buy some time – what do you do?

These problems are not easily solved, but we hope this book may help in some small way. Research for this book has been difficult because the information on the outpatient management of patients, especially follow-ups, is difficult to obtain. There is no standard management of each condition in every patient and this book does not aim to set one. The aim of this book is to describe a reasonable line of management suitable for most patients, but one which the reader should modify to take account of individual patient factors and local variations and preferences in practice.

Michael Gaunt
Tjun Tang
Stewart Walsh
Cambridge, UK
August 2008

About the editors

Tjun Tang graduated from Cambridge University in 2000 with distinction in surgery. He undertook house jobs and his basic surgical training in Cambridge and he joined the East Anglian specialist registrar rotation in General Surgery in 2004. He is currently completing his MD thesis on imaging carotid plaque inflammation using contrast-enhanced MRI, and he wishes to sub-specialise in vascular surgery. He has published over 50 peer-reviewed manuscripts and has co-written several revision books for the MRCS examination. He is actively involved in undergraduate teaching at Addenbrooke's Hospital in Cambridge and has been an examiner for the Final MB.

Stewart Walsh graduated from University College Dublin in 1997. After completing house jobs in Northern Ireland, he undertook basic surgical training in the north-west of England. He joined the Cambridge specialist registrar rotation in General Surgery in 2002. In 2006, he obtained an MSc from the University of Liverpool. He has published over 50 peer-reviewed papers and, at present, is completing his Master of Surgery thesis on the peri-operative care of vascular surgery patients. He teaches on both the Basic Surgical Skills course and the Care of the Critically Ill Surgical Patient course.

Michael Gaunt qualified in medicine with distinction at Leicester University in 1988 and undertook his surgical training in hospitals around the Midlands. He was elected Fellow of the Royal College of Surgeons of England in 1992 and undertook a period of research leading to the award of a doctorate of medicine with distinction. During his training he received a number of research awards, including the Moynihan Medal of the Association of Surgeons of Great Britain and Ireland the Founders Prize of the Vascular Society of Great Britain and Ireland, and the European Vascular Surgery Prize. Mr Gaunt was elected Hunterian Professor of Surgery of the Royal College of Surgeons of England in 1996.

In 1999 he was appointed consultant vascular surgeon at Addenbrooke's Hospital and associate lecturer at Cambridge University. Mr Gaunt has published over 100 peer-reviewed research papers and is actively involved in both undergraduate and postgraduate medical education.

List of contributors

Miles Banwell PhD, FRCS
Specialist Registrar in Plastic Surgery
Eastern Deanery

Satyajit Bhattacharya MS, FRCS
Consultant Surgeon
Hepato-Biliary and Pancreatic Surgery Unit
The Royal London Hospital, London

Edward Cheong BSc(Hons), BMedSc, MD, FRCS (Gen Surg)
Specialist Registrar in Upper GI Surgery
Norfolk and Norwich University Hospital, Norfolk

David Cooper MA, MS, FRCS
Specialist Registrar in Vascular Surgery
Cambridge Vascular Unit
Cambridge University Hospitals NHS Foundation Trust, Cambridge

Bill Fleming FRACS, FRCS
Consultant Endocrine Surgeon
Hammersmith Hospital
Imperial College Healthcare NHS Trust, London

Richard Hardwick MD, FRCS
Consultant Surgeon and Lead Clinician for Upper GI Cancer
Cambridge Oesophago-Gastric Centre
Cambridge University Hospitals NHS Foundation Trust, Cambridge

Michael Irwin FRCS, FRCS (Plast)
Consultant Plastic and Reconstructive Surgeon
Department of Plastic and Reconstructive Surgery
Cambridge University Hospitals NHS Foundation Trust, Cambridge

Neville Jamieson MD, FRCS
Consultant Hepatobiliary and Transplant Surgeon
Cambridge University Hospitals NHS Foundation Trust, Cambridge

Fiona MacNeill MBBS, FRCS, MD
Consultant Breast Surgeon and Breast Tutor
Royal College of Surgeons of England
Royal Marsden Hospital, London

Adrian O'Sullivan MB, FRCSI
Specialist Registrar
Hepato-Biliary and Pancreatic Surgery Unit
The Royal London Hospital, London

Umar Sadat MRCS
Clinical Research Associate
Cambridge Vascular Unit and University Department of Radiology
Cambridge University Hospitals NHS Foundation Trust, Cambridge

Paris Tekkis BMedSci, BM BS, MD, FRCS
Senior Lecturer and Consultant Colorectal Surgeon
Imperial College London

Henry Tilney MBBS, MRCS
Specialist Registrar in General Surgery
South West Thames Higher Surgical Training Rotation

Alastair Windsor MD, FRCS, FRCS(Ed)
Consultant Surgeon and Honorary Senior Lecturer
University College London Hospitals, London

List of abbreviations

^{131}I	radio-iodine
^{131}MIBG	meta-iodobenzylguanidine
5-ASA	5-aminosalicylate
5FU	5-fluorouracil
5-HIAA	5-hydroxyindoleacetic acid
5-HT	5-hydroxytryptamine
^{99m}Tc	technetium-99m
AAA	abdominal aortic aneurysm
ABPI	ankle-brachial pressure index
ABS	Association of Breast Surgery
ACE	angiotensin-converting enzyme
ACTH	adrenocorticotropic hormone
ADH	atypical ductal hyperplasia
AFP	alpha-foetoprotein
AIDS	acquired immunodeficiency syndrome
ALP	alkaline phosphatase
ALT	alanine transaminase
ANA	antinuclear antibodies
ANCA	antineutrophil cytoplasmic antibody
ANCA	antineutrophil cytoplasmic autoantibodies
APA	aldosterone-producing adenoma
APT	prothrombin antigen
ARDS	acute respiratory distress syndrome
ASCA	anti-*Saccharomyces cerevisiae* antibodies
AST	aspartate aminotransferase
AXR	abdominal X-ray
BASO	British Association of Surgical Oncology
BBC	benign breast change
BC	breast cancer
BCN	breast care nurse
beta hCG	beta human chorionic gonadotropin
BP	blood pressure
BT	Breslow thickness
BU	breast unit
C&S	culture and sensitivity test
C14	glycocholate
CA 19-9	carbohydrate antigen 19-9
CAD	cystic adventitial disease
CBD	common bile duct
CBT	carotid body tumour
CCA	common carotid artery
CE	capsule endoscopy
CEA	carcinoembryonic antigen
CHOP	cyclophosphamide, doxorubicin, vincristine and prednisone
CML	chronic myeloid leukaemia
CRP	C-reactive protein
CT	computed tomography
CTA/MRA	computed tomography angiography/magnetic resonance angiogram
CTD	connective tissue disease/disorders
CWD	continuous wave Doppler

CXR	chest X-ray
CXR-PA	chest X-ray, posterior anterior view
DCIS	ductal carcinoma in situ
DF118	dihydrocodeine
DMSA	dimercaptosuccinic acid
DSA	digital subtraction angiography
DVT	deep-venous thrombosis
ECA	external carotid artery
ECG	electrocardiogram
EHIDA	99Tcm-diethyl-IDA
ELISA	enzyme-linked immunosorbent assay
ENT	ear, nose and throat
EPO	evening primrose oil
ERCP	endoscopic retrograde cholangiopancreatography
ER/PR	oestrogen/progesterone receptors
ESR	erythrocyte sedimentation rate
EUA	examination under anaesthetic
EUS	entoscopic ultrasound
EVAR	endovascular repair
EVLA	endovenous laser
F/A	fibroadenoma
FACS	follow-up after colorectal surgery
FAP	familial adenomatous polyposis
FBC	full blood count
FHH	familial hypercalcaemic hypocalciuria
FMD	fibromuscular dysplasia
FNAC	fine-needle aspiration cytology
FNH	focal nodular hyperplasia
FOB	faecal occult blood test
GA	general anaesthetic
gamma GT	gamma-glutamyl-transpeptidase
GIST	gastrointestinal stromal tumour
GnRH	gonadotropin-releasing hormone
GOJ	gastro-oesophageal junction
GORD	gastro-oesophageal reflux disease
GTN	glyceryl trinitrate
H2RA	H2-receptor antagonist
Hb	haemoglobin
HBsAg	hepatitis B surface antigen
HCC	hepatocellular carcinoma
HDL	high-density lipoprotein
HHT	hereditary haemorrhagic telangiectasia
HIB	*Haemophilus influenzae* type b
HNPCC	hereditary non-polyposis colorectal cancer
HPV	human papillomavirus
HPZ	high-pressure zone
HRT	hormone replacement therapy
IBD	inflammatory bowel disease
ICA	internal carotid artery
IgA	immunoglobulin A
IgG	immunoglobulin G
IgM	immunoglobulin M
IMA	inferior mesenteric artery
INR	international normalised ratio

IPA	idiopathic hyperaldosteronism
IPSID	immunoproliferative small intestine disease
IVC	inferior vena cava
LCIS	lobular carcinoma in situ
LDL	low-density lipoprotein
LDS	lipodermatosclerosis
LFT	liver function test
LIF	left iliac fossa
LN	lymph node
LUQ	left upper quadrant
MALT	mucosa-associated lymphoid tissue
MAOI	monoamine oxidase inhibitor
MC&S	multi culture and sensitivity
MCV	mean corpuscular volume
MDM	multidisciplinary meeting
MDT	multidisciplinary team
MEN	multiple endocrine neoplasia
MI	myocardial infarction
MIBG	meta-iodobenzylguanidine
MLD	manual lymphatic drainage
MRCP	magnetic resonance cholangiopancreatography
MRI	magnetic resonance imaging
MST	morphine sulphate
MTBE	methyl tert-butyl ether
MTC	medullary thyroid cancer (medullary carcinoma of thyroid)
NAC	nipple areolar complex
NHSBSP	National Health Service Breast Screening Programme
NICE	National Institute for Health and Clinical Excellence
NIDDM	noninsulin-dependent diabetes mellitus
NP59	6-beta-iodomethyl-19-norcholesterol
NSAID	non-steroidal anti-inflammatory drug
OA	osteoarthritis
OCP	oral contraceptive pill
OGD	oesophago-gastro-duodenoscopy
OPD	outpatient department
OPSI	overwhelming post-splenectomy infection
PAIR	percutaneous fine-needle puncture, aspiration, injection of hypertonic saline and reaspiration
PAN	polyarteritis nodosa
PAS	p-aminosalicylic acid
PDT	photodynamic therapy
PEC	percutaneous endoscopic colostomy
PET	positron emission tomography
PG12	prostacyclin
PGE1	prostaglandin E1
PID	pelvic inflammatory disease
P-J	Peutz-Jeghers syndrome
PPAM	post-amputation mobility
PPI	proton-pump inhibitor
PPPD	pylorus-preserving pancreatoduodenectomy
PTC	percutaneous transhepatic cholangiography
PTFE	polytetrafluoroethylene
PTH	parathyroid hormone (parathormone)
PV	polycythaemia vera

PV/ESR	plasma viscosity/erythrocyte sedimentation rate
PVD	peripheral vascular disease
RA	rheumatoid arthritis
RAS	renal artery stenosis
RET	proto-oncogene reticuloendothelium
RFA	radiofrequency ablation
RT	radiotherapy
RUQ	right upper quadrant
SBE	small bowel enema
SBFT	small bowel follow through
SCC	squamous cell carcinoma
SeHCAT test	75-selenium homotaurocholic acid retention test
SFA	superficial femoral artery
SFJ	saphenofemoral junction
SGOT	serum glutamic oxaloacetic transaminase
SGPT	serum glutamic pyruvic transaminase
SLE	systemic lupus erythematosus
SMA	superior mesenteric artery
SOB	shortness of breath
SOD	sphincter of Oddi dysfunction
SPECT	single photon emission computed tomography
SS	systemic sclerosis
SSV	short saphenous vein
TAA	thoraco-abdominal aneurysms
TACE	transarterial chemoembolisation
TART	transanal resection of tumour
TBPI	toe-brachial pressure index
TED	thromboembolic disease
TEM	transanal endoscopic microsurgery
TENS	transcutaneous electric nerve stimulation
TIA	transient ischaemic attack
TIPS	transjugular intrahepatic portosystemic shunt
TOCS	thoracic outlet compression syndrome
TPN	total parenteral nutrition
TSH	thyroid-stimulating hormone
U&E	urea and electrolyte
UC	ulcerative colitis
UCSF	University of California, San Francisco
USS	ultrasound scanning
UTI	urinary tract infection
VNUS®	radiofrequency ablation procedure developed by VNUS
VIPoma	vasoactive intestinal peptide tumour
VBI	vertebrobasilar ischaemia
VA	vertebral artery
VLDL	very low-density lipoprotein
WCC	white cell count
ZE	Zollinger-Ellison syndrome
ZN	Ziehl-Neelsen

General outpatient·issues

Michael Gaunt, Tjun Tang and Stewart Walsh

ONE

The outpatient consultation
Purpose of the outpatient consultation
It is worth emphasising the simple but fundamental point that each consultation has a purpose. If the doctor cannot identify a purpose for another consultation then the patient should be discharged. Discharging a patient does not mean casting them off into the wilderness. Patients should be discharged with a plan and instructions for re-referral if appropriate.

The structure of the consultation
Each consultation should have a structure, which becomes routine. In this way important stages and information are not overlooked. Doctors develop their own routine, but a simple structure might consist of the following.
✧ Read the referral letter.
✧ Read the previous clinic letters and old notes.
✧ Be clear about the purpose of the consultation before entering the room.
✧ Introduce yourself and who you work for.
✧ Put the patient at ease; ascertain who has accompanied the patient.
✧ Explain what you are going to do, e.g. take a history then perform an examination.
✧ Take the history.
✧ Perform the relevant examination.
✧ Have a think and decide what to do.
✧ Discuss any investigations or treatments with the patient.
✧ Answer any questions.
✧ Give concluding remarks and instructions.
✧ Insert a handwritten entry in the notes, include diagrams etc.
✧ Dictate the clinic letter.

The referral letter
The consultation begins before the patient is seen, when the doctor reads the referral letter in the case of new patient or the last clinic letter in the case of follow-ups. For new patients, the referral letter usually contains the reason the patient has been sent to the clinic and other useful information such as a list of co-existing medical conditions and a list of current medication. The referral letter sets the scene and provides useful information, but this should n.ot be allowed to unduly influence the consultation. Once patient contact is made the diagnostic process starts again from scratch with the history and examination.

The previous clinic letter and notes
The previous notes are in the clinic for a purpose – they are there for you to read. In general it is better to have as much information as possible before starting a consultation. Reading the notes puts the current presenting illness in context and prevents any repetition of investigations. An apparently successful consultation can be undermined by the patient informing you that they have already had the investigations you were proposing and they were all normal. You are embarrassed and the patient leaves with the impression that you didn't know what you were doing. Reading a very large set of notes during a busy clinic is not feasible. This is where a detailed previous clinic letter is invaluable in summarising what has gone before.

Purpose of the consultation
New patients
In the case of new patients the objectives of the consultation are either to reach a diagnosis or to exclude any serious pathology related to that speciality. If it is suspected that the patient's symptoms may be caused by a potentially serious or malignant condition, investigations will need to be performed and reviewed promptly.

Follow-up patients
Seeing the follow-up patients is a task often delegated to junior staff, who may lack a clear understanding of the consultation objectives. In surgery, follow-up patients fall into three categories: those with new undiagnosed conditions who are returning for the results of investigations; those with chronic conditions that are being monitored; and post-operative patients.

New conditions under investigation
These patients are returning to clinic to receive the results of investigations performed so far. The patient will have been seen previously, either by you or by a colleague. Read the previous clinic letter and review the notes to remind yourself of the case. It is useful to ensure that the results of all investigations are available before you meet the patient. This may involve telephoning for the results, out of earshot of the patient. Decide whether the results are diagnostic or whether further investigations are necessary. If the results are diagnostic and the outcome is bad news, e.g. cancer, plan how you are going to break the news. If the results are equivocal it may be necessary to repeat the history and examination to detect new features that may have developed and will aid the diagnosis. Think about possible further investigations and the timescale for obtaining these results. It may be that the results are not diagnostic but serious causes have been excluded and the need to obtain a diagnosis is less urgent. If the results are diagnostic and good news, decide whether further follow up will be required or whether the patient can be discharged with advice.

Chronic conditions
The purpose of the consultation in the case of these patients is to detect whether the patient's condition is stable, improving or deteriorating and to detect any complications of the underlying condition or treatment. Ideally the previous clinic letter should contain the reason for the follow-up, what to look for and an objective description of the clinical condition at that time to allow comparison with the present. It may be time for a routine investigation to be performed, e.g. yearly mammogram, three-monthly FBC. If the patient's condition has been stable for some time it may be appropriate to decrease the frequency of outpatient consultations or to discharge the patient, with clear instructions to the GP and the patient on when to re-refer. Do not automatically bring the patient back at the same time interval as did the last clinic doctor.

Another useful option is the 'open appointment'. With an open appointment the patient is not given another clinic date but has open access to make an appointment directly if his or her condition recurs. This system works best for sensible patients, familiar with their clinical condition, who have been stable for a long period but who may relapse and require prompt treatment. Usually, open appointments have a time limit, e.g. a year, after which a new referral through the GP is required if the condition recurs. Open appointments must be used sparingly; otherwise the clinic can become overloaded and open to abuse. Some patients make appointments for an opinion on unrelated conditions or even for other members of their families! Never underestimate the importance of the GP as gatekeeper to the proper functioning of the health service.

Post-operative patients

The purpose of these consultations is to decide whether the operation has been successful in achieving its objectives, e.g. relieving the patient's symptoms or completely removing a tumour. Prior to seeing the patient, read the notes to determine the operation performed and whether there were any intra-operative or post-operative complications that require long-term follow-up, e.g. damage to the common bile duct. If tissue was removed at the time of operation and sent for histology, make sure you read the histology report even if this was routine. Occasionally, routine histology can reveal occult cancer that was never suspected but that may necessitate further management.

If the operation was to remove cancer, determine whether this was all removed or whether the tumour extended to the radial or longitudinal resection margins, indicating residual disease requiring further surgery or adjuvant therapy. The histological grade of the tumour and any evidence of lymph node spread or vascular invasion may indicate that adjuvant radiotherapy/chemotherapy is required. Decide on the outlines of a treatment plan before breaking any bad news to the patient. The patient may modify the plan according to their own preferences, but uncertainty on the part of the doctor at this difficult time is to be avoided.

Meeting the patient

Thoroughly prepared, the doctor enters the consultation room. Ascertain which person in the room is the patient, and introduce yourself. Many patients will be expecting to see the consultant, because that is the name on their appointment card. Who you are and your position in the hierarchy needs to be explained. Determine the relationship of other people in the room to the patient. Do not automatically assume they are relatives. In this way you will avoid an embarrassing exposure of a patient in front of a neighbour or volunteer driver.

It may be appropriate to put the patient at ease with some friendly comments before launching in to the consultation proper, e.g. apologise for the long wait. It is often useful to explain the structure of the consultation to the patient: 'What I'd like to do is to ask you some questions, then examine you and then we'll discuss what we are going to do.'

History and examination

Obtain the relevant history and perform the relevant examination. Examination in the outpatient clinic can be difficult. The patient may be relatively immobile and encased in numerous layers of clothing, which take a long time to remove. It is frustrating to wait – but more frustrating to miss an obvious and vital clinical sign due to inadequate examination.

Have a think: the management plan

Many doctors seem embarrassed to be seen thinking, but it is actually what we are paid to do. Once the history and examination are complete and the patient is getting dressed, there is time to record and reflect on the findings and formulate a management plan. For simple and routine problems this will be brief, but for more complicated problems this may be the time to obtain more senior advice or consult a helpful text.

Medicine is a partnership between patient and doctor. The more the patient understands about what you are trying to achieve, the more likely they are to comply with the investigations or treatment. Therefore, although you have a management plan, you must be prepared to modify it depending on the patient's preferences. Always allow time for the patient to ask any questions, and answer them as fully as you can.

Concluding remarks

The consultation has to be brought to an end. Ideally this occurs when all questions are answered and everyone understands what is involved. However, there may be occasions when a more formal signal that the consultation is drawing to a close is needed. Usually standing up and closing the notes folder is taken as the relevant cue. Final remarks may consist of: 'You'll receive an appointment for the ultrasound scan through the post in a few weeks' time and we'll see you again in the clinic a week after the scan to discuss the results.'

Handwritten entry in the notes
A handwritten entry in the notes is necessary as a contemporaneous record of the consultation and the management plan. Diagrams can be included to illustrate clinical findings, which are difficult to incorporate in the typed letter. Also, a detailed handwritten note is invaluable some days later when the audio-typist reports that the tape from the clinic is corrupted and you need to dictate the letters again.

Dictating the clinic letter
Matters concerning the composition of clinic letters and other forms of communication are covered in the next section.

Communication
Good communication is at the heart of good medicine, and this is particularly the case in outpatient medicine. A doctor needs to communicate effectively with the patient and the patient's relatives at the time of the consultation. The importance of this has been recognised in most medical schools, and communication with patients, in particular breaking bad news, now forms part of most courses. However, a more neglected area is communication with other healthcare professionals. The most common means of communication in the clinic is the outpatient letter.

Communication with the patient
This consists mainly of verbal communication during the consultation itself. The importance of introductions and determining the relationship to the patient of any accompanying person has already been emphasised. If the patient is accompanied by a member of staff from a nursing or residential home, this person may be a useful source of information and may be able to relay instructions back to the nursing home. Relatives may be another useful source of information but, alternatively, may try to dominate the consultation with their own interpretation of events. Generally if the patient is capable of answering questions they should be allowed to do so without interference, and relatives should be encouraged to keep quiet. However, the relative may be an important carer for the patient, so it is worth avoiding alienation. Explaining that you wish the patient to answer their own questions at this point in the consultation – but you would be interested in the relative's observations at the end – may control the situation.

Breaking bad news
This usually means a diagnosis of cancer or other serious disease. Prior to the consultation decide how certain the information is or whether further investigation is needed. If there is no reasonable doubt, then a plan of how to break the news is needed.

There are numerous helpful texts on the subject of how to break bad news, which cover the subject in more detail than can be given here. But several basic principles, which are applicable to the outpatient setting, will be described. If possible a patient should not be given bad news in isolation. Ideally a relative or close friend should be there when the news is given. Hospitals vary in their provision for these circumstances, but a trained counsellor or nurse in attendance is also useful for providing comfort and further explanation if required.

Another principle is that bad news should be tempered with good news. One of the first questions a patient tends to ask after receiving an adverse diagnosis is, 'Is there anything that can be done?' It is reassuring to be told that reasonably effective treatment is available and that the hope of cure exists. The best interpretation should be put on the situation without instilling false hopes. Uncertainty on the part of the doctor at this stage will make a bad situation worse. Therefore, the management plan needs to be decided before the consultation begins. This may involve talking with the consultant and deciding on the best course of action before meeting the patient.

Answer as many questions as you can and then withdraw, giving the patient some time to come to terms with what has been said and to receive the comfort and reassurances of relatives and nurses. During this time further queries may occur and the nurse can relay these so that you can return to answer them. The nurse should also determine how the patient is getting home. Probably no patient should be allowed to drive immediately after receiving this kind of news. They are unlikely to be concentrating fully on their driving. It may be more sensible to order a hospital taxi and for the patient or relative to arrange for the car to be picked up the following day.

The outpatient letter

This letter is unusual because one letter is written to several different potential readers who require different information and may interpret the same information differently.

The first person you are writing the letter to is yourself. This letter is your record of what happened during the consultation, which you can refer to if a query arises. The letter is best dictated immediately after a consultation, when all the details are fresh in your memory. There may be the temptation not to record certain facts in the belief that you will remember them. This may be true for a week or two, but six months and possibly a thousand patients later this will not be the case. If you think that something might be relevant, note it down.

The next person you are writing to is the GP, who receives a mountain of mail every week and does not have the time to wade through a lot of flowery prose. The GP basically wants to know the diagnosis and the management plan, including further investigations, treatment and timing of the next outpatient appointment. The GP also wants this information as soon as possible after the consultation – not two months down the line. Some GPs prefer letters that consist of a list of headings, such as diagnosis, investigations, treatment, follow-up; this removes the need to compose a letter at all.

The next person to read the letter is the next outpatient doctor, who has never seen the patient before. This doctor requires a summary of the original complaint or symptoms, what has happened in terms of investigations or interventions and an outline of the current management plan. The alternative to a letter summarising this information is the task of wading through the whole set of notes trying to read other people's handwriting and trying to find pathology/radiology reports – a considerable waste of time that could have been spent with the patient.

Finally, remember this letter may be read by a hospital manager investigating a complaint, or ultimately by a prosecution lawyer. Humorous or apparently witty statements, which seemed funny at the time, may appear at best insensitive and at worst patronising and disparaging when read in the light of subsequent adverse events.

Most letters are dictated onto tape (dictaphone) and typed some time after the clinic by an audio-typist.

Dictating the letter

There are many different makes and models of dictating machine around, so before dictating a whole clinic's worth of letters make sure you know how the machine operates. Check that the tape and the machine are compatible, and that what you are saying is recording and can be played back in an intelligible form. Nothing is worse, after a long clinic, than to find that none of your carefully composed letters have been recorded and you have to do it all again.

Decide whether you are going to state the punctuation as you dictate (comma), or leave it to the secretary to put in the punctuation based on your sentence construction and voice intonation (full stop). If possible, discuss this with the secretary who is going to be typing the letters to find out what the secretary prefers. Some secretaries are expert at making sense of the worst dictation. Secretaries can also advise you as to the preferred style of your consultant.

Start the tape by stating the date; the title of the clinic, e.g. Mr Big's Endocrine Clinic; and who you are, e.g. Mr Small dictating. Then say: 'The first patient is . . . etc.' This enables the tape to be identified even if it becomes separated from the notes.

At the start of each letter state the patient's name and hospital identification number or date of birth. Next, state to whom the letter is being sent, e.g. letter to the GP Dr Good, with a copy to the stoma care sister.

The style of the letter may be largely determined by the 'house style' of the firm you are working for. It may be a structured letter under set headings, with or without a section of text. For text it is a good idea to allocate a new paragraph to the introduction, history, examination, investigations and treatment.

Letter to the general practitioner

The GP wants to receive answers to the following questions: What is the diagnosis, or which investigations are being performed to reach a diagnosis? When do you expect to make a diagnosis? What should be done about the symptoms in the meantime? What have you told the patient? If the diagnosis has been made, what is the treatment plan and what is the prognosis?

As stated earlier, the average GP receives a mountain of mail every week, so short, concise communications are appreciated. Try to limit one consultation to one sheet.

The style of letter varies from hospital to hospital. The style you adopt will be determined largely by the preferred format of the department you are working in. Increasing in popularity is the formulated letter, consisting of a series of headings such as diagnosis, investigations awaited, results, medications and so on. This is a very efficient letter, but some consider it too impersonal and not sufficiently explanatory. At the other end of the scale is flowery prose consisting of long sentences and paragraphs, which many GPs skip to read the bottom line. A combination of the two exists. It starts with a structured summary under relevant headings and then includes a section of text explaining how the diagnosis was reached and why a series of investigations has been requested. Whatever the style, all good letters contain the following information:

✧   a summary of why the patient was referred
✧   a summary of the history
✧   a summary of examination findings
✧   a list of differential diagnoses
✧   a list of investigations
✧   the treatment plan
✧   the time course for investigations or treatment
✧   what the patient and relatives were told
✧   arrangements for follow-up, open appointment, or, if the patient has been discharged, the conditions under which the patient should be re-referred.

Follow-up patients

For follow-up patients, letters should include the following information:

✧ a summary of the course of the illness and any interventions so far, which sets the consultation in context
✧ a reason why the patient is being followed
✧ current history and examination findings
✧ results of recent investigations
✧ an explanation of the symptoms and signs to look out for
✧ how long the follow-up is likely to continue
✧ when the patient is likely to be discharged.

Letter to the next OPD doctor

It is important to write the OPD letter bearing in mind that the next doctor to see the patient may not be yourself. In the case of new patients returning for the results of investigations, the needs of the next clinic doctor are the same as the GP and a letter containing the information outlined in the previous section is adequate.

Follow-up letters, which consist of: 'I have reviewed Mrs Smith and her condition is unchanged and we will see her again in three months' time,' are completely unhelpful.

Each letter should start with a summary, which sets the consultation in context, e.g. 'I reviewed this 43-year-old lady who, in April 1996, underwent a right simple mastectomy with a level 1 axillary node clearance. Her prognostic factors revealed this to be a 1cm tumour, which was a moderately differentiated (Bloom & Richardson grade II) ductal carcinoma with 3 out of 8 axillary lymph nodes involved. Following surgery she was treated with a full course of adjuvant CMF chemotherapy, from which she made a good recovery and on her last two outpatient visits she has been well with no signs of recurrence . . .'.

The next doctor now knows exactly what the original problem was without having to search for the operation note, the oncology notes or the several histology reports. Once this trend is established it is a simple matter for the next doctor to use the same paragraph, modified appropriately, to start the next letter.

Referrals to other clinicians

There may be occasions when referral of a patient to another speciality is indicated, either because the original complaint is not your speciality or the original complaint is your speciality but there is a co-existing condition which merits treatment in its own right. Many GPs have their preferred referral pathways, and therefore non-urgent cases should be referred back to the GP with reasons why a referral is indicated. However, on other occasions a referral may be urgent, or closely related to surgical treatment, e.g. a cardiology assessment prior to a surgical procedure in a patient with an existing heart condition. In these instances it is probably advisable to refer the patient yourself, but send a copy of the referral letter to the GP.

Prior to referring to another speciality, it is wise to discuss the case with your consultant, who can confirm a referral is indicated and advise you as to the correct referral pathway. In this case the referral letter should start by indicating that your consultant has been involved in the decision to refer. Then outline the reason why the patient was referred to your speciality and what your main findings have been. Explain why a referral to another speciality is indicated and how this affects the condition, if at all. Finally, express a time by which you would like the patient seen and explain how this fits in with your own timetable for follow-up and treatment.

Ordering investigations

Investigations tend to be classified as either urgent or routine. Difficulty arises in the case of patients who are not urgent – but if the result was positive the surgeon would want to know immediately. For example, in an investigation of rectal bleeding the decision may be made to investigate the condition further with a barium enema. The investigation is performed to exclude a colonic carcinoma. There may be an eight- to ten-week waiting list for routine barium enemas. If the result is negative there are few consequences, but if a colonic cancer is detected two months have been wasted, during which potentially life-saving treatment could have been administered. When deciding on whether a case is urgent or not, one must always consider the consequences of a positive result.

Routine investigations

Routine investigations are usually arranged by completing the relevant request form. An experienced clinic nurse can usually advise you as to the correct form. If not, you can always telephone the relevant department and ask their advice. One assumes there is no pressing need to know the results as long as they are available for the next consultation. However, for certain investigations there may be very long waiting times indeed – once again, contact the relevant department for more advice.

Urgent investigations

Obtaining urgent investigations is an art-form. Just writing 'urgent' on the request form is no guarantee that the request will be treated as urgent. Clearly stating when the result is needed helps investigating departments plan and prioritise their work appropriately. However, many departments have set procedures for dealing with urgent requests and unless these procedures are followed precisely the request fails. This information is often known to the people who have worked in the hospital for many years, but is a labyrinthine mystery to newly rotated doctors. A telephone call to the relevant department to obtain advice regarding these procedures, or a specific appointment time, is useful. Always record the name of the person you spoke to, in case of future difficulties. Telephone calls can use up a lot of time in the clinic and it may not be possible to contact the relevant person. It may be possible to delegate such calls to the clinic clerk and get involved only if difficulties arise.

In very difficult cases, admitting the patient to the hospital and performing the investigations with them as an in-patient is one option. However, in many cases it may be inappropriate and it is often wasteful of hospital resources.

In the end, a dictated letter to the consultant in charge of the department in question, explaining the clinical features and asking them to ensure the investigation is performed within a certain time, tends to ensure the right result – even if you get a less than friendly written reply.

Performing procedures in clinic

Performing procedures in clinic may be an integral part of the investigation or treatment of the patient's condition. Procedures commonly performed in the OPD include fine-needle aspiration, Tru-cut biopsy, rigid sigmoidoscopy, proctoscopy, injection of haemorrhoids and rectal biopsy. Other procedures may be performed depending on the speciality. Details of these procedures are given in the relevant chapters.

Obviously one should never perform an invasive procedure unless one has been trained to do so. Also, consider the issue of consent. It is unusual for patients to sign a consent form prior to these procedures. However, there may be occasions when this is appropriate. Usually, informed verbal consent is sufficient, but this situation may change in the future.

The discharge plan

Discharging patients from clinic can be a contentious issue. On the one hand, if all patients were followed up indefinitely, the clinics would soon become overburdened and cease to function. On the other hand, if discharge is handled insensitively there can be criticism that the patient has been abandoned, or that an unfair onus of further management has been placed on the GP.

The decision to discharge a patient from the clinic is easy when the patient originally presented with a relatively simple condition, which was treated and the symptoms resolved. However, with other patients the decision to discharge can be more difficult. Earlier in the text, I emphasised that if a reason for follow-up cannot be identified the patient should be discharged. This seems like common sense and for an experienced clinician it is a relatively simple decision. But junior surgeons may fear that they cannot identify a reason for follow-up because their knowledge is deficient – they suspect a good reason does exist, but they fear they are ignorant of it. In this situation there is a strong temptation to 'play safe' and follow the course of the previous clinic doctor, reviewing the patient in the clinic at the same interval as before. Inappropriate outpatient visits are wasteful of NHS resources and cause an inconvenience for patients and their carers, so every effort should be made to reserve outpatient consultations for those patients who really need them.

Another problem with multiple inappropriate clinic visits is that some patients become accustomed to attending the hospital and may actually look forward to their appointments. These patients may have adopted the sick role, and frequent hospital visits legitimise their 'illness'. There may be certain sociological and economic benefits, e.g. people are excused from work, or receive social security benefits that they feel may be threatened if they are discharged. These can be difficult patients to manage. To avoid conflict it may be necessary to delay discharge until they have seen the consultant at the next appointment.

For some chronic conditions or after major surgery, follow-up intervals become very long, e.g. yearly. In these situations the doctor should question whether further hospital follow-up is appropriate. After all, it is unlikely that the occurrence of new symptoms will coincide with the next appointment date. It is more likely that if new symptoms arise within that time the patient will seek the advice of their GP, who in turn will ask for the appointment to be brought forward. The original appointment will become irrelevant. If the patient had been discharged with instructions to consult their GP if new symptoms arose, the same procedure would have been followed and the patient seen in the same time but without the inconvenience of the original clinic appointment.

An alternative arrangement is the time-limited open appointment, where the patient has open access to the clinic to make their own appointment if the symptoms recur within a certain time after discharge, e.g. one year.

Patients should be discharged with a plan, which includes instructions as to when they should seek a medical opinion. The instructions should be included in the clinic letter, stating what the patient was told and giving additional instructions to the GP.

TWO

Breast

Fiona MacNeill

Introduction

In the United Kingdom, the female breast has a cultural, psychological and sociological significance far beyond its function as a milk-producing organ. As well, breast health issues have become increasingly politicised as a consequence of powerful advocacy and lobbying and high media involvement.

Although the incidence of breast cancer is rising slowly (especially in those aged over 70), mortality is declining rapidly (13 000 deaths per annum) and many patients now survive their cancer in extended remission. The five-year survival for screen-detected cancers is more than 95%.

The team

Breast cancer is a high-stake diagnosis: women fear a diagnosis that is associated with reduced life expectancy and disfiguring surgery, with a perception of reduced feelings of femininity and sexuality. They may also fear rejection from their husband or partner. Patients with a breast symptom or breast change are often terrified they might have breast cancer – no matter how low the likely risk – and the time spent waiting for a breast clinic appointment or results of breast investigations is stressful and full of uncertainties. Consequently, modern breast units have developed a specialist, streamlined and efficient breast assessment service. Specialist multidisciplinary care has been shown to improve patient outcomes as well as to enhance the quality of care and overall patient experience.

The core multidisciplinary team (MDT) consists of individuals who specialise, often exclusively, in 'breast', especially breast cancer: surgeons (breast/general, oncoplastic, plastic), radiologists and imaging teams, pathologists, oncologists, breast care nurses and an extensive clerical and management staff. The delivery of high-quality care is rarely dependent on the skills of one clinician; it is mainly the result of good organisation and a functional, patient-focused team.

Practical tips for the trainee

It is suggested that trainees take note of the following tips.

- Be aware of the National Institute for Health and Clinical Excellence (NICE) Breast Cancer Outcome guidelines: www.nice.org.uk.
- Read and understand the Association of Breast Surgery (ABS) and National Health Service Breast Screening Programme (NHSBSP) symptomatic assessment guidelines and Quality Assurance (QA) standards: www.baso.org.uk.
- Find out the latest government diagnostic and treatment targets for breast services, e.g.:
  - ∝ all women with a symptomatic breast problem to be assessed within two weeks
  - ∝ thirty-one days from referral to diagnosis and 62 days from referral to treatment.
- Multidisciplinary meetings (MDM) have a strong educational value and are a powerful learning resource for new team members. You will be able to learn how to function within a MDT and watch the complexity of team dynamics and leadership styles. Collaborative working represents the future model of healthcare. Working within the MDT means you will never be making decisions in isolation.
- Draw from the experience of the whole team.
- Each unit will have its own protocols for breast triple assessment. Ask if these are available, as they are a useful guide.

- ✧ At your first clinic, ask if you can sit in and watch someone more experienced or senior do the first few assessments.
- ✧ If possible, in the early days of your attachment follow a patient through the whole process of triple assessment. It will give you the opportunity to:
  - ∝ understand the process from the patient's perspective
  - ∝ see the rest of the unit and introduce yourself to the whole team
  - ∝ attend as many different types of breast clinic as possible.

Breast assessment

Breast referrals are made for a wide variety of breast/chest wall and axillary problems, pain being the most common symptom and a lump the most common sign. Most patients (90%) will have normal breasts: the breast is a dynamic organ under constant hormonal influence, especially from puberty to menopause, so the majority of breast changes are functional or physiological alterations secondary to puberty, pregnancy/lactation or the menopause. From 35 years onwards the breast starts to involute. This accelerates after the menopause.

Pain is not a symptom of breast cancer (BC) but is usually what draws the patient's attention to their breast. A lump is more likely to be breast cancer as the age of the woman increases. In the teenage to twenty-year age group most breast lumps are fibroadenomas (F/A). In the thirty to forty-year age group, as the breast involutes, a focal area of benign breast change (BBC) is the commonest cause. Above the age of fifty, BC is more common, and in the sixty-plus age group most breast lumps will be cancer.

The safest course of action is to assume each lump might be a cancer whatever the patient's age, until proven otherwise by triple assessment. Table 2.1 shows the percentage of symptoms that turn out to be cancer.

TABLE 2.1

SYMPTOM	% BC
Breast lump	36
Painful lumpiness	33
Pain alone	17.5
Nipple discharge	5
Nipple retraction	3
Family history of breast cancer	3
Others	2.5

TABLE 2.2

AGE	RISK OF BREAST CANCER
20	1:20 000
30	1:2000
40	1:200
50	1:50
60	1:25
70	1:15
80	1:10
90	1:8

Table 2.2 shows the age-related risk of breast cancer in the general population. (These risks are likely to be slightly higher in a symptomatic breast-clinic population.)

Triple breast assessment

Triple assessment (clinical assessment, mammography/ultrasound and cytology/biopsy) is the core of breast assessment. The principles of triple assessment underpin all breast assessment. It allows rapid and accurate diagnosis of cancer prior to surgery and, conversely, reliable exclusion of cancer, allowing most patients to be discharged back to their GP after one clinic visit.

The appropriate use of these three modalities will reduce *but not eliminate* the chance of missing a cancer, as no modality is 100% sensitive or specific. Not all cancers present as discrete changes or with classical clinical or radiological features; this is especially true now that women are more breast aware and present with early-stage disease with minimal signs.

Clinical skills and experience remain an important aspect of triple assessment, especially when reviewing the *concordance* of the assessment process.

The cancer most commonly 'missed' is lobular; clinical and radiological presentation can be subtle and cytology may have a bland appearance. The most common cause of a delay in BC diagnosis (and therefore of litigation) is failure to use triple assessment appropriately and failure to recognise non-concordance. This is usually due to poor departmental processes and procedures rather than poor individual competence.

The following notes describe the use of triple assessment in the symptomatic breast clinic. Symptomatic cancers are usually larger than 2.5cm but screen-detected cancers may be smaller than 15mm and are usually asymptomatic. Women with solid, screen-detected lesions (that are usually impalpable) also undergo full triple assessment in separate NHSBSP assessment clinics.

Triple assessment scores

As shown in Table 2.3, each modality of triple assessment is scored 1–5, i.e. normal to malignant. The aim is to try to bring objectivity into a subjective area. If there is any diagnostic doubt, repeat investigations or further 'second stage' investigations are arranged.

TABLE 2.3

	CLINICAL (P – PATIENT)	IMAGING (R – RADIOLOGY) (U – ULTRASOUND)	BIOPSY C – CYTOLOGY B – CORE BIOPSY
Normal	1	1	1
Benign	2	2	2
Uncertain	3	3	3
Suspicious	4	4	4
Malignant	5	5	5a Ductal carcinoma in situ (DCIS) 5b Invasive disease

A score of '1' can also indicate inadequate assessment, so it needs to be interpreted with caution.

No definitive cancer treatment should be undertaken unless *two of the three* triple assessment modalities are positive for cancer, one of which must be cytology or, ideally, histology. A false positive diagnosis of cancer is rare, but may result in unnecessary cancer treatment with far-reaching physical and psychological consequences.

Triple assessment stage one: Clinical

Breast history

Introduce yourself and explain your status. It is important the patient understands you will see them first and then discuss their management with the senior doctor/consultant, who may also wish to see them.

You and the patient should ideally be seated during the history taking. The patient's breasts must not be exposed at this stage of the consultation. They must be covered, either with the patient's own clothes or with a specially designed Breast Unit (BU) top.

Whilst taking a history you have the opportunity to assimilate other 'softer' issues, for example, your patient's concerns and fears: what drove them to report their symptoms and come to see you? What do they want from you? It is not always the obvious.

Try to establish rapport, as the patient may already be nervous and embarrassed about the intimacy of the forthcoming breast examination. Make lots of eye contact, smile, and try to appear friendly and relaxed as well as confident and calm, as patients are often very scared and tearful.

Occasionally a female patient will refuse to see a male doctor. Usually the nursing staff will have anticipated and managed the situation. This can be hurtful and seem personal. It isn't – be sensitive, not offended.

The stressful consultation

Sometimes the consultation is tense and stressful – usually because the patient is terrified of what you may find. A patient may scrutinise your face, and over-interpret (usually negatively) words and actions. Alternatively, they may be cold and withdrawn or angry and aggressive. Occasionally they may cry continuously. Patients may ask repeatedly if it is all OK. You may feel intimidated and pressurised, but try not to give bland reassurances or distance yourself. Try to understand their vulnerabilities, but be honest. If it feels OK, say so; if you are not sure, say so; if you are concerned, express your concerns. Explain that the examination is one part of the assessment process and you may not be able to confidently tell what the problem is until the imaging has given you some clues – hence the importance of a thorough assessment.

Taking the history

Age is the most important factor in assessing the likelihood of a new breast change being cancerous.

Pain may be cyclical or non-cyclical. Note when the pain first started, duration, site, severity, relieving and exacerbating factors and associated symptoms.

Cyclical breast pain is related to ovarian function. Breasts are swollen and tender and/or lumpy 3–10 days (can be longer) prior to menstruation, with pain relieved by menstruation.

Non-cyclical breast pain is pain caused by specific conditions of the breast not related to ovarian function, e.g. trauma and fat necrosis, infected cyst, mastitis (periductal or lactating), abscess, fistula.

Reasons for *non-breast pain* include angina, cholelithiasis, cervical spondylosis, hiatus hernia, nerve entrapment, Tietze's syndrome, oesophageal lesions and lung conditions.

If there is a *lump*, get the patient to describe it to you – 'pea', 'marble', 'grape' and 'torpedo' are useful comparisons. How was the lump noticed? How long has it been present?

Nipple discharge may be spontaneous or on stimulation (e.g. after the bath). Ask about colour (blood, bloody, watery, yellow/sticky, pus-like, green). Is it associated with pain? (Consider papilloma, infection, ectasia.)

History of presenting problem: determine the time course of each symptom and any variation within the menstrual cycle, as this is often a clue to the diagnosis. Getting bigger or smaller, varies in size with periods? Associated pain or tenderness?

Any previous breast imaging: date and location of last mammogram.

General: general health and co-morbidities. Smoking is important in breast sepsis.

BC risk factors: the most powerful risk factor is family history.
- ∝   Family history: maternal and paternal, first- and second-degree.
- ∝   Past history of radiation to the chest wall (mantle radiotherapy (RT) for Hodgkin's).
- ∝   Any previous breast problems – nature, investigation and outcome.
- ∝   We ask about other risk factors but in reality these are of little help in assessing an individual's risk in the symptomatic breast clinic. However, such information helps to build a picture of your patient and if your unit runs a database the information may be useful for future analysis.
- ∝   Endogenous oestrogen exposure: menarche, menopause, age at first pregnancy, number of pregnancies, breast-feeding history.
- ∝   Exogenous oestrogen exposure: oral contraceptive pill (OCP), hormone replacement therapy (HRT).

Breast examination

Always have a chaperone, regardless of your gender. The room and your hands must be warm. Explain at each stage what you are going to do and why and obtain verbal consent. There are many breast examination techniques. You need to watch a variety and develop your own. Consistency and reliability are the objectives.

A common technique is to imagine the breast as a clock and work your way around the clock face from 12 to 12, examining the breast from the outer margin towards the nipple (*see* Figure 2.1).

The signs of locally advanced cancer are difficult to miss when a patient undresses: ulceration; fixation to chest wall (ribs, muscles); erythema of the skin; satellite nodules; peau d'orange; invasion of the skin; matted, fixed axillary lymph nodes; lymphoedema. Try not to look shocked: remain professional. The patient already knows the diagnosis and is gauging your reaction. However, it is unusual to see advanced breast cancer (fewer than 10% present with stage IV disease).

- ✧   Ask the patient to expose their whole torso, displacing long hair and jewellery, and to sit on the right side of the couch facing you.
- ✧   Ask them to point to the area they are concerned about: the patient's use of hand and fingers will give you a clue to whether it is a focal or generalised problem.
- ✧   *Look* for asymmetry, visible lumps, skin dimpling or peau d'orange. Inspect the nipple areolar complex (NAC).
- ✧   *Look* for skin dimpling or distortion as the patient slowly raises both hands above the head.
- ✧   Ensure the patient is lying supine but not flat, with a pillow under the head, arms elevated with elbows flat on the bed and hands tucked under the head.
- ✧   Examine the asymptomatic breast first to gain some idea of the normal texture of the breast.
- ✧   Palpate breast tissue.
    - ∝   Palpate all breast tissue with the flat of the fingers. Focus on the area of patient concern, remembering the axillary tail and the NAC.

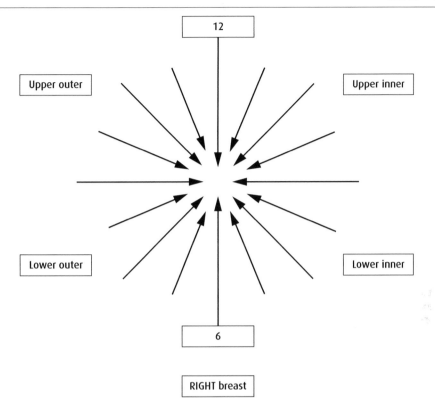

FIGURE 2.1 Breast quadrants. Most breast glandular tissue lies in the outer quadrants, especially the upper outer quadrant.

- ∝ If you find a lump consider its site, size, consistency, surface and skin/muscle tethering.
- ∝ If the problem is nipple discharge, ask the patient to massage the breast/nipple to demonstrate the discharge: assess colour, and number of ducts involved (uniduct or multiduct).
- ∝ Palpate the axilla for enlarged lymph nodes (with the patient's arm supported in your non-examining hand to allow better access to the axilla).
- ∝ Palpate infraclavicular and supraclavicular fossa for lymph nodes.

Repeat the process for the opposite side.

What is a lump?

Do not agonise over whether tissue is a lump or not. If the patient feels her breasts have changed and/or she thinks there is a lump, you need to prove she doesn't have a cancer. A lump is tissue or an area that feels prominent or asymmetric. Clinical examination, although helpful, is unreliable and subjective. All women's breasts feel very different so it is important to compare the two breasts, since asymmetry is a useful guide for proceeding to imaging.

Lumps can be obviously discrete and circumscribed, e.g. an F/A, cyst, lipoma or cancer; or they can just feel like an area of asymmetric lumpiness, e.g. BBC, F/A, cyst, lipoma or cancer. A discrete lump deep in the breast will feel like lumpiness because it elevates the surrounding tissue. The texture of the patient's tissue and skin and the proportion of fat to glandular tissue will also affect your ability to feel a lump. A young breast with low fat content and a tight skin envelope has little laxity and feels generally hard (dense), so it can be difficult to feel even a superficial discrete lump. An older breast with a greater fat to glandular tissue ratio and a more lax skin envelope (ptosis) is softer, so lumps are usually more obvious.

✧ *Benign breast changes* may show generalised islands of nodularity, occasionally focal or asymmetric.

✧ *Fibroadenoma* lumps are firm, round, very mobile and may be multiple. They usually cannot be compressed.

✧ *Breast cyst* lumps are firm, round, mobile and may be multiple: as the fluid is compressed, they may have a 'bouncy' feel. They are sometimes tender.

✧ *Breast cancer* has some classical signs such as hardness, irregularity, dimpling, tethering, ulceration and so on, but now we are seeing smaller, earlier cancers that do not demonstrate these signs. Virtually any type of breast change can indicate a cancer.

The nipple
Nipple discharge

Pre-menopausal discharge is common and usually settles with the menopause: therefore all post-menopausal discharge must be regarded as suspicious. In the younger woman, watery discharge can be a sign of DCIS. There are a number of *physiological* causes of nipple discharge.

✧ Multi-duct, multi-coloured (yellow to dark greeny-brown) discharge is common and normal. It is often secondary to nipple massage or a hot bath/shower. It is occasionally spontaneous. It is usually seen pre-menopausally.

✧ Ectatic ducts produce a sticky yellow fluid or toothpaste-like material on massage.

✧ Milk-like fluid can be expressed by most pre-menopausal women who have lactated. True galactorrhoea (pituitary adenoma – raised prolactin levels) is rare and the discharge is spontaneous and copious.

Pathological discharges are usually watery (blood-stained), single duct, spontaneous and persistent. They may be pre- or post-menopausal.

✧ Intraduct papilloma usually presents with pure blood discharge.

✧ Cancer (especially a presenting feature of DCIS) discharge is usually watery, with intermittent pinkish staining.

Nipple inversion/retraction

Understand the differences between inversion (benign) and retraction (malignant). Inversion and retraction look very different.

Inversion is usually slit-like (letterbox appearance) and often congenital. It is due to fibrosis and shortening of the periductal tissue and major ducts. The nipple can often be gently everted with manipulation and the areola is soft and healthy.

Retraction is due to a retro/periareolar cancerous process or mass pulling the NAC inwards. Often the nipple is visible but distorted and the surrounding areolar tissue is hard, inflexible and indrawn in a saucer-like manner.

Eczema and Paget's disease

Eczema and Paget's can look identical, especially in the early stages of Paget's. Eczema usually spares the nipple and affects the areola and surrounding skin. It can be bilateral and associated with a generalised eczematous skin change.

Paget's usually starts centrally, destroying the nipple architecture and spreading outwards onto the areola. However, these signs are not pathognomic and a scaling/excoriated NAC should undergo a punch biopsy.

Record the examination

Record examination findings and score your clinical impression (*see* Figure 2.2).

✧   Always mark the site of patient concern.
✧   There are standard ways of illustrating your findings.
✧   Imagine the breast as a clock face: describe the site of the lesion accordingly.
✧   Record the distance of the lesion from the nipple.
✧   Give the size of the lesion.

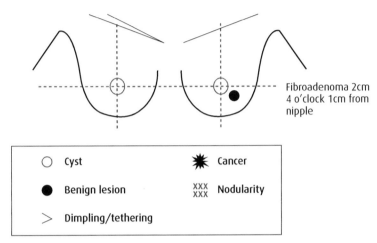

Fibroadenoma 2cm
4 o'clock 1cm from
nipple

○	Cyst	✸	Cancer
●	Benign lesion	XXX XXX	Nodularity
>	Dimpling/tethering		

FIGURE 2.2 Recording the examination.

Triple assessment stage two: Primary imaging

Most women who attend a rapid diagnostic clinic will be offered imaging regardless of their presenting symptom or sign: clinical examination is poor at discriminating between cancer and normal changes, particularly in the pre-menopausal woman with a dense nodular breast.

Indications for imaging

First you should *check your local protocols*. However, the following recommendations are commonly used. All women with symptoms who are more than 35 years of age should have:

✧   mammography: to screen both breasts
✧   targeted ultrasound – focused on the symptomatic area.

Women younger than 35 who have focal lumps, nodularity, pain or tenderness should have:

✧   targeted ultrasound – focused on the symptomatic area.

Results are scored M1–5 (or R1–5) for mammography and U1–5 for ultrasound. Results must always be interpreted in combination with the rest of the triple assessment.

Mammography

Mammography uses soft-tissue X-rays to image the breast. The breast is compressed between two plates while the image is made. Mammography is the gold-standard breast imaging and screening tool because of its high sensitivity and specificity. Usually two views (oblique and cranio-caudal) are obtained using 1 mGy of radiation. The breast is more radio-dense before the age of 35, making mammography less sensitive. Mammography is particularly good at detecting early non-palpable lesions, microcalcification and multifocality. It is not very useful for women under 35 (breasts are too dense).

Ultrasound
Acoustic water-based gel, which is a good medium for the transmission of ultrasound waves, is applied to the breast and an ultrasound probe is manipulated over the breast by the sonographer. There is no radiation. This is the best imaging for those under 35, and it looks at retroareolar tissue, which is not well seen using mammography. Ultrasound gives an accurate size and an indication of how well circumscribed a lesion may be. It is operator dependent, not as sensitive as mammography and not used as the sole investigation for those over 35. Because it is a poor screening tool, scanning an asymptomatic breast is not recommended.

Other breast imaging modalities (secondary imaging)
If a patient has changes that are suspicious or diagnostic for cancer, the sonographer will usually scan the axilla. If a node appears to be suspicious for cancer (local criteria), fine-needle aspiration cytology (FNAC) is performed. Pre-operative identification of axillary nodal disease will allow for more appropriate management of the axilla and cancer, for example axillary clearance, than sentinel node biopsy will.

There are many other breast imaging techniques whose roles are unclear or still in the research or developmental arena, e.g. positron emission tomography (PET) scanning and scintiscanning. Magnetic resonance imaging (MRI), with its high sensitivity, is especially useful in imaging the difficult breast (very young and dense, post surgery and radiotherapy) or in assessing multifocality, but a low specificity and difficulty in MRI biopsy restrict use to very specific indications. You should see your local protocols.

Triple assessment stage three: Tissue diagnosis
Techniques for tissue diagnosis include:
✧ fine-needle aspiration cytology (FNAC)
✧ nipple aspiration cytology
✧ punch biopsy
✧ percutaneous wide-bore needle (core) biopsy.

In general you should only proceed to obtaining tissue if there is a focal or discrete *solid* change, either on imaging, clinical examination or, as is more usual, both modalities. Random aspiration of a lumpy area is to be avoided.

Most units prefer to perform FNAC or core biopsy after the clinical exam and imaging, as any invasive procedure can cause tissue inflammation/bleeding and can reduce the accuracy of clinical and radiological findings.

Increasingly, core biopsy is the preferred technique for obtaining tissue, as it gives histology rather than cytology. Histology is the gold-standard diagnostic modality. Core biopsy will give a definitive diagnosis of benign lesion (e.g. it will confirm if the lesion is a fibroadenoma and can be safely ignored) and will give more information about the cancer, so allowing better pre-operative planning.

Aspirate cysts only if they are symptomatic or if patients request aspiration. Asymptomatic cysts do not require aspiration. After aspiration, cyst fluid can be discarded if there is no blood-staining or residual mass – which can indicate a papilloma, intracystic carcinoma or necrotic cancer with cystic degeneration.

Occasionally, on aspiration you will perforate an unseen vessel and blood will enter the cyst fluid in your syringe. If you are in doubt, request cytology.

Tissue/cyst drainage can be performed either freehand (usually by the surgeon or nurse practitioner) or under image control (by the radiologist, sonographer or surgeon).

Image guidance (ultrasound or stereotactic mammography) is the preferred method, especially for smaller lesions. It reduces the risk of missing the lesion and limits false negative results, which can result from poor sampling. This means that the opportunity to perform FNA and core biopsies now lies in the imaging department. Take advantage of this training opportunity.

Results are scored C1–5 for cytology and B1–B5a, b for histopathology. Always interpret the results in combination with the rest of the triple assessment.

Fine-needle aspiration cytology

FNAC requires a 10 ml syringe and a green or blue needle. The patient is positioned as for examination of the breast and the procedure is explained. Verbal consent is usually sufficient. Clean the skin and infiltrate with local anaesthetic. The lesion is fixed with one hand while the other inserts the needle, applying suction to the syringe and passing 5–6 times through the lesion. Suction is released and the needle withdrawn. The sample is deposited either onto glass slides or into cytological preservative fluid (*check your local protocol*).

As soon as the needle is withdrawn, pressure is applied with a cotton wool ball to the area of aspiration for 3–4 minutes to minimise bruising. A sticking plaster or other covering is applied to prevent staining of the patient's garments.

The technique is quick to perform, gives almost immediate results and samples a wide area. Information provided is limited to 'cancer' or 'benign'. It can be difficult to get an adequate number of epithelial cells. The results are very dependent on the experience of the clinician doing the FNAC and on the cytologists interpreting the result. FNAC is not useful for assessing microcalcifications. ABS standard: less than 20% of FNAC reported as C1 (inadequate).

Nipple fluid cytology

Nipple fluid can be smeared on a slide and cytology requested. This can be helpful in distinguishing physiological from pathological discharge.

Punch biopsy

Punch biopsy is useful for the breast skin or very superficial lesions in the skin (e.g. skin tumour deposit), especially in the area of the NAC if you want to exclude Paget's disease. Explain the technique (verbal consent is usually sufficient) and position the patient as for a breast examination. Clean the NAC skin and infiltrate under the NAC with local anaesthetic.

Punch biopsy cutting blades are provided on a handle, in a range of sizes from 2–6mm. Using a screwing motion, push the round cutting blade through the skin and underlying tissue. Lift the tissue above the skin using forceps or a needle, and cut the tissue free with scissors. Place the tissue in a formalin pot. Sutures are not required. Apply a suitable dressing.

Percutaneous wide-needle (core) biopsy

After explaining the technique (verbal consent is usually sufficient), position the patient as for a breast examination. Clean the skin and infiltrate with local anaesthetic. Make a small incision with a number 11 blade in the skin over the lesion. Fix the lesion between thumb and forefinger and insert the special biopsy needle (gun) up to the lesion. After the gun is fired the needle is removed in the closed position and opened to deposit the core of tissue into a formalin pot.

As soon as the needle is removed, pressure is applied to the biopsy site with a cotton wool ball to minimise bleeding and bruising. Take 3–4 cores. A core containing sufficient breast tissue will sink in the pot. Apply a suitable dressing.

Histological diagnosis is so much more informative, especially if cancer is found: it gives morphology, grade, oestrogen/progesterone receptors (ER/PR) and HER2 status. It takes slightly longer to perform than does FNAC, it is slightly more traumatic (more bruising) and results take 24–48 hours to obtain.

Excision biopsy

This is surgical excision of a lesion or microcalcification, with or without a localising guidewire. It is performed when triple assessment is non-concordant and biopsy, or repeat biopsy, is not possible.

Microdochectomy or Hadfield's procedure (major duct excision) may be useful to diagnose the underlying cause of a bloody/watery nipple discharge. Microdochectomy retrieves a large amount of tissue for histology. If the lump is benign the procedure provides both diagnosis and treatment. The procedure requires a formal operation, which leaves a scar. If a lump proves to be malignant, a second operation may be needed for staging and wider excision. Only a small number of lesions require formal surgical excision to make a diagnosis – usually the smaller screen-detected cancers or small foci of microcalcification.

Frozen section

This is used *only in exceptional circumstances* and after full discussion with the pathologist and patient.

A frozen section involves surgical excision of the lump and immediate processing of tissue for histological diagnosis while the patient is still anaesthetised. If a lump proves to be malignant, a further surgical procedure is performed without waking the patient from anaesthesia, removing the need for a second operation. The procedure has now fallen into disuse – tissue is no longer available for future, more detailed analysis; and accurate histological diagnosis is more difficult on frozen sections (especially for subtle lesions, DCIS, lobular carcinoma in situ (LCIS), and atypical ductal hyperplasia (ADH)). It is difficult to advise and gain consent from the patient pre-operatively.

Other diagnostic breast investigations

These are determined by the presentation, history and examination, but in general very few other diagnostic investigations are required (*see* gyneacomastia).

Multi culture and sensitivity (MC&S)

If the patient has breast sepsis, try to obtain pus for culture before starting treatment.

Staging

If the patient is diagnosed with breast cancer they may require staging. Each unit will have a specific protocol, but routine pre-operative staging is not recommended and is reserved for those with advanced disease or specific symptoms and signs that may indicate metastatic disease.

Staging tests include full blood count (FBC), liver function tests (LFT), chest X-ray (CXR), bone scan and liver scan.

Triple assessment: Concordance

There are two main questions to answer concerning concordance.
✧ Do the assessment results fit the clinical picture? If not, investigate further, repeat tests.
✧ Is each aspect of the 'triple' assessment in agreement? If not, investigate further, repeat tests.

The rapid diagnostic clinic

Assessment results must be discussed with the senior/responsible clinician during the rapid diagnostic (RD) clinic *especially before discharging* a patient. If you are uncertain about what to do, a follow-up appointment is not the solution – discuss the problem with the senior clinician, who will be pleased to provide guidance.

The multidisciplinary meeting

Patients who have undergone full triple assessment are usually discussed further at the weekly MDM. The process and details vary from unit to unit, but in general most units will discuss the triple assessment results of that week's new cancers, and will review all cases that had FNAC or cores. This is to confirm concordance and appropriate management, be that discharge, definitive treatment or further investigations.

Occasionally review of the assessment process will throw up uncertainties and surprises, resulting in complex diagnostic problem solving. Try to understand the MDT decision-making process. If it is not clear – ask.

After triple assessment: what to do next

Advice and education

After appropriate assessment and diagnosis you need to formulate a management strategy with your patient. This will be mainly in the form of advice and education regarding BBC and normal age-related breast changes; and guidance on breast awareness and the use of breast screening. Make sure patients know they are always welcome back if they have further problems, and explain the local referral mechanisms – usually via the GP. If you make a patient feel they have wasted your time because they have normal breasts, they will not report future changes for fear of being made to look foolish.

Most patients do not understand the complex nature of a breast and the hormonal influences that cause breast changes. Understandably, patients think pain is a sign of disease rather than function. A simple explanation will transform understanding. A well-informed patient will have greater confidence in managing their own breast signs and symptoms in the future, which will help reduce the number of clinic attendances for minor breast problems such as cyclical breast pain and lumpiness. The breast care nurse will have copious literature available. Use leaflets judiciously: handing out information sheets is no substitute for a careful face-to-face explanation.

Breast awareness is more than breast self-examination and looking for a lump. It is about knowing your breasts, so if there is a change – any change – you will know there has been a change and can report it to the doctor or nurse. They can then review the change at a different stage of the menstrual cycle (in a pre-menopausal woman) or refer straight to a breast clinic (in a post-menopausal woman).

The anxious patient

Occasionally you will meet a patient who finds it difficult to accept they have normal breasts. Often all that is required is more time and a careful repeat explanation of the results. Sometimes a patient may have a cancer phobia or other underlying psychological/psychosocial problems. These patients need to be identified early and seen by the senior clinician and breast care nurses rather than to have large numbers of unnecessary investigations or treatments.

The dissatisfied patient

Occasionally a patient will not be satisfied that the assessment has been carried out properly. This requires careful handling. Always involve the senior clinician and do not be dismissive. Listen to concerns with courtesy and sympathy – you might be wrong and the concerns justified. Remember, no test is infallible.

Breaking bad news

You may need to explain the diagnosis of cancer; this is difficult for you, but remember it is even more difficult for the patient. It is normal for a patient to be distressed at a diagnosis of breast cancer. Allow them the time to weep. To begin with, sit in with a more experienced clinician and take guidance from the breast care nurses. Develop your own style and approach: it is possible to be honest, clear and humane.

Management of specific breast conditions

Each unit has its own protocols – *know these*.

Breast cancer

The management of breast cancer is beyond the scope of this book.

Normal or benign lumps

Fibroadenoma

If you have histological proof of an F/A (B2) nothing further need be done. The majority of F/As involute and have no increased cancerous potential. Some women prefer to have the lump removed. However, this is at the expense of a scar, the possibility of chronic pain and the risks of surgery. Some F/As will grow. Explain that the patient can always return.

Cysts

After investigations confirm cysts, nothing further needs to be done unless there is a dominant cyst that is troublesome (pain, infection). Aspiration with a fine needle (blue or orange) is all that is required. Cytology is not requested unless the fluid is blood-stained (perhaps from intracystic carcinoma or papilloma) or the lump doesn't disappear (consider necrotic cancer with cystic degeneration).

Benign breast change

BBC is normal. Once you have confirmed BBC no further action is required.

Other benign lumps

For other benign lumps, e.g. lipomas, if assessment shows the lump is benign, no further action is required.

Pain

Most patients with pain have hormonally mediated breast pain. They are usually happy to cope and self-manage after cancer has been excluded and they have been given an explanation of the condition. Giving some helpful advice such as trialling the wearing of a bra 24 hours a day or taking evening primrose oil (EPO) (prescription not required) does seem to help some women, but the evidence base is flimsy. Simple analgesia is generally not helpful.

Complementary therapies such as acupuncture or reflexology are non-evidence based, but help some women cope with their symptoms.

It is possible to reduce breast pain with medication that alters the breast hormonal axis, e.g. danazol, bromocriptine, tamoxifen and GHRH analogues, but these are powerful drugs that should never be recommended without consultation with the senior clinician and a careful and detailed risk-benefit discussion.

Surgery *never* offers a solution for chronic breast pain.

Nipple inversion

Gentle manipulation may encourage the nipple to evert to allow breast-feeding. Surgery will provide a permanent solution, but at the expense of division of the major ducts, which will prevent feeding.

Breast sepsis

Pain, redness and swelling are the usual symptoms of breast sepsis, but these symptoms can also be caused by rare inflammatory breast conditions that are often diagnosed by exclusion, e.g. granulomatous mastitis.

Inflammatory breast carcinoma may present with the history and appearance of an acute breast infection.

Breast infections may be present in lactating or non-lactating women.

Breast infection during lactation

Puerperal mastitis/abscess occurs during breast-feeding and weaning. There may be a history of cracked nipples, allowing bacteria (*Staphylococcus aureus, S. epidermidis,* streptococci) to enter.

Breast infection without lactation

There are a number of possible causes.

✧ *Periductal mastitis* affects young/middle-aged women who have a history of smoking, which damages the periareolar ducts. Infection of the damaged ducts causes periareolar inflammation with or without a mass (caused by enterococci, anaerobic streptococci, *Bacteroides* and *S. aureus*).

✧ *Mammary duct fistula* is a communication between the skin, usually in the periareolar region, and a major duct. It usually follows a history of periductal mastitis with periareolar inflammatory mass, which discharges spontaneously. It is occasionally seen after a biopsy of an area of inflammation, or incision and drainage of a non-lactating abscess.

✧ *Infected sebaceous cysts* are common in the sternal and inframammary regions of the breast.

✧ *Variations of Hidradenitis suppurativa* can be seen in the breast, especially around the nipple and axilla.

Other rare causes of sepsis or breast inflammation need to be considered if the sepsis doesn't settle with appropriate treatment.

Treatment

If infection is suspected (redness, heat, pain, swelling, fever) it is justified to start treatment based on clinical judgment and modify according to the results of investigation. If the patient is toxic they may require admission for intravenous (IV) antibiotics (flucloxacillin or augmentin).

✧ *Abscess* – regardless of aetiology, most can be treated in the clinic or A&E with ultrasound-guided aspiration under local anaesthetic. Overlying thinned or necrotic skin needs removal to allow free drainage, but this can also be done in the clinic or A&E. Prescribe antibiotics. Encourage manual expression of milk and/or feeding. Repeat aspirations every 24–48 hours as required. Surgery is indicated for refractory or multiloculate abscesses.

✧ *Periductal mastitis* – try flucloxacillin. If persistent or if anaerobes are cultured, add metronidazole. If ultrasound shows an abscess, repeat aspiration is better than incision and drainage, which results in a mammary fistula in up to one-third of patients. The patient should stop smoking.

✧ *Mammary duct fistula* requires antibiotics and surgical excision.

Follow-up

Follow-up is determined by the diagnosis and course of the condition. Periductal mastitis is difficult to treat and may have a relapsing course. Treatment for recurrent disease is surgical excision of the diseased duct system under antibiotic cover. The cosmetic outcome can be very poor. Periductal mastitis usually resolves after the menopause.

Male breast problems

Gyneacomastia and breast cancer

More men are attending breast clinics because of increased awareness of male breast cancer – there are 300 cases in the United Kingdom each year – and because they are distressed by the appearance of gyneacomastia.

The male breast does not have lobules (glandular) tissue. Gyneacomastia is diffuse, often tender (in the early stages) enlargement of the breast ductal/stromal tissue behind the male nipple. The tissue becomes enlarged due to alterations in the male oestrogen/testosterone ratios.

Causes

The two most common causes of true gyneacomastia are puberty and senescence. Other causes include virtually anything that will alter the oestrogen/testosterone ratio: antiandrogen drugs (cimetidine, digoxin, spironolactone), cirrhosis, malnutrition, primary hypogonadism, secondary hypogonadism, hyperthyroidism, renal disease, lung cancer and, finally but rarely, testicular tumours.

History and examination

Male breast patients require a full general history with a detailed drug, alcohol and smoking history. A full examination including the genitalia is mandatory. Male BC can mimic gyneacomastia but usually presents with all the classical features of female BC, i.e. an asymmetric lump with dimpling and so on. In general the diagnosis of male BC is straightforward, as there is no surrounding glandular tissue to cause diagnostic uncertainty.

Investigations

Male BC is rare, especially in men in the under-50 age group with no family history of the condition, but you should proceed to assessment if concerned. Mammography of the male breast is possible. If tissue is required, core biopsy is the preferred technique because cytology can be misleading in the male breast.

There are numerous causes of gyneacomastia. It can be difficult to settle on a realistic investigative algorithm, as the yield from a series of diagnostic trawling tests is very low. The history and examination will in general guide any further investigations. Contrary to what is written in the textbooks, gyneacomastia is often asymmetric and painless.

Treatment

Male BC is treated in a similar fashion to female BC.

Physiological gyneacomastia requires no specific treatment other than explanation and reassurance. Surgery for gyneacomastia is essentially aesthetic: expectations are very high and outcomes often poor. Since men go topless far more frequently than women, surgery should be undertaken only by an appropriately trained and experienced surgeon (oncoplastic or plastic).

Breast follow-up clinics

The purpose of triple assessment is to exclude cancer and confirm a normal/benign breast, thus allowing prompt discharge of the patient. Women with normal breasts do not require regular checkups. Ask yourself – why do I want to bring this patient back? If you are not confident about the concordance of the initial assessment, then go with your instincts. Repeating tests or getting further tests needs to be done now, not in three months' time at review. Discuss with a senior clinician. However, there are exceptions, of which the following are examples.

✧ Occasionally a patient with a cancer phobia may respond to a structured follow-up schedule over a few years, until her underlying fears have been addressed through counselling or other appropriate interventions.

✧ Women who are at high risk of BC due to their family history or to other factors should be part of a regular quality-assured high-risk screening programme. The process will vary from unit to unit.

✧ Women with known cysts who get recurrent lumps can find an open-access clinic for a mini assessment useful.

The post-surgery 'results' clinic

The composition of a results clinic may vary, but usually in attendance are the surgeon and the breast care nurse with or without the oncologist(s).

Histology results are available on average from 7 to 14 days after surgery. Results clinics should be held after the weekly MDM, with all the necessary information and a management plan.

Patients can become distraught whilst awaiting results, especially if there is uncertainty about the diagnosis. The breast care nurses bear the brunt of this distress. Patients with benign lesions can be contacted by letter or phone to save them a journey or relieve anxiety before the clinic appointment. However, you need to have a reliable mechanism in place to ensure this happens.

Procedure at the clinic

Examine the patient for possible complications of surgery before discussing the results.

✧ Once you have completed the examination you can ask the patient to dress.

✧ Ensure the patient is comfortable and sitting next to their partner.

✧ Explain the results.

✧ It can be very helpful to have the breast care nurse (BCN) present, especially if the information is complicated or the results indicate a poor prognosis.

Never give the results whilst the patient is undressed.

During the consultation, assess your patient's physical and emotional recovery. Emotional recovery may be more difficult to judge in the acute stages of recovery, but the BCN may have invaluable insight.

Pain

Breast and axillary surgery is not painful; pain is generally mild and controlled with simple analgesia. Neurogenic pain can be difficult to manage, so early involvement of the pain team is essential to prevent a chronic pain syndrome developing.

✧ If pain has been difficult to control since surgery, consider nerve damage.

✧ If pain was mild but is getting worse, consider infection.

✧ Poor mobility can increase pain due to disuse atrophy and stiffness, so consider intensive physiotherapy.

Wound

Infection occurs in 5–10% of breast surgery wounds. It is normally minor and self limiting. Take swabs or aspirate fluid for culture and prescribe antibiotics.

✧ Abscess formation is rare, but needs prompt drainage in the clinic.
✧ Delayed haematoma can occur – the wound will be bulging and oozing blood. The clot requires evacuation, which can often be done in the clinic.

Seroma formation

This is common after any breast and axillary surgery (>50%). It requires aspiration only if it is very large and uncomfortable (stretching the wound to dehiscence) or looks infected. Most seromas will reabsorb over a few weeks. If aspiration is required, use aseptic technique, insert the needle or trocar through the insensate wound and keep the needle parallel to the chest wall.

Lymphoedema

Early, very mild, post-operative oedema of the arm or breast is common after axillary node dissection and improves as other routes for lymph flow are established.

Cording (lymphatic thrombosis) is common and can be traced from the axilla, down the inner aspect of the arm, across the elbow to the wrist. It is self limiting.

Nerve damage

Intractable pain or hyperparesthesia in the nerve distribution is often the clue. Physiotherapy may help to lessen any disability.
✧ Intercostobrachial – sensation altered for the inner aspect of the arm, axilla and posterior axillary fold.
✧ Serratus anterior (long thoracic nerve) – may see winging of the scapula.
✧ Latissimus dorsi (thoracodorsal nerve) – wasted posterior axillary fold.

Shoulder mobility

It is normal to have slightly restricted movements in the first few weeks after axillary surgery, but the importance of physiotherapy exercises must be reinforced to prevent the development of a frozen shoulder as the scar tissue starts to mature and contract. Early identification and referral for intensive physiotherapy of potential shoulder problems is crucial.

The joint breast/oncology clinic

Patients who have completed their cancer therapy are reviewed on a regular basis in the joint breast/oncology clinic. The schedule is determined by local protocols, which you should *know*, as they can sometimes be very complex. The minimum is usually a yearly examination and mammography for 2–5 years or whilst the patient is on active treatment.

The value of routine clinical examination in detecting recurrent or new cancers is debatable, as most recurrences are screen- or patient-detected. It is clear patients value follow-up consultations, as they provide reassurance and the opportunity to discuss concerns and worries. The trend is to nurse-led follow-up. In the future this might be community based.

Once again the structure of the clinics and who performs the follow-up varies from unit to unit.

Use the clinic to gain a better understanding of cancer treatment protocols – reading and summarising the patient's history on the GP letter is a powerful learning tool.

History

The following are a few prompts that may be useful.
✧ How are they? How is their general health? How is life?
✧ Are they menstruating?
✧ Are they taking their prescribed anti-cancer treatment?

✧ Do they have any side effects?

✧ Have they noticed any new symptoms or breast changes?

Examination

The examination is mainly focused on checking for loco-regional recurrence in the breasts and nodal basin, but take general note of the patient's state of health – advanced metastatic disease is usually obvious.

✧ Skin and chest wall: local recurrence may present as scattered skin lesions in the vicinity of the previous surgery or on the chest wall.

✧ Breasts: local recurrence after breast-conserving surgery may be difficult to detect because of the fibrous changes that occur following surgery and radiotherapy. Contralateral cancers occur in 5% of patients.

✧ Nodal basin: axillae, infra and supraclavicular fossae, intramammary chain (sternal intercostal spaces).

✧ Other sites for clinical examination such as the abdomen or chest will be determined by the history.

Investigations

If the patient is asymptomatic and well, routine follow-up investigations such as bone scan, CXR or tumour markers are not recommended.

✧ Suspected local recurrence needs to be proven, ideally with targeted imaging and histology. Systemic recurrence is diagnosed mainly on imaging appearances and pattern, as histology can be difficult to obtain.

✧ On confirmation of recurrence it is necessary to restage the disease – *use local protocols.*

Treatment

Results are discussed at the MDM and a treatment plan is instituted; the details are beyond the scope of this handbook.

When a patient relapses it is a demoralising experience, and their fears about dying will resurface. Most patients regard the diagnosis of recurrence as a greater psychological blow than the original diagnosis. It is important to be honest about the implications of relapse, especially if the patient has very advanced disease with poor prognosis. Honesty can be delivered with humanity and is usually appreciated. Realism must always be tempered with hope – a difficult balance even for the experienced clinician. Considerable psychological support will be needed and time should be allocated during the clinic to dealing adequately with all these aspects.

✧ A local relapse may predict for an early systemic relapse in the next year or so, or it may indicate that the original local control was inadequate and further treatment may still be curative.

✧ A systemic relapse indicates the disease is not curable. Further treatment is to control and contain. However, depending on response to second-line treatment, remission can be measured in terms of years, especially if the disease is bony rather than visceral. Newer targeted therapies are offering extended remissions.

Finally

In conclusion:

✧ never forget your duty of care is to the patient

✧ do not make decisions beyond your level of training or competence. If you are not sure check and check again – a patient may pay a very high price for your uncertainty

✧ never be afraid to ask for help or advice. Do not work in isolation – you are a member of the MDT, and the MDT is there to both train and support you.

Enjoy your time with the breast team. It will be a demanding, but rich and stimulating, professional and personal experience.

GP guidelines
'Urgent' referrals
Fewer than 5% of breast cancers occur in women under 40 years of age.
  Urgent referrals should be made for those:
✧ older than 35 years whose symptoms/signs are *highly* suggestive of breast cancer
✧ between 35 years and menopause for any discrete lump that persists over a menstrual cycle
✧ after menopause for any discrete lump.

Referral criteria for symptomatic breast clinic
Signs of breast cancer
Signs of breast cancer are:
✧ lump with dimpling/ulceration
✧ nipple retraction (new), distortion, ulceration (unilateral)
✧ others – change in skin contour, peau d'orange, dimpling and fungation.

Lumps
Please do not needle a lump with no recent/proven history of cysts. Signs include:
✧ discrete lump – lumps in post-menopausal women not using HRT are usually cancers
✧ asymmetrical, discrete nodularity that persists and does not change with cycle
✧ post-menopausal abscess/infection – refer for urgent treatment and investigation.

Nipple discharge
Multi-duct or multi-coloured discharge is innocent – duct ectasia.
  Signs of cancer include:
✧ any post-menopausal discharge
✧ bloodstained discharge (although 85% of bloody nipple discharge is benign, e.g. intraduct papilloma)
✧ persistent single duct discharge, especially if watery
✧ excessive discharge, sufficient to stain clothes (i.e. socially embarrassing)
✧ 'eczema': Paget's ulcerates the nipple then the areola. Eczema usually affects the areola only.

Pain
(Fewer than 5% of breast cancers *present* with pain and no lump. Pain is important if it is:
✧ associated with a lump (usually benign breast changes or cyst)
✧ intractable (but first try reassurance, well-supporting bra, dietary or lifestyle changes, EPO)
✧ unilateral, persistent (more than three months) pain in post-menopausal women.

Women who can be managed by a GP/practice nurse
The following conditions can be managed by a GP or practice nurse.
✧ Recurrent cysts: GP cyst aspiration should be performed only in women with proven cystic changes (previous triple assessment at Breast Unit). Always request cytology.
✧ Starting HRT: mammography is not indicated.

- Most women aged under 30 years: especially with cyclical, tender, lumpy breasts or symmetrical nodularity, with no focal or discrete abnormality.
- Most breast pain: explain its hormonal nature.
- Most nipple discharge: especially if multi-duct/multi-coloured.
- Most family history: asymptomatic women with average risk.
- Simple lactational sepsis that responds to antibiotics.

Breast screening eligibility

Breast screening is suitable only for *asymptomatic* women.

Familial breast cancer (up to 50 years of age)

Refer www.nice.org.uk.
   The following are the minimum referral criteria for moderate or higher risk.
- Mantle radiotherapy for Hodgkin's.
- One first-degree relative younger than 40 years with breast cancer or with bilateral breast cancer at any age.
- Two first-degree relatives younger than 50 years with breast cancer.
- Three first- or second-degree relatives at any age with breast cancer.
- Male relative (first-degree) with breast cancer or with a family history of ovarian/breast cancer.

NHSBSP (over 50 years of age)

Tel: 01206 744749
- Women aged between 50 and 70 receive an automatic invitation to have a three-yearly mammogram. There is no examination. The first invitation is sent at 49 to 52 years, depending on the local screening cycle. It is not sent at the fiftieth birthday.
- Women aged over 70 should be encouraged to self-refer to NHSBSP if they are asymptomatic.

Neck and endocrine

Bill Fleming

THREE

Introduction

The referral pattern of endocrine problems and neck lumps is variable, so general surgery trainees are likely to see these conditions during their training. Endocrine problems may be seen initially by an endocrinologist who refers suitable cases for surgery, or may present directly to general or specialist endocrine surgical clinics. In some centres patients may be referred to multidisciplinary endocrine clinics incorporating both physicians and surgeons. Neck lumps may be referred to almost any speciality and later be referred to appropriate specialist surgical clinics for investigation and treatment. Excisional biopsy may not be the correct course of action. Therefore, the surgical trainee needs a working knowledge of endocrine conditions so that the patient is managed appropriately.

Assessment of endocrine disorders

If a patient is referred with a lump in an endocrine gland there are certain principles that need to be followed.

✧ Make the endocrine diagnosis.
✧ Make the patient safe for surgery, if necessary.
✧ Localise the tumour.
✧ Decide whether the patient needs an operation.
✧ Decide what operation is appropriate.
✧ Replace any deficit.

How these principles are applied depends on the particular gland being assessed, and will be dealt with later in the chapter. In the first instance a careful history and examination are required, followed by targeted endocrine investigations to make the endocrine diagnosis.

Endocrine history

Most endocrine problems are found in the thyroid or parathyroid glands, but the adrenal and endocrine pancreas can also be affected. Unlike most other conditions, there is no single endocrine history. The symptoms vary widely according to the affected endocrine system, but the objectives of each consultation are similar: determining whether that lump is associated with an endocrine abnormality, or with any other lumps elsewhere, and whether the lump is benign or malignant.

It is not proposed to discuss pituitary disorders in this chapter, and pancreatic endocrine lesions and the Zollinger-Ellison syndrome are described in the pancreatic chapter. The carcinoid syndrome is described in the chapter about small intestinal disorders.

Endocrine examination

The examination is generally directed towards the specific endocrine system, but any endocrine gland mass may be associated with an endocrine syndrome, producing widespread effects on the patient, e.g. Cushing's syndrome. Endocrine masses are generally palpable only in the neck, as the pancreas and adrenals are relatively out of reach.

Investigation of endocrine disorders

As with the history and examination, investigations are targeted towards the endocrine gland in question, in order to firm up the diagnosis. In general, laboratory investigations aim to estimate hormone levels in either serum, urine or both, while imaging is used to localise the tumour, assess function and possibly determine the likelihood of malignancy.

Tissue biopsy, usually in the form of fine-needle cytology, may help in diagnosis of malignant lumps and direct the appropriate surgical approach. This is particularly important in the diagnosis of thyroid lumps.

Some of the specific investigations used in endocrine diagnosis will be described below.

Laboratory investigations

Biochemistry

Serum tests

Biochemical assays are available to determine the levels of most hormones in the serum as a measure of disease. Thyroid, parathyroid, adrenal and gut hormones can all be measured directly to determine over- or under-activity.

In addition, other disease markers can be estimated. Tumour markers are available, such as thyroglobulin in papillary thyroid cancer, and calcitonin and carcinoembryonic antigen (CEA) in the case of medullary carcinoma of the thyroid. These are particularly useful in the follow-up after total thyroidectomy and can act as an early warning of recurrence.

Urinary tests

These are particularly useful in patients with hyperparathyroidism, when 24-hour urinary calcium excretion may be elevated. Low excretion of calcium (less than 2 mmol/day) may indicate the rare condition of familial hypercalcaemic hypocalciuria (FHH), which can mimic hyperparathyroidism.

Functioning adrenal tumours may well be detected by excess hormone in the urine. Elevated 24-hour urinary catecholamines are indicative of phaeochromocytoma, while estimation of urinary cortisol excretion is used in the assessment of Cushing's syndrome. Conn's syndrome is associated with a low serum potassium and elevated excretion of potassium in the urine.

Provocation tests

Sometimes the standard measurement of serum levels does not accurately identify the disease or identify the ectopic production of a hormone. Provocation tests involve administering an agent that stimulates production of the hormone in question. Serum levels are monitored to determine whether levels of the hormone rise in response to the stimulus. For example, most ectopic sources of adrenocorticotropic hormone (ACTH) are not responsive to corticotropin-releasing hormone (CRH), while most pituitary lesions remain so. Administration of CRH produces a rise in serum ACTH if there is a pituitary source but no rise if there is an ectopic source.

A provocation test can be combined with selective venous sampling to localise the site of the lesion producing the hormone. For example, gastrinomas and other pancreatic or gut tumours can be stimulated to release hormones by administration of calcium into the arterial supply of the affected part. Selective venous sampling can then localise the tumour to the area of highest stimulated hormone excretion, even if no lump is visible on other imaging.

Immunology

Antibodies to thyroid peroxidase (thyroid microsomal antigen) are found in most patients with Graves' disease and in those with Hashimoto's thyroiditis. Thyroid-stimulating hormone receptor antibodies are found in 90% of patients with Graves' disease.

Genetic tests

Genetic tests are used mainly to screen first- and second-degree relatives of patients with multiple endocrine neoplasia (MEN) syndrome. MEN 1 is caused by an abnormality on the long arm of chromosome 11, while MEN 2 shows an abnormality on chromosome 10. Referral to a medical genetics department is essential, as pre-test and post-test counselling is an important part of the process.

Fine-needle aspiration (FNA) cytology

FNA is simple, safe and the most cost-effective method of assessing thyroid lumps. It is a quick technique that is well tolerated by the patient and well suited to busy clinics. Results are always interpreted in combination with the clinical and imaging assessments. Reports may use terms such as malignant, benign, suspicious or inadequate, or may be classified using the THY numbered classification. Results depend on the experience of the person performing the technique and the cytologist interpreting the result. Inadequate results occur infrequently if the FNA is performed by the cytologist or cytology technician. Generally inadequate FNA means the test must be repeated, with ultrasound guidance if the lesion is difficult to locate. The technique provides a tissue diagnosis, and in thyroid disease can accurately diagnose colloid nodules, thyroiditis, papillary carcinoma, medullary carcinoma, anaplastic carcinoma and lymphoma. Small numbers of cells are obtained. Follicular lesions on cytology cannot be separated into follicular adenomas and carcinomas, and usually require excision.

Imaging techniques
Ultrasound

This non-invasive technique is good at differentiating cystic and solid lesions, and it can detect nodules less than 0.5mm. Fine-needle aspiration can also be performed under ultrasound control for cytological examination, and the wall of cysts can be aspirated for cytology. It is a critical part of the localisation of parathyroid tumours. It is also possible to increase diagnostic yield by the use of contrast agents or microbubble techniques. Ultrasound is operator dependent and usually cannot distinguish between benign and malignant disease.

Thyroid isotope scan

The most common agents used in the assessment of the thyrotoxic patient are ^{123}I and technetium pertechnate ^{99m}Tc. The technique can differentiate hot from cold nodules, but overall it has a very limited role. Detection of metastases in patients after total thyroidectomy for medullary carcinoma of the thyroid can be achieved using pentavalent dimercaptosuccinic acid (DMSA), octreotide or meta-iodobenzylguanidine (MIBG).

In a low dose (2–5 mCi), ^{131}I can be used to detect metastatic disease after total thyroidectomy for the more common forms of thyroid cancer. The patient must have stopped thyroxine replacement some weeks beforehand or have recombinant thyroid-stimulating hormone (TSH) administered prior to the test. Detected metastases can then be treated with a therapeutic dose (150–200 mCi) of ^{131}I. It may be useful, in the assessment of the thyrotoxic patient, to differentiate single toxic nodules, toxic multinodular disease and Graves' disease.

Most metastatic follicular carcinomas and more than 80% of papillary carcinomas can be imaged. The technique uses radioactivity. Differentiation of nodules into 'hot' and 'cold' does not identify or exclude malignancy and therefore has a limited role assessing thyroid nodules. Twenty per cent of papillary carcinomas are not imaged by [131]I.

Parathyroid isotope scan

Technetium-sestamibi is the investigation of choice in the localisation of parathyroid tumours, superseding the older method of technetium-thallium ([210]Tl-chloride) subtraction scanning. Sestamibi accumulates in the mitochondria of parathyroid cells and has a more favourable emission spectrum, improving the sensitivity of the technique. Single photon emission computed tomography (SPECT) is also possible with this technique, allowing better spatial resolution.

Adrenal isotope scan

MIBG is taken up by catecholamine granules and is used mainly for localising phaeo-chromocytomas in the adrenal and in extra-adrenal sites and for the detection of metastases. Multiple gland involvement can be found in MEN syndromes. Therapeutic doses of MIBG can be used to treat some lesions. MIBG is very specific for catecholamine tumours with very few false positives, although false negatives occur in 5–10%.

Computerised tomography (CT) scans

CT scans are particularly useful in the assessment of large retrosternal goitres, to determine the relationship to other structures. They may also be used to locate ectopic or mediastinal parathyroid glands. Most adrenal lesions larger than 3cm can be detected with CT scanning. It uses ionising radiation.

Magnetic resonance imaging (MRI) scan

MRI scans are particularly useful in the assessment of large retrosternal goitres, to determine the relationship to other structures. The scan is also useful in detecting small pituitary, adrenal and pancreatic lesions and in detecting ectopic sites of hormone production or metastases. MRI is a useful technique for locating ectopic parathyroid glands, although angiography and venous sampling are more accurate. The technique is expensive and generally of limited availability. Many patients find the experience unpleasant.

Selective venous sampling

The technique is usually performed under local anaesthetic. The femoral vein is cannulated using the Seldinger technique, and vascular catheters are inserted and manipulated under radiological control until positioned correctly. Samples of blood are withdrawn from the catheter and from a peripheral vein simultaneously and the serum concentrations of hormone are compared. Sometimes an injection of a substance, such as calcium, is used to stimulate hormone release.

Selective venous sampling is used in difficult or recurrent cases to identify the site and side of secretion of the particular hormone. It is used in assessment of pituitary lesions and parathyroid lesions, but it can be used in the assessment of adrenal lesions and of ectopic production of hormones from other body sites. It is an expensive, time-consuming and invasive technique with a small but definite morbidity and mortality, so it is confined to redo surgical patients and some adrenal patients in general.

Neck lumps

The causes of neck lumps can be considered in four main groups: salivary gland lumps, thyroid lumps, lymph nodes (thyroid lumps and lymph nodes form the bulk of neck lumps referred to the general surgeon) and then non-thyroid lumps, which contain well-known but relatively rare causes that everyone learns for exams. The majority of thyroid lumps can be palpated in the region of the thyroid gland and move on swallowing, while non-thyroid lumps are in other locations and do not move on swallowing. Differentiating non-thyroid lumps from lymph nodes requires knowledge of their different characteristics, and these will now be described. If you are unsure of the extent of any of these lumps, especially recurrent lesions or extensive primary lesions, a high-resolution ultrasound or MRI scan is extremely helpful.

Lymphangiomas

Lymphangiomas are abnormal collections of lymph-filled tissue that are classified into three main groups:
✧ lymphangioma simplex (one-third occur in the floor of the mouth, e.g. as a ranula)
✧ cystic hygroma
✧ cavernous lymphangioma (mainly affects the tongue).

The smaller lymphangiomas occur in the lips and cheek, where the tissue planes are tighter, whereas cystic hygroma has more room to expand in the tissue planes of the neck. Two-thirds are noted at birth and 90% before the end of the second year. They usually transilluminate. Cystic hygromas can recur in adulthood at the margins of previous surgical excision.

Midline dermoid tumours

These are lumps caused by elements of one dermal layer trapped in another, either congenitally or by trauma.
✧ Epidermoid cysts contain cheesy contents of squamous epithelium only.
✧ True dermoid cysts contain squamous epithelium and skin appendages such as hair.
✧ Teratoid cysts contain endo, meso and ectoderm elements such as nails, teeth and brain.

These lumps tend to present as solid or cystic masses in the midline of the neck or lateral to the submandibular gland. Painless swelling is the only symptom, usually presenting in the second and third decades.

Thyroglossal duct cysts

These are a remnant from the descent of the thyroid from the back of the tongue. They can occur anywhere from the foramen caecum to the manubrial notch. They are found in an age range from four months to 70 years, but mean age at presentation is five years. Most are midline, but up to 10% may be deviated to one side (usually left).

History

Most patients complain of a painless cystic lump. Some present with tenderness and rapidly increasing size due to infection, while others present with a fistula discharging fluid.

Examination

Mobile in all directions; usually transilluminates; moves on swallowing or protruding tongue. Suprahyoid cysts may be mistaken for submental adenitis or a dermoid. Prehyoid cysts tend to be dumbbell or bar shaped and if large can push the tongue upwards, causing dysarthria.

Investigations

This is usually a clinical diagnosis. In doubtful cases ultrasound scanning (USS) will confirm the cystic nature. FNA is usually unnecessary and may introduce infection, but it may help in difficult cases.

Treatment
These cysts are prone to recurrent infection and are best treated by complete surgical excision.

Follow-up
Review at short intervals (1–4 weeks) until diagnosis is obtained. Arrange surgical excision promptly to prevent further episode of infection.

Post-operative follow-up
Review with histology to confirm diagnosis and to exclude the extremely rare thyroglossal duct carcinoma. Examine for general complications of neck surgery. The most common specific complication is a thyroglossal fistula, which results from infection or failure to remove the whole cyst. It usually presents as an opening in the lower neck, discharging clear fluid. Treatment is by further surgical excision.

Thyroglossal duct carcinoma is rare but should be excluded. It is always papillary. Ten per cent have metastases. Treatment is by local excision, thyroidectomy, radioactive iodine therapy and tumour suppressive doses of thyroxine.

Lingual thyroid
Lingual thyroid results when an embryological remnant of thyroid fails to descend to the normal position in the neck. They may be asymptomatic and unnoticed unless enlargement of the thyroid tissue occurs. The lingual thyroid may be the patient's only thyroid tissue, so excision may render the patient hypothyroid.

History
Patients may complain of a lump at the back of the tongue or of respiratory or swallowing difficulties.

Examination
Examination may be normal, or ear, nose and throat (ENT) examination reveals the swelling.

Investigations
The diagnostic investigation is ^{123}I scan, which differentiates lingual thyroid from other causes.

Treatment
It is possible to shrink an enlarged lingual thyroid with thyroxine therapy. If this fails, therapeutic radio-iodine (^{131}I) should be used. There is seldom any need to resort to surgery.

Follow-up
Follow-up is at short intervals (1–4 weeks) until diagnosis is obtained and relief of symptoms is achieved. Then intervals are increased (1–6 months) until the condition is stable and the patient is symptom-free. Monitor thyroid function tests to ensure adequate T4 replacement and TSH suppression. The patient may then be discharged, with advice to return if symptoms recur and for the GP to monitor the thyroid function tests.

Branchial cysts
The exact aetiology is unknown. The cysts may be remnants of branchial clefts, pouches or squamous metaplasia of a lymph node. Age range is 1–70 years, but peak incidence is in the third decade. Most occur on the left side and appear anterior to the sternomastoid muscle in the upper third of the neck.

History

Most patients complain of a continuous swelling, though in some patients the swelling can be intermittent. Pain affects up to a third of patients but infection occurs in less than 15% and some patients may complain of pressure symptoms.

Examination

Most feel cystic on palpation but do not transilluminate. Approximately one-third are solid. They tend to not have any attached sinus or fistula track, as branchial fistula is a separate disease. Branchial fistulas extend from an internal opening in the tonsillar bed, through the carotid artery bifurcation to an external opening in the lower part of the anterior triangle of the neck. Sinuses have similar external openings, but no internal openings. Fibrous tracts can also occur.

Investigations

A CT/MRI scan may be needed to differentiate from a chemodectoma if there is direct or transmitted pulsation and the cyst feels solid. If there is no pulsation, FNA can be performed and will reveal aspirates rich in cholesterol.

Treatment

Optimal treatment consists of primary excision surgery. Try to avoid excision drainage of infected tissue unless there is an obvious cyst that is going to discharge through the skin. If infection seems to be a problem, pre-operative antibiotics to reduce the amount of inflammatory tissue are worthwhile.

Follow-up

Review with results at 1–3 months and decide on management.

Post-operative follow-up

Review with results of histology (which, rarely, may contain squamous carcinoma) to confirm diagnosis and detect complications of the operation. Uncomplicated cyst removal not complicated by infection can be discharged. If there is doubt about complete excision, recurrence would normally occur within the first year. Thereafter advise and discharge.

Laryngocele

This is a rare, air-containing sac arising from the laryngeal saccule. Incidence is one in 2.5 million people per year, with a 5:1 male to female ratio. Peak incidence is 50–60 years. It may be external, presenting through the thyrohyoid membrane, or internal. The most important causative factor to exclude is a *co-existent carcinoma of the larynx*.

History

There may be hoarseness, neck swelling, stridor, dysphagia, sore throat, pain or cough. Ten per cent are infected.

Examination

There is a large swelling over the thyrohyoid membrane, which can be emptied easily by squeezing – but do not do it before the X-ray! Arrange for a full ENT examination of the larynx.

Investigations

Soft tissue neck X-ray shows an air-filled sac.

Treatment
Surgical excision – try to avoid emptying the sac before it is identified.

Follow-up
Review with results. Once cancer is excluded, arrange excision if fit for surgery.

Post-operative follow-up
Review once with histology and to detect any complications, e.g. wound infection. Reassure and discharge if uncomplicated.

Chemodectomas (paragangliomas)
These are tumours of neural crest tissue that occur in the carotid body, the jugular bulb and the ganglion nodosum of the vagus nerve in the neck.

Carotid body tumours (*see* vascular section) are rare, with an age range of 35–50 years. Five per cent are bilateral; 10% are malignant. There is a strong family history and they may be associated with phaeochromocytomas.

History
There is a long history of a painless lump (typically 4–7 years). Other symptoms include headache, neck pain, dizziness, hoarse voice and dysphagia caused by local invasion or cranial nerve compression. Occasional flushing, arrhythmias and hypertension are caused by neuroendocrine secretion by the tumour.

Examination
There is a lump up to 4–5cm in size that moves from side to side, but not up and down. It exhibits a transmitted but not an expansile pulse. Bruit may be present and may reduce in size with carotid compression. Large tumours may involve IX, X, XI and XII nerves and occasionally the sympathetic chain, causing Horner's syndrome.

Investigations
Duplex ultrasound and angiogram shows a splayed bifurcation and a 'tumour blush' circulation. There may be a feeding vessel from the external carotid or vertebral artery. CT/MRI may be useful to define the relationship of the tumour to other structures, especially if local invasion is suspected.

Treatment
Treatment involves surgical excision by an experienced vascular surgeon, in case vascular reconstruction is required.

Follow-up
Follow up in short intervals of 1–4 weeks, until diagnosis is obtained.

Post-operative follow-up
Review with histology to confirm diagnosis and complete excision and to detect any complications of wound healing. Exclude bilateral tumours and phaeochromocytoma. Arrange for genetic counselling and screening if there is a strong family history.

Glomus vagale tumour is a rare cause for a mass at the angle of the jaw. Angiography may show an abnormal circulation from the external carotid artery.

Neck lymph nodes
The first objective is to determine whether the enlarged lymph node is due to a localised problem in the head and neck or whether it is part of a generalised lymphadenopathy.

If the cause is localised to the head and neck, the second objective is to determine whether the cause of enlargement is non-malignant (e.g. infection – acute/chronic) or malignant (i.e. metastatic from a head and neck carcinoma). Any patient over the age of 50 presenting with a single enlarged lymph node in the upper part of the neck must have a full examination of the naso-, oro- and hypopharynx before biopsy of the neck node to exclude occult carcinoma in these areas.

History

Ask about local head and neck symptoms, nasal symptoms, voice change, cough, hoarseness and dysphagia. Ask about recent bouts of sore throat or tonsillitis, which may have given rise to enlarged draining nodes. General symptoms include weight loss, respiratory symptoms, abdominal symptoms and night sweats.

Examination

Examine the lump, noting size and consistency. Try to determine whether the node is isolated or part of generalised enlargement. Site the node in one of the anatomical triangles of the neck. The anterior triangle is formed by the midline of the neck, the anterior border of the sternomastoid muscle and the lower margin of the mandible. The posterior triangle is formed by the posterior border of the sternomastoid, the anterior border of the trapezius and the upper border of the clavicle. A thorough examination by an ENT specialist needs to be performed, of the mouth, naso-, oro-, and hypopharynx. A thorough examination of the thyroid, breast, lung, abdomen (including spleen and liver) and lower extremities needs to be performed for the site of possible primaries, especially if the enlarged nodes are in the supraclavicular fossae. All other lymph node sites need to be examined (axillae, groins, mediastinum and abdomen).

Investigations

Excision biopsy of the enlarged lymph node is not the first investigation. Laboratory tests include FBC and film (haematological abnormalities), polycythaemia vera/erythrocyte sedimentation rate (PV/ESR) and Monospot/Paul Bunnell (for glandular fever). Perform FNA of non-pulsatile lumps for cytology.

If lymphoma is a possibility, ask the laboratory for advice regarding the transport of specimens for tumour markers and flow cytometry.

Imaging with ultrasonography is useful for the differentiation of solid and cystic lumps, and for the diagnosis of vascular lumps such as carotid artery aneurysms or chemodectomas.

FNA is also useful for potentially infective lumps/lymph nodes, when a sample should also be sent for microbiology. If tuberculosis (TB) is suspected, a sample should be sent for Ziehl-Neelsen (ZN) stain and culture.

If no primary can be found in the head and neck for a malignant lymph node, the search has to be continued into the chest. A chest X-ray may indicate a bronchial neoplasm, TB or hilar/mediastinal pathology. Assessment of the gastrointestinal tract (GIT) may be indicated, with upper and lower gastrointestinal (GI) endoscopy. Consider ultrasound of the abdomen and occasionally CT scan of retroperitoneum and pancreas; consider breast mammogram for impalpable breast neoplasms.

Treatment

Management depends on the results of investigations. The assessment of all lumps depends on the clinical assessment, imaging and cytology. In children and young people, once lymphoma has been excluded the causes are usually related to infective episodes and will settle in time with antibiotics. Similarly, the management of TB lymph nodes is the relevant chemotherapy and referral to an infectious disease specialist.

In cases related to generalised lymphadenopathy, e.g. lymphoma/leukaemia or glandular fever, the management is of the underlying condition.

Occasionally FNA does not supply sufficient histological information, and surgical excision biopsy is indicated. This should not be undertaken without multidisciplinary input from ENT or a head and neck specialist.

For a single malignant lymph node presenting in the neck, a primary will be found on examination in approximately one-third of cases. The primary sites in order of frequency are: nasopharynx, tonsil, base of tongue, thyroid gland, supraglottic larynx, floor of mouth, palate, pyriform fossa, bronchus, oesophagus, breast and stomach. In a further third of patients no primary is evident at the time of presentation but becomes apparent on follow-up in the following sites: oropharynx, nasopharynx, thyroid, hypopharynx, lung, abdomen and miscellaneous (10%).

For a head and neck cancer, treatment is of the primary lesion with block dissection of the relevant lymph node field as indicated. If excision biopsy is necessary this should be performed by the surgeon who would perform the definitive head and neck surgery.

Follow-up

Follow-up intervals should be short until cancer has been excluded or the primary site identified.

Post-operative follow-up

Review at 1–2 weeks with the results of the histology and arrange further treatment if appropriate. Complications include wound infection, which usually responds to antibiotics. If the lymph node resection reveals TB, infection may be long term and chronic until antibiotic therapy is effective. Persistent lymph leak can occur, especially if the lymph node was neoplastic. Most will settle over 4–6 weeks. Some persistent or copious leaks may be associated with neoplastic lymphatic obstruction, which may respond to local radiotherapy.

Salivary gland lumps

Causes of salivary gland enlargement are divided into:
- enlargement of more than one gland (mumps, echo, coxsackie viruses, Sjögrens)
- generalised enlargement of one gland (sialectasis)
- localised enlargement of part of one gland
  - benign tumours – pleomorphic adenomas, monomorphic adenomas (Warthin's), oncocytoma
  - malignant tumours – adenoid cystic carcinoma, adenocarcinoma, squamous carcinoma, malignant pleomorphic adenoma
  - potentially malignant tumours – mucoepidermoid, acinic cell, rare tumours.

Twenty per cent of parotid tumours are malignant; 45% of submandibular tumours are malignant; 65% of minor salivary gland tumours are malignant.

History

The following should be considered.
- Age: mumps is more common in children, but if it occurs twice it is more likely to be congenital sialectasis.
- Does the swelling affect one gland or more than one: tumours are unilateral (Warthin's is occasionally bilateral).
- Is swelling related to eating: calculous disease secondary to sialectasis.
- Pain is generally due to duct obstruction from calculous disease. Occasionally adenoid cystic carcinoma with nerve involvement will be the cause of pain.

✧ Systemic disorders which can cause painless salivary gland enlargement include myxoedema, diabetes, Cushing's, cirrhosis, gout and alcohol abuse, sarcoid and TB, as well as certain drugs, such as thiouracil and high-oestrogen pills.

Examination

Examine all salivary glands. Is one gland affected, or more than one? Is enlargement due to a localised mass within the gland or is there a generalised enlargement of the gland? Is there skin involvement? Is there facial weakness? Is the lesion solid or cystic? Is the lesion irregular? (However, benign pleomorphic adenomas are often irregular and knobbly.) Benign tumours are usually mobile.

Investigations

If indicated, use laboratory tests to exclude myxoedema, diabetes, Cushing's, rheumatoid arthritis.

If sarcoid is suspected, a Kveim test is needed. FBC and ESR may be needed.

Plain X-rays are used if calculous disease is suspected. However, remember that parotid stones are radiolucent; submandibular stones are radiopaque. Intraoral films may be required.

Sialography (cannulation of the salivary duct and injection of contrast) is useful for a diagnosis of sialectasis. Congenital saccular sialectasis gives a snowstorm appearance. Advanced cystic disease shows large collections of dye. Pure duct stenosis is nearly always an iatrogenic artifact caused by traumatic cannulisation.

CT scans are useful for determining the extent of spread of malignant salivary tumours and for planning the surgical approach.

FNA for cytology is mandatory in every case. Avoid excision biopsies unless there is diffuse enlargement of the gland and no diagnosis has been reached by other methods.

Diagnosis of minor salivary gland tumours is by incisional biopsy performed by the surgeon who will eventually remove the lesion.

Treatment

The following treatments are used.

✧ Benign parotid tumours are treated by superficial parotidectomy if the tumour is located in the superficial part of the gland, which happens in 80% of cases. Benign submandibular tumours are rare and the treatment is removal of the whole gland. Minor salivary gland tumours are diagnosed by incisional biopsy and then excised.

✧ Malignant parotid tumours are treated by total parotidectomy. If the facial nerve is involved this is also excised and a decision is made at operation regarding nerve grafting. If neck nodes are palpable, total parotidectomy is combined with a radical neck dissection. Post-operatively, radiotherapy is given if the resection margins are in doubt.

✧ Malignant submandibular tumours are treated by excision of the gland and, if necessary, the mandible, skin and adjacent nerves if involved. Reconstruction is possible. Post-operative radiotherapy is used if there are doubtful resection margins.

✧ Minor salivary glands are treated by wide excision and reconstruction of the oral cavity.

✧ Mucoepidermoid and acinic cell tumours are often diagnosed on post-operative histology after excision of an apparently benign mass. Tumours are graded as either high grade or low grade, with prognosis determined by the grade. For low grade, 90% have five-year survival; for high grade, it is 20%. Many surgeons give immediate post-operative radiotherapy. Some surgeons prefer to follow up patients monthly or bi-monthly for 4–5 years to detect recurrence, and then to treat by wide field excision and post-operative radiotherapy. Refer for an oncology opinion in every case.

◇ Sialectasis has mild and infrequent symptoms, so advise the patient to finish each meal with a citrus drink and massage the duct to expel debris from it. Many patients have no further trouble after the diagnostic sialogram, which flushes the ducts.

◇ Submandibular duct stones are treated by surgical removal via the intraoral route and marsupulisation. Stones in the body of the gland are treated by removal of the whole gland.

◇ Parotid duct stones are removed intraorally. Persistent severe symptoms are treated by total parotidectomy (superficial parotidectomy is often insufficient).

Follow-up

Follow-up intervals are short (1–4 weeks) until cancer has been excluded. Generalised causes of salivary gland enlargement are referred to the relevant specialist. Mild sialectasis can be discharged with the relevant treatment advice and a plan to return if symptoms deteriorate. More severe cases can be reviewed at three-monthly intervals or greater until the patient and surgeon feel that surgery is indicated.

Post-operative follow-up

The success of the operation is determined by the histology, the wound healing and the absence of complications. Review the histology report to ensure that presumed benign lumps were benign and did not contain any malignant elements. If the operation was performed for malignant disease, confirm that the resection margins were clear of tumour. If not, or if resection margins were very close to the tumour, refer for an oncology opinion regarding radiotherapy.

◇ Complications of parotidectomy: Frey's syndrome consists of discomfort, sweating and redness of the skin over the parotid area during and after eating. This is caused when the severed ends of parasympathetic secretomotor nerve fibres in scar tissue are stimulated (as they formerly were to produce saliva) causing vasodilatation and sweating. Spontaneous resolution within six months is usual. Treatment for severe persistent cases is an ipsilateral tympanic neurectomy to divide the parasympathetic pathway.

◇ Facial nerve injury causing facial muscle weakness may respond to rehabilitation. Occasionally tarsorrhaphy, fascial sling procedures, nerve grafting or a unilateral face lift are required.

◇ Salivary fistula tends to occur where a sialectatic deep lobe is left in situ with a cut surface. Most cases settle with time. Anticholinergic drugs may help, as may radiotherapy for persistent cases. Alternatively, further surgery to remove the deep lobe is indicated.

Thyroid lumps

Goitre

There is visible or palpable enlargement of the thyroid gland. Causes of thyroid disease can be divided into diffuse enlargement of the thyroid gland such as physiological goitre (pregnancy, menarche); endemic goitre (iodine deficiency, Derbyshire neck); sporadic goitre (goitrogens include cabbage, p-aminosalicylic acid (PAS) and lithium drugs); autoimmune (Graves' disease, Hashimoto's); and focal lumps in the thyroid (non-toxic nodular goitre, adenomas, carcinomas, lymphoma and medullary cell carcinoma).

History

History of the lump and history of thyroid symptoms are required. Most patients give a history of painless enlargement. Look at rate of growth and if there has been sudden recent enlargement. Ask about voice change. Look for symptoms of tracheal compression, including inspiratory stridor. Hyperthyroid symptoms include sweating, palpitations, heat intolerance, menstrual irregularities, weight loss, anxiety, diarrhoea and muscle weakness. Hypothyroid symptoms are the opposite of these. Painful enlargement of the gland may indicate Hashimoto's thyroiditis.

Examination
Examination of the lump
Inspect to see if the enlargement is visible, and, if so, whether it moves on swallowing or protrusion of the tongue. Palpate to determine whether the whole gland is enlarged or just part of it. Is the enlargement confined to one lobe? Does the gland feel regular (Graves') or irregular (nodular goitre)? Are draining lymph nodes enlarged? A thyroid swelling firm to palpation, either diffuse or one-sided in a post-menopausal female, usually raises the suspicion of Hashimoto's.

Undifferentiated thyroid cancers and medullary cancers can present with an enlarging neck mass involving other neck structures, e.g. recurrent laryngeal nerve. ENT examination may be required if recurrent laryngeal nerve palsy is suspected.

Examination of thyroid status
Over-activity is indicated by hand tremor, palmar sweating and tachycardia; under-activity by slow pulse, hoarse voice and slow relaxing tendon reflexes. Features of Graves' disease include exophthalmos, lid lag, lid retraction and pretibial myxoedema. Destruction of the thyroid tissue by the autoimmune process in Hashimoto's usually renders patients hypothyroid eventually, although they may be thyrotoxic in the early stages.

Investigations
Management should follow the principles outlined earlier, determining the diagnosis, localising the lesion and then determining if the patient needs an operation and, it so, which one.

As with lumps in other body sites, thyroid lumps should undergo triple assessment consisting of clinical assessment combined with imaging and cytology from FNA and biochemical assessment of thyroid status: T4, T3 and TSH. Thyroglobulin is available as a tumour marker, but it is only of use after total thyroidectomy, when it should fall to zero in the absence of metastases.

Ultrasound examination of the thyroid will determine whether lumps are solid or cystic and whether lumps are single (suspicious) or multiple (e.g. part of a multinodular goitre).

^{123}I isotope scanning can identify thyroid tissue and determine whether nodules are hot or cold, but this is rarely useful except in the toxic patient. A CT or MRI scan of the neck and upper chest can identify tracheal deviation and retrosternal extension of thyroid. FNA biopsy for cytology should be performed in every case.

If medullary carcinoma is suspected, serum calcitonin levels are very high and can be used as a tumour marker. A rise in levels after treatment may indicate recurrence. If medullary carcinoma is confirmed, patients should be screened for co-existing parathyroid adenoma (calcium, phosphate and serum parathyroid hormone (PTH)) and phaeochromocytoma (urinary catecholamine levels).

Tests for thyroid autoantibodies are performed if Hashimoto's thyroiditis is suspected, and they can confirm a diagnosis of Graves' disease.

Results
- ✧ Diffusely enlarged gland, euthyroid: physiological and endemic goitre.
- ✧ Diffusely enlarged gland, hyperthyroid: Graves' disease. The early stages of Hashimoto's may give this appearance but this is rare. In contrast to Graves', Hashimoto's does not demonstrate increased uptake in a radioisotope scan.

- Focally enlarged gland, euthyroid: diagnosis includes simple cysts; a single dominant nodule in a multinodular goitre; benign adenomas; and malignant tumours.
  - ∝ Malignant tumours can be classified as papillary, follicular, medullary and anaplastic. FNA cannot differentiate between follicular adenomas and carcinomas and all should be regarded as potentially malignant.
- Focally enlarged gland, hyperthyroid: thyrotoxic adenoma, thyrotoxic nodule in a multinodular goitre.

Treatment

All suspicious and malignant lumps require surgery. Cystic lumps which are malignant, greater than 4cm in size, contain blood or recur after 2–3 aspirations require surgery. Most retrosternal goitres require surgery.

Benign lumps

- Benign cysts should be aspirated and reviewed at six weeks. This can be repeated on two or three occasions. If they recur, surgery is required. If there is no recurrence, review at six months, and if there is still no recurrence, discharge.
- For a solitary thyroid nodule that is euthyroid and benign, surgery is required only for treatment of pressure symptoms or from patient preference. Repeat FNA once or twice over the next 12 months, and if there is no change, the patient could be discharged.
- A solitary thyroid nodule, hyperthyroid, benign and less than 3cm in size can be treated by radio-iodine or surgery. Those greater than 3cm require surgery.
- For a multinodular goitre, euthyroid, if no dominant nodule or pressure symptoms are present patients should be observed for 12–18 months, then discharged with advice, unless surgery is indicated for large lesions or the patient is worried by the cosmetic appearance.
- For a multinodular goitre, euthyroid, with a dominant nodule that is benign on FNA and shows no pressure symptoms, observation is acceptable. If the dominant nodule is suspicious or malignant, surgery is indicated.
- A multinodular goitre, hyperthyroid, for small glands can be treated with ^{131}I. Large glands are treated with antithyroid drugs and surgery.

Malignant thyroid tumours

These tumours can be classified as papillary, follicular, medullary and anaplastic.

- Differentiated thyroid cancer: prognosis is determined by age. Children and young adults have a 90% five-year survival. The same tumour occurring in mid-life is associated with a 60% five-year survival. Prognosis is worse if there is a history of prior neck irradiation. Treatment generally consists of total thyroidectomy, which will treat frequently multifocal disease, decrease local recurrence and allow post-operative treatment with ^{131}I and monitoring of thyroglobulin levels. Local enlarged lymph nodes should also be excised, followed by radio-iodine ablation and suppressive doses of thyroxine. The patient is then monitored for recurrence using ultrasound and by measurement of thyroglobulin levels. Metastases are treated with therapeutic doses of radio-iodine. Treatment of low-risk microcarcinomas (smaller than 1cm) by total lobectomy is adequate, followed by TSH-suppressive doses of thyroxine.
- Undifferentiated thyroid cancer: frequently symptoms of rapid swelling, voice changes and stridor may require total thyroidectomy to relieve or prevent respiratory obstruction, but prognosis is grave. Adjuvant radiotherapy can be given but chemotherapy has no role.
- Medullary carcinoma of the thyroid arises from parafollicular cells and has no benign variant. Calcitonin levels are high and can be used as a tumour marker. Medullary

thyroid cancer (MTC) is sporadic in 80% of patients, but 20% have MEN-2 syndrome, associated with phaeochromocytoma and parathyroid adenomas, which should be excluded by estimations of serum PTH and urinary catecholamine levels. Treatment consists of total thyroidectomy and excision of central compartment lymph nodes. This tumour is not responsive to radiotherapy, chemotherapy or TSH suppression, so thyroxine is given in replacement doses.

✧ Lymphoma: primary lymphoma is rare and usually of the non-Hodgkin's B-cell type, and it tends to complicate cases of Hashimoto's thyroiditis of 10–15 years' duration. This responds well to radiotherapy and chemotherapy, and if diagnosed early enough thyroidectomy can be avoided. Surgery is reserved for tracheal decompression. Stridor can sometimes be successfully managed with dexamethasone and radiotherapy.

Other thyroid conditions

✧ Autoimmune thyroiditis in practice means Hashimoto's, since other variants, such as Riedel's and de Quervain's, are so rare that some experienced thyroid surgeons have never seen a case. Surgical intervention is avoided and the condition responds well to T3/T4 therapy to suppress TSH-stimulated enlargement of the gland.

✧ Graves' disease: three treatment options are available, but choice depends on individual circumstances.

   ∝ Antithyroid drugs such as carbimazole or propylthiouracil can be given for 18 months, which cures fewer than 50% of patients. Nearly 45% relapse in the first year after stopping, and 20% of the remaining patients relapse in each of the subsequent five years. Drug toxicity is not uncommon. Beta blockade can also be used for control of symptoms and is especially useful in patients being prepared for surgery when given in combination with an antithyroid drug.

   ∝ Radio-iodine treatment ablates the thyroid tissue and will cure most patients, although repeat doses may be needed. More than 60% will become hypothyroid in the first year. Radio-iodine is the favoured method of treatment, but may not be suitable in young women of child-bearing age or in those with young children. Others simply prefer to avoid radiation exposure and opt for surgery.

   ∝ Indications for surgery include patients with recurrence of thyrotoxicosis after medical therapy; patient preference; pressure symptoms; and the presence of unsightly goitres. Generally the author favours total thyroidectomy to guarantee cure and prevent possible recurrence. Subtotal thyroidectomy, leaving approximately 5 ml of tissue on each side, is difficult to judge successfully, resulting in a small recurrence rate or hypothyroidism. The patient should be euthyroid before surgery, so antithyroid drugs are continued up to the day of surgery.

Follow-up

In the diagnostic phase, follow-up intervals should be short (1–2 weeks) until malignant causes have been excluded. Similarly, any thyrotoxic patient should be reviewed within 1–2 weeks with the results of the thyroid function tests, and at 2–4-weekly intervals to assess the effect of antithyroid drug therapy. When putting patients on the waiting list for operation, patients with focal thyroid lumps should be operated on within 4–6 weeks to exclude malignancy. Known malignant tumours should be removed quickly, as should those with non-malignant causes but with symptoms of tracheal compression.

Post-operative follow-up

Review the patient with the histology report to confirm the diagnosis and adequate excision and to detect any complications of thyroidectomy. All patients should be referred to a multidisciplinary team for further assessment and management.

Differentiated thyroid cancer

For those patients who have undergone total thyroidectomy, surveillance for recurrence is required using either regular estimations of serum thyroglobulin levels, or ultrasound, or both.

If tumour size is greater than 1cm, the patient undergoes a ^{131}I total-body scintiscan 4–6 weeks post-operatively. If there is evidence of uptake in the neck or elsewhere, therapeutic radioactive iodine is administered. The scintiscan is repeated six-monthly for the first two years and then annually for five years.

In the absence of metastases, thyroglobulin falls to zero after total thyroidectomy. Any rise post-operatively is an indicator of functioning thyroid tissue, either as a local recurrence or as distant metastases, which requires ablation with radio-iodine. All patients receive TSH-suppressing doses of thyroxine.

Undifferentiated thyroid cancer

All patients receive TSH-suppressing doses of thyroxine. Patients should be referred to an oncologist for consideration of adjuvant radiotherapy.

Medullary carcinoma

There is a 90% five-year survival in the absence of lymph node involvement; 45% if lymph nodes are involved. Patients are monitored for recurrence with regular calcitonin and CEA levels. A rise in levels can indicate recurrence, which can be detected by USS, CT/MRI, DMSA, MIBG or selective venous sampling. Recurrences can be treated by re-operation or radiotherapy, but response rates are poor.

Voice change due to inadvertent damage to the recurrent laryngeal nerve occurs in less than 1% of cases. Damage to the external laryngeal nerve supplying the cricothyroid muscle causes difficulty in tensing the vocal cords. It affects the quality of the voice and may be particularly significant to singers. Damage to the internal laryngeal nerves – usually during mobilising the upper pole – desensitizes the appropriate side of the larynx and can cause aspiration or coughing. Referral for an ENT opinion is appropriate. Hypoparathyroidism occurs in approximately 1%. Temporary hypocalcaemia is common in the first few days, especially after thyrotoxicosis, due to a combination of venous congestion and hungry bones demineralised by the thyrotoxic state. Long-term treatment with vitamin D may be necessary.

Other problems of the wound include haematoma formation, keloid formation and suture granuloma. Haematomas are uncommon but can be life-threatening if large. Because sudden respiratory difficulty after thyroid surgery may be due to haematoma formation, sutures should be removed in the ward to evacuate the clot, including deep sutures. Most minor haematomas detected in outpatients can be handled conservatively. Suture granulomas respond to removal of the suture, while keloid scars can be excised after a year, but can recur.

Parathyroids and disorders of calcium metabolism

The dominant hormone regulating calcium metabolism is parathormone (PTH), and the total absence of calcitonin has little effect on calcium homeostasis. A fall in serum calcium level stimulates an increase in PTH secretion, as do a fall in magnesium and an increase in phosphate. PTH increases serum calcium concentration by increasing resorption of bone, decreasing excretion by the kidney and increasing absorption from the intestines. PTH mediates the production of the active 1,25-dihydroxycholecalciferol from vitamin D precursors in the kidney. The effects of PTH on the bones and intestine do not occur in cases of vitamin D deficiency.

Hypercalcaemia

The main cause of hypercalcaemia of interest to the surgeon is hyperparathyroidism. Other causes include bone metastases, excess vitamin D ingestion, milk alkali syndrome, hyperthyroidism, multiple myeloma, reticuloses, leukaemias, sarcoidoses, Addison's disease, Paget's disease of bone, renal failure, thiazide diuretics and ectopic secretion of PTH.

History

This usually involves vague symptoms of tiredness, lethargy and muscle pains; it is rare to see 'bones, moans, stones and groans'. There may be a change in mood, especially depression; a history of dyspepsia or peptic ulceration; or polyuria, nocturia or polydipsia. There may be a history of renal stones; constipation; thiazide diuretic therapy; or vitamin D ingestion. Symptoms are related to the possible underlying causes.

There may be a family history of hypercalcaemia, e.g. MEN syndrome. There is also the condition known as familial hypercalcaemic hypocalciuria (FHH), which is due to a resetting of the sensitivity of the calcium receptor and is unrelated to parathyroid disease. A low urinary calcium excretion, combined with a family history, should alert the clinician.

Examination

Parathyroid adenomas seldom produce lumps in the neck large enough to palpate. A general physical examination is performed, looking for signs suggesting other diagnoses, e.g. Paget's. Hypercalcaemia may produce few signs apart from dehydration, myopathy and, rarely, a calcified ring around the cornea.

Investigations

Confirm the hypercalcaemia. Repeat the serum calcium levels corrected for serum albumin, and measure the PTH and vitamin D levels. A low serum phosphate and a raised alkaline phosphatase and chloride suggest a parathyroid cause. A plain CXR, full blood count and film, urea and electrolytes and serum electrophoresis will exclude many non-parathyroid cases. A normal or raised PTH level, in the presence of a raised calcium level, indicates hyperparathyroidism.

Treatment

Mild to moderate hypercalcaemia (2.6–3 mmol/l) usually responds to medical measures such as avoiding bed rest, keeping well hydrated and consuming a diet containing a moderate amount of calcium. This is combined with treatment of the underlying cause. Moderate to severe hypercalcaemia (more than 3 mmol/l) cannot be easily controlled by these medical measures and may require the use of bisphosphonates or even admission to hospital for intravenous saline. Investigation and surgical therapy if indicated should be expedited.

Follow-up

Mild hypercalcaemia can be reviewed at short intervals (1–4 weeks) to monitor serum calcium levels in response to treatment and to establish the diagnosis. More severe hypercalcaemia may require admission to hospital for further management.

Hypocalcaemia

Causes include uraemic osteodystrophy; post-operative parathyroid and thyroid surgery; and vitamin D deficiency. Ureamic osteodystrophy occurs in chronic renal failure, where calcium is not reabsorbed by the kidneys and phosphate is not secreted, leading to accumulation. PTH is secreted in excess, the parathyroid glands become hyperplastic and calcium is resorbed from the bones, leading to osteitis fibrosa cystica.

History

Hypocalcaemia gives symptoms of paraesthesia of the fingers and around the mouth. Long-term hypocalcaemia may lead to the development of epilepsy. There may be a history of recent neck surgery; of inadequate diet, poor in the fat soluble vitamins; or of religious clothing preventing adequate exposure to sunlight.

Examination

Signs of hypocalcaemia include positive Chvostek's sign and positive Trousseau's sign. In the long term, hypocalcaemia leads to the development of cataract. There may be signs of osteomalacia and rickets; of recent neck surgery; or of chronic renal failure.

Investigations

Test for serum calcium, albumin, urea and electrolytes and PTH level. Carry out liver function tests and a renal ultrasound scan.

Treatment

- ✧ Uraemic osteodystrophy: correction of hypocalcaemia, then total parathyroidectomy.
- ✧ Osteomalacia and rickets: Vitamin D (1-alpha-cholecalciferol).
- ✧ Post-surgery hypocalcaemia: temporary hypocalcaemia is common after thyroidectomy for thyrotoxicosis, due to venous congestion of parathyroid glands and hungry bones. In the acute situation, intravenous injection of 10 ml of 10% calcium gluconate is rarely needed and should only be given via a central line. Patients can generally be controlled acutely and in the longer term with oral calcium supplements and 1-alpha-cholecalciferol. Regular checking of serum calcium and PTH is essential, as parathyroid recovery may lead to iatrogenic hypercalcaemia.

Hyperparathyroidism

Primary hyperparathyroidism is due to a parathyroid adenoma or, more rarely, primary hyperplasia. Secondary hyperparathyroidism is caused by a reactive hyperplasia of the glands in response to chronic calcium losing states such as malabsorption or chronic renal failure. Tertiary hyperparathyroidism occurs when a secondary gland becomes autonomous. Exclude other associated neoplasms (MEN 1, MEN 2). Hyperparathyroidism pathology consists of a single adenoma (85%), two adenomas (5%), carcinoma (1%) and hyperplasia (5–10%).

History

Secondary and tertiary causes can generally be excluded if there is no history of malabsorption or chronic renal failure. A family history of other endocrine neoplasms should raise the possibility of the multiple endocrine neoplasia syndromes.

Examination

Look for evidence of hypercalcaemia, malnutrition or chronic renal failure.

Investigations

Following the principles of endocrine assessment, diagnosis of hyperparathyroidism is confirmed on finding a normal or raised PTH level in the presence of hypercalcaemia. Once the diagnosis has been made, and the patient has a safe calcium level (below 3 mmol/l), the tumour needs to be localised to allow minimally invasive surgery.

Localising investigations consist of high-resolution ultrasound and technetium-sestamibi scanning, which will find the affected gland in about 75% of cases. For redo cases, other imaging with MRI or CT scanning and angiography with selective venous sampling are required.

Treatment

If the tumour has been localised with concordant scans, a minimally invasive surgical approach is indicated, removing only the affected gland. If the tumour is not localised or hyperplasia is suspected, surgical exploration of all glands is undertaken and the abnormal glands are removed. Intra-operative frozen section should always be used to confirm the appropriate tissue has been removed, and intra-operative PTH measurement is very useful if available.

- ⬥ Primary parathyroid adenoma: surgical excision by minimally invasive approach.
- ⬥ Secondary parathyroid hyperplasia (four glands): usually excision of all four glands, or three glands, and leave half of the fourth marked with a metal clip.
- ⬥ Tertiary hyperparathyroidism, autonomously functioning hyperplastic or adenomatous: usually total parathyroidectomy and lifelong maintenance on calcium and vitamin D therapy; or total parathyroidectomy and reimplantation of gland fragments in the brachioradialis muscle of the forearm.
- ⬥ Parathyroid carcinoma: if recognised pre- or intra-operatively it is treated by parathyroidectomy, ipsilateral thyroid lobectomy and lymph node dissection (if nodes present), followed by radiotherapy.

Follow-up

Bone disease caused by excess reabsorption of calcium by hyperparathyroidism (osteitis fibrosa cystica) is particularly severe with secondary and tertiary hyperparathyroidism, and it requires calcium and vitamin D therapy for months.

Post-operative follow-up

Review with histology to confirm the diagnosis. Confirm the biochemical success of the operation. Persistent hyperparathyroidism is diagnosed if hypercalcaemia recurs within six months of operation. Recurrent hyperparathyroidism occurs after six months. The common cause of persistent hyperparathyroidism is unrecognised multiple gland disease. The source of persistent or recurrent tumour can be localised with angiography and selective venous sampling. Reoperation is indicated but technically can be very difficult.

Parathyroid carcinoma is monitored with frequent estimations of serum calcium and PTH to detect recurrence or metastases. Recurrence in the neck is treated by en bloc resection if possible, otherwise palliation of hypercalcaemia with calcimimetics.

Multiple endocrine neoplasia (MEN) syndromes

Multiple endocrine neoplasia syndromes are rare, but require screening of family members for the genetic abnormalities and the appropriate investigation of possible tumours if the genetic defect is found. Family members without the genetic defect do not need to be screened.

MEN 1

MEN 1 is an autosomal dominant disease consisting of hyperparathyroidism, pituitary tumours and pancreatic tumours. It is caused by a defect on the long arm of chromosome 11.

- ⬥ Hyperparathyroidism occurs in 90% of patients, characteristically hyperplasia.
- ⬥ Pancreatic islet tumours occur in 30–75% and tend to be multiple. Gastrinomas occur in 30–60% and insulinomas in 35%. Others consist of glucagonomas and vasoactive intestinal peptide tumors (VIPomas).
- ⬥ Pituitary adenomas occur in 15–40%. Prolactinomas are the most common, with acromegaly (growth hormone) and Cushing's syndrome (ACTH hypersecretion) less common.

✧ Carcinoid tumours and thyroid neoplasia are more common, and adrenocortical adenomas are also found, although tending to be non-functional.

Investigations

Screening of affected family members consists of genetic screening, biochemical tests and imaging. In family members carrying the defective gene on chromosome 11, biochemical screening is performed yearly after puberty and consists of measuring serum calcium, PTH, prolactin and gut hormones every 1–3 years. Suspected insulinomas are investigated by measuring serum glucose, insulin and pro-insulin levels during symptomatic episodes. MRI scans of the pituitary are performed every five years and combined with estimations of serum prolactin levels.

Treatment

✧ Hyperparathyroidism is treated by total parathyroidectomy.
✧ Gastrinomas: medical therapy is effective, but needs to be lifelong. Enucleation is performed for lesions in the head of the pancreas or duodenum. Distal pancreatectomy is performed for lesions in the body or tail. Recurrent or metastatic disease occurs in 50% and is treated symptomatically.
✧ Insulinoma: enucleation is performed for suitable lesions. Inoperable disease is treated with diazoxide and chemotherapy. Octreotide is effective.
✧ Pituitary lesions: hypophysectomy and external beam radiotherapy are used. Bromocriptine and its derivatives are effective for treatment of prolactinomas and acromegaly.

MEN 2

This is an autosomal dominant condition with a chromosomal defect in the RET proto-oncogene on chromosome 10. Three forms exist.
✧ MEN 2A represents approximately 90% of cases of MEN 2, consisting of medullary carcinoma of thyroid (MTC)(25%), phaeochromocytoma (50%), and hyperparathyroidism (15%).
✧ MEN 2B represents 5% of MEN 2, with an association of MTC, phaeochromocytomas (often bilateral), a general lack of parathyroid disease, and a Marfanoid body habitus, multiple mucosal neuromas and gut ganglioneuromas (which can cause severe constipation and diarrhoea).
✧ FMTC or familial MTC – patients with inherited MTC but no other endocrine abnormalities.

Investigations

Genetic screening of all first- and second-degree relatives is performed. Affected individuals undergo yearly biochemical screening, consisting of calcitonin levels and screening for phaeochromocytoma (urinary catecholamine levels) and hyperparathyroidism (serum calcium, phosphate and albumin, PTH).

Treatment

Total thyroidectomy is performed in all affected children aged 5–7 to prevent metastatic medullary carcinoma, but it should be done as early as possible in genetic carriers, as MTC can occur as early as the first year of life. The parathyroids are examined at the same time and removed if enlarged. Phaeochromocytomas are treated appropriately if they are detected.

The adrenal gland

The main disorders of the adrenal gland requiring surgical intervention include Cushing's syndrome and Conn's syndrome, which affect the adrenal cortex, and phaeochromocytoma, which affects the medulla.

Cushing's syndrome

Excess amounts of cortisol in the blood lead to the characteristic features of Cushing's syndrome, which is most commonly caused by long-term steroid treatment. True Cushing's disease is adrenocortical hyperplasia caused by a pituitary lesion. The diagnosis of Cushing's syndrome is suspected in patients with the characteristic clinical features and confirmed by finding an inappropriately raised serum and urinary cortisol level. Once this has been obtained the next objective is to determine whether this is due to a pituitary lesion, adrenal lesion (adenoma or carcinoma), or ectopic production of ACTH by oat cell carcinoma of bronchus, branchial carcinoid tumours, thymic tumours, islet cell tumours or phaeochromocytomas. If an adrenal lesion is implicated the next objective is to localise it.

History/examination

Look for obesity, especially of face and trunk, with thin extremities, moon face, menstrual irregularities, osteoporosis, striae, glucose intolerance, myopathy, hirsutism, bruising and oedema. In ectopic ACTH syndrome the clinical appearance is dominated by the effects of malignancy – pigmentation and severe proximal myopathy. Patients may also present with symptoms of diabetes mellitus, polyuria and hypertension.

Investigations

A simple screening test is to measure the cortisol in a 24-hour urine collection.

For definitive diagnosis the patient generally needs more extensive investigation in hospital, with determination of 24-hour urinary free cortisol and then serum cortisol to demonstrate loss of circadian rhythm. Low- and high-dose dexamethasone suppression tests are undertaken as well. Morning serum ACTH levels are measured. They will be high in pituitary tumours, very high in ectopic production and low in adrenal tumours.

Localisation

If ACTH is not raised, this indicates an adrenal lesion – a CT or MRI scan of the abdomen localises the adrenal tumour or tumours.

If ACTH is raised, this indicates either a pituitary lesion or ectopic production. A CXR may reveal a bronchial lesion or a widened mediastinum caused by a thymic tumour. An MRI scan of the chest for ectopic sources is more sensitive. Similarly, an MRI scan of the pituitary fossa will identify most pituitary lesions. Most ectopic sources are not CRH dependent, so an injection of CRH will not cause a rise in ACTH, whereas most pituitary lesions remain CRH dependent and a rise does occur. Similarly, high-dose dexamethasone will decrease cortisol levels in pituitary lesions but not in ectopic lesions. If this does not resolve the site of ACTH secretion, selective venous sampling of the inferior petrosal sinuses and the chest, measuring the ACTH levels in response to a dose of CRH injected, helps to localise pituitary lesions to one side or the other. A rare cause of Cushing's is ectopic CRH production.

Treatment

✧ Cushing's disease: transphenoidal adenectomy or transphenoidal hemihypophysectomy (based on inferior petrosal venous sampling). Radiotherapy – recurrence rates at two years are 50%. If these treatments are unsuccessful then bilateral laparoscopic adrenalectomy may be considered.

- ⋄ Autonomous adrenal tumour: surgical excision, usually by laparoscopic approach. Because of suppression of the normal gland, steroid replacement therapy may be needed for up to two years. Testing of the hypothalamic-pituitary-adrenal axis (short synacthen test) at regular intervals over that period is indicated.
- ⋄ Ectopic ACTH: excision of primary tumour if the primary is benign or pancreatic. For oat cell – palliation. For indolent metastatic carcinoids, bilateral adrenalectomy is occasionally indicated.

Adrenocortical carcinoma (10% of adrenal tumours) often presents late, with large tumours and pulmonary metastases. It is often malignant if it occurs in children. Treatment is surgical debulking of the tumour and/or control of metastatic disease with mitotane. Partial remissions can be obtained with chemotherapy (fluorouracil (5FU), doxorubicin, cisplatin).

Follow-up
Follow up at short intervals until diagnosis is obtained. In many cases a planned admission to hospital is required to perform the investigations in consultation with an endocrinologist.

Post-operative follow-up
Review with histology to confirm the diagnosis and excision and to detect any complications of surgery. Exclude adrenal insufficiency and confirm adequate cortisol replacement under joint management with an endocrinologist. A combination of hydrocortisone and fludrocortisone is required after bilateral adrenalectomy. Counsel the patient regarding the need for increased steroid therapy during illness or further surgical procedures. A patient receiving chemotherapy may also become hypothyroid and require thyroxine.

Cushing's should gradually improve over a year after surgery. Scaly desquammation of the scalp is a sign of improvement. Weight loss occurs, muscle strength improves and diabetes often resolves. Urine and electrolytes return to normal.

Conn's syndrome
This syndrome consists of hypertension and hypokalaemia caused by an adrenocortical adenoma secreting aldosterone. Approximately 60% of cases are due to a benign adrenal adenoma (aldosterone-producing adenoma (APA)) and 40% are due to bilateral hyperplasia (idiopathic hyperaldosteronism (IPA)). The occasional case is due to carcinoma.

Secondary causes of hyperaldosteronism include stimulation by angiotensin in response to decreased circulating volume, which may be caused by cirrhosis, nephrotic syndrome, diuretic therapy and cardiac failure. Other causes include renal artery stenosis or a renin-secreting tumour.

History
Patients present because a raised blood pressure has been noticed, which either fails to respond to treatment or is associated with accompanying symptoms of muscle weakness, tetany, polyuria, nocturia and thirst.

Examination
May be normal or there may be a raised blood pressure with evidence of muscle weakness and tetany.

Investigations
Suspect Conn's in any hypertensive patient with hypokalaemia; however, a third of Conn's patients have a normal potassium. Potassium excretion in the urine is inappropriately

high. If hyponatraemia co-exists this may indicate secondary hyperaldosteronism. Hypernatraemia is more typical of primary aldosteronism. Morning renin and aldosterone levels are measured from a blood sample taken from an arm vein between 9 and 10am (after fasting from 10pm the night before). Ideally the patient should have been off all medications for four weeks prior to the blood test.

Conn's is diagnosed by an elevated plasma aldosterone level in the presence of a low plasma renin level. High plasma aldosterone levels are not suppressed by increased intake of sodium chloride. Glucocorticoid levels should be normal. Secondary hyperaldosteronism is characterised by high plasma renin levels with hypertension and often renal disease or sodium depletion.

Localisation

CT scanning plus ^{131}I 6-beta-iodomethyl-19-norcholesterol (NP59) scintigraphy can distinguish between adenoma and hyperplasia. Occasionally MRI scanning and selective venous sampling is useful in localising difficult cases.

Treatment

✧ Adrenal tumour: unilateral laparoscopic adrenalectomy. Precede surgery with 1–6 weeks of spironolactone to return serum potassium to normal. Patients will need cortisone cover peri-operatively.
✧ Adrenal hyperplasia: medical therapy. Treat hypertension with spironolactone 100 mg/ day rising to 400 mg/day until potassium returns to normal, then reduce the dose. Resistant hyperplasia requires total or subtotal adrenalectomy.

Follow-up

Follow up at short intervals until diagnosis is obtained, hypertension is controlled and potassium returns to normal. Admission to hospital is often required. Spironolactone can cause gynaecomastia, decreased libido, impotence and menstrual irregularities but still not control the hypertension. Second-line therapy with amiloride or triamterene may be required.

Post-operative follow-up

Review with histology to confirm the diagnosis and excision and to detect any post-operative complications. Confirm a biochemical return to normal. Exclude adrenal insufficiency and treat with steroid replacement as required.

Phaeochromocytoma

Ten per cent are malignant, 10% are bilateral and 10% can occur anywhere along the sympathetic chain from the neck to the pelvis. Phaeochromocytomas may be familial and associated with other tumours such as neurofibromatosis (10%), acoustic neuroma, meningioma, glioma, astrocytoma and cerebellar haemangioma (14%). In MEN 2, phaeochromocytoma is associated with medullary carcinoma of thyroid and parathyroid adenomas. Adrenal hyperplasia can occur as a precursor of phaeochromocytoma.

History

History includes palpitations, fear, facial flushing; abdominal symptoms such as nausea and vomiting; diarrhoea and weight loss; glucose intolerance; and cardiac failure. Also look for attacks of high blood pressure with headaches; nausea and vomiting; chest and abdominal pain; anxiety; pallor; sweating and palpitations – lasting a few minutes to several hours.

Examination

Hypertension can be sustained or paroxysmal, with periods of normotension or hypotension, so single blood pressure readings can be normal. If the phaeochromocytoma secretes noradrenaline or dopamine, hypotension can be the presenting sign. Examine for tachycardia and palpitations, evidence of cardiac failure, dehydration and recent weight loss.

Investigations

Measuring catecholamines and metanephrines in a 24-hour urine collection is 90% sensitive. Plasma catecholamine levels are raised, but tests can be rendered inaccurate by calcium channel blockers, monoamine oxidase inhibitors (MAOIs), phenothiazine, tricyclic antidepressants and beta-blockers.

Extra-adrenal and malignant phaeochromocytomas tend to secrete noradrenaline, while benign adrenal phaeochromocytomas tend to secrete adrenaline.

Localisation

Most tumours are usually greater than 3cm in diameter. Take a CT scan of adrenal, para-aortic and pelvic areas. Meta-iodobenzylguanidine (^{131}MIBG) is taken up by catecholamine granules and is extremely useful in confirming the site of the tumour and in diagnosing extra-adrenal and bilateral phaeochromocytomas. It can also be used therapeutically for treatment of metastases.

Treatment

Phenoxybenzamine (alpha-blocker, 20–80 µg daily) is started when diagnosed, for at least two weeks prior to surgery or longer in the presence of electrocardiogram (ECG) abnormalities. Additional therapy with beta-blockers (20–40 µg, 6-hourly) can be used to control tachycardia. Labetalol (an alpha- and beta-blocker) can also be used.

When hypertension is controlled, unilateral laparoscopic adrenalectomy is performed.

Follow-up

Follow up at short intervals (1–4 weeks) until diagnosis is achieved. There is a clinical association with MEN 2, so medullary carcinoma of the thyroid and hyperparathyroidism should be excluded in all cases of phaeochromocytoma.

Post-operative follow-up

Seventy per cent of patients are cured of hypertension by surgery. Review with histology to confirm diagnosis and excision and to detect complications of surgery. Patients with malignancy should be followed up long term to detect recurrence. Recurrence is suspected by recurrence of symptoms, and confirmed biochemically. Metastases are localised by an MIBG scan, which is then given in a therapeutic dose. Malignant phaeochromocytomas that recur can also be treated by surgical debulking. Chemotherapy has been used with a 50% response rate.

Childhood adrenal tumours

These include neuroblastoma, ganglioneuroma and neurofibroma.

Adrenal incidentaloma

With the increasing availability of abdominal CT scanning, apparently asymptomatic adrenal masses are being referred for surgical opinion. Over 50% are metastases from a known primary, 30% are cortical adenomas with potential endocrine symptoms (phaeochromocytoma, Cushing's, Conn's), 5% are metastases from an occult primary and 5% are adrenal malignancies. Other causes include cysts, haematomas and myelolipomas.

History/examination

Take a history to elicit symptoms of endocrine conditions, and examine for relevant clinical signs. In particular, determine any known primary malignancy.

Investigations

Often the CT scan appearance is diagnostic or suggests malignancy due to an irregular outline, invasion of adjacent structures or lymph node metastases. If not, perform biochemical tests for phaeochromocytoma, Cushing's and Conn's: e.g. urinary catecholamines, serum and urinary potassium and serum and urinary cortisol estimations. Ultrasound/CT-guided biopsy may be justified.

Treatment

All adrenal masses greater than 4cm require surgical excision because of malignant potential. Even with metastatic masses, surgical excision may be justified. Cysts are very rarely malignant and do not require surgery unless large. Haematomas may occur spontaneously and resolve over time, but can occur within primary or metastatic tumours. Myelolipomas are benign and surgery is indicated only if they become large.

Follow-up

Follow up at short intervals (1–4 weeks) until diagnosis is achieved. If all investigations are normal and surgery is not indicated because of size or other features, serial MRI scan observation performed every six months initially is justified.

Post-operative follow-up

Review with histology to confirm diagnosis and excision and to detect any complications of surgery. Follow-ups for specific lesions are described under their relevant sections.

Hirsutism

Plasma testosterone and urinary 17-oxysterol are elevated when there is a virilising adrenal tumour, but may be elevated in other virilising syndromes such as ovarian tumour. Most patients have congenital adrenal hyperplasia, which may present as virilisation in male and female children.

History

Determine the onset of hirsutism. Patients may complain of oily skin, acne and increasing facial and other body hair. The voice may deepen. There may be menstrual irregularities or amenorrhoea.

Examination

Perform a general examination. Examine for the male pattern of body hair and acne. Abdominal examination may reveal an abdominal or pelvic mass. Rectal and vaginal examination may reveal an ovarian mass.

Investigations

Adrenal imaging by CT or MRI is essential. Simultaneous imaging of the ovaries is also helpful. Measure plasma testosterone and 17-oxysterol. Serum ACTH is high in congenital adrenal hyperplasia.

Treatment

Benign adrenal tumours are excised, which improves acne and restores menstruation, ovulation and fertility. Hirsutism usually persists. Malignant tumours may require chemotherapy.

Congenital adrenal hyperplasia is treated by replacement of deficient adrenal steroids to reduce the stimulation of the adrenals and the production of virilising by-products caused by the high levels of ACTH.

Follow-up

Review at short intervals (1–4 weeks) until adrenal or ovarian tumours are excluded. Monitor the effect of hormone replacement in collaboration with an endocrinologist. Gynaecological referral is indicated for treatment of ovarian tumours.

Post-operative follow-up

Review with histology to confirm diagnosis and excision and to detect complications of surgery. Exclude adrenal insufficiency.

Surgical management of obesity

Determine whether the patient is clinically obese, exclude underlying metabolic disorder, detect complications of obesity and select appropriate patients for surgery.

Surgery should be considered prophylactic in relatively young or middle-aged patients.

History

Look at types of abnormal eating or binge eating; types of diet; impact of obesity on life; and psychological upsets. Trials of medical therapy, i.e. diet and exercise.

Examination

Determine the body mass index (BMI): weight (kg)/height^2 (m^2). A BMI of 20–25 is a desirable weight. Morbid obesity is defined as a BMI greater than 40–45, or more than 100 lbs (45 kg) overweight.

Examine for conditions caused by obesity, including cardiovascular disease, diabetes mellitus, osteoarthritis, cancer and respiratory disease.

Examine for underlying metabolic conditions that can cause obesity, include Cushing's syndrome and hypothyroidism. Excess weight gain can also be associated with fluid retention secondary to cardiac, renal or hepatic disease.

Investigations

Look at height, weight, BMI, BP, ECG, full blood count (FBC), lipid levels, CXR, spirometry, blood gases, glucose tolerance tests, ultrasound gall bladder and thyroid function tests.

Treatment
Selection of patients suitable for surgery

Criteria are five years or more presence of morbid obesity and BMI greater than 40–45 kg/m^2; patient has made serious attempts at losing weight through diet; increasing immobility; intelligent and working; strongly motivated; mentally stable with no history of alcoholism, drug addition or attempted suicide; not a high operative risk.

Relative indications include hypertension, hyperlipidaemia, noninsulin-dependent diabetes mellitus (NIDDM) and osteoarthritis (OA).

Contraindications include unwilling patient, unfit for general anaesthetic (GA), psychological instability, unable to lose weight on dieting.

Team approach

The team will include the anaesthetist, surgeon, dietitian, and physiotherapist.

Surgical procedures include Lap Band, vertical banded gastroplasty and gastric bypass with Roux-en-Y leaving a 150 ml reservoir. The patient is then fed on a diet of solid food requiring chewing and is required to exercise. Operative mortality is approximately 2%. Morbidity consists mainly of pulmonary atelectasis, venous thrombosis and wound infection.

Results

Reducing BMI to less than 35 is successful in 40–70% of vertical gastric stapling procedures.

Follow-up

Review at regular intervals until underlying metabolic disorder is excluded and the need for surgery is determined.

Post-operative follow-up

Review to detect any complications of surgery and to determine success in terms of weight reduction.

Oesophagus
Edward Cheong

FOUR

The oesophagus

On a simple level, the oesophagus is a tube whose function is to transport food from the mouth through the chest and diaphragm into the stomach. Successful completion of this task requires the co-ordinated function of brain, nerve, muscle and mucosa. Disorders affecting any of these systems can result in oesophageal symptoms, as may disorders originating in the chest or the diaphragm.

A particular diagnostic difficulty is the differentiation of pain, which may be cardiac or oesophageal in origin. Because cardiac pain may represent a potentially life-threatening disorder, investigation of the cardiovascular system may take priority over oesophageal investigation in this situation.

Abnormalities in gastric function, such as acid hypersecretion, may first present with oesophageal reflux rather than gastric symptoms, as may conditions associated with increased intra-abdominal pressure.

Therefore, the assessment of oesophageal conditions may require the consideration of a number of different body systems to arrive at the correct diagnosis.

Oesophageal history

Start with a general gastrointestinal history. When the responses indicate a possible oesophageal problem, a more detailed oesophageal history is required to differentiate oesophageal problems from cardiac or pulmonary disorders and gastric problems.

Dysphagia

Dysphagia strongly suggests an oesophageal problem and can be due to mechanical or motility disorders. The site and time course of onset are useful points.

Are symptoms intermittent, and helped by sipping fluids or repeated swallowing (motility), or are they persistent and progressive, suggesting a mechanical stricture of the lumen, e.g. carcinoma?

Dysphagia for solids suggests a mechanical cause; dysphagia for fluids only suggests a motility disorder.

Regurgitation

There is a sour taste in the mouth, it may occur most at night, and in the morning the fluid has stained the pillow.

Postural regurgitation that is increased by a supine posture or that is worse after large meals, bending or straining suggests reflux disease.

Overflow at night causing coughing or aspiration might be due to a constricting lesion, but is more common in a motility disorder, e.g. achalasia.

Odynophagia

Localised pain, usually in the lower sternal region immediately the patient swallows certain foods and liquids such as hot drinks, suggests organic disease, e.g. oesophagitis.

Heartburn

Due to gastro-oesophageal reflux causing chemical inflammation to the oesophageal mucosa.

Oesophageal anterior chest pain

Angina-like, it can radiate to the back, jaw and arm and may be difficult to differentiate from cardiac pain. Often relieved by nitrates. Seen in both reflux and motility disorders, it can be precipitated by meals, emotion and exercise.

Water brash

Excess secretion of saliva, which tastes salty; often experienced in reflux disease.

Atypical presentations

✧ Anaemia.
✧ Haemetemesis.

Twenty to forty per cent of patients with chest pain and normal coronary angiograms have oesophageal pain.

Oesophageal examination

Perform a general examination. In particular look for:

✧ signs of weight loss
✧ pallor due to anaemia
✧ neck swelling (e.g. pharyngeal pouch)
✧ enlarged lymph nodes in left supraclavicular fossa, which may represent metastatic spread from a gastrointestinal malignancy.

Percussion and auscultation of the lungs should be performed to detect aspiration pneumonia.

The presence of an epigastric mass and/or hepatomegaly may represent the presence of advanced malignant disease.

Perform an examination of the cardiovascular system to detect any cardiac disease if the presentation includes atypical chest pain.

Investigation of oesophageal disorders
Laboratory investigations
Haematology

✧ Full blood count (FBC) may indicate microcytic anaemia.
✧ Leucocytosis may suggest infection.

Biochemistry

Abnormal liver function tests (LFT) may indicate liver metastases in malignancy.

Microbiology

Microbiology may show candidiasis of the mouth/oesophagus.

Cytology/histology

Cytology is of brushings, or histology of biopsies taken at endoscopy.

Imaging techniques
Chest X-ray

All patients who have oesophageal symptoms should have a chest X-ray (CXR) to look for:

✧ aspiration pneumonia
✧ mediastinal widening due to lymph node metastases

✧ suspicious soft tissue shadows (infection or metastatic disease)
✧ fluid/gas levels (large hiatus hernia with intrathoracic stomach, dilated oesophagus in achalasia).

Oesophago-gastro-duodenoscopy (OGD)

Except for suspected pharyngeal pouch (do a water-soluble contrast study), this should be the first investigation in all patients with oesophageal symptoms. It allows direct visualisation of mechanical obstructions and enables biopsies to be taken for histological diagnosis. It can also visualise oesophagitis, ulceration, varices and so on.

Certain therapeutic manoeuvres, e.g. dilatation of benign strictures, can be performed.

However, it is an invasive procedure that is unable to diagnose early motility disorders, which require oesophageal manometric study. Some patients may find it unpleasant and are unable to swallow the scope. Complications include:
✧ aspiration
✧ trauma to the oesophagus, stomach and duodenum, which may cause bleeding, pain or occasionally perforation.

Barium swallow/meal

This is the first-line investigation if oesophageal web, oesophageal motility disorder or pouch is suspected. It is the second-line investigation if OGD fails to provide a diagnosis.

It is also useful after oesophageal or gastric surgery in symptomatic patients to exclude a mechanical cause or herniation. The investigation is good for diagnosing:
✧ hiatus hernia
✧ oesophageal perforations (use water-soluble contrast)
✧ abnormalities of the upper oesophageal sphincter and swallowing mechanism.

Double contrast (barium-air) barium meals are useful for the evaluation of oesophageal cancer, especially the length of the lesion, which may correlate with depth of invasion and resectability. They are not reliable in the diagnosis of reflux. (Approximately 20% of normal people exhibit reflux in the Trendelenburg position, but only reflux demonstrated when upright is significant.)

Computerised tomography (CT) scanning

CT scanning is used in staging oesophageal malignancy to demonstrate:
✧ extent of mural invasion
✧ involvement of adjacent structures
✧ mediastinal lymph node involvement
✧ distant metastases.

It tends to underestimate early mediastinal spread and lymph node metastases, and it is not totally reliable in differentiating direct metastatic spread from reactive inflammation surrounding a tumour.

Ultrasound

Ultrasound is mainly used non-invasively with the ultrasound probe applied to the outside of the body after applying acoustic water-based gel.

Endoluminal ultrasound is a specialised technique where a specialised probe is placed into the oesophagus to provide images of the oesophageal wall and adjacent lymph nodes. It is good for determining intramural spread, tumour size (T stage) and lymph node involvement.

Laparoscopic ultrasound is another specialised technique that uses a special probe inserted into the abdomen at laparoscopy. It may be applied directly to organs, e.g. liver, and used to give more detailed information on suspicious liver lesions or suspected nodal spread. It is operator dependent. CT is required to confirm findings.

Radioisotope scans

These scans are used to assess gastro-oesophageal junction (GOJ) incompetence in patients with reflux and to evaluate the transit of liquid or solid boluses in motility disorders.

The patient swallows technetium-99m-labelled liquid or solids (e.g. eggs) while the process of swallowing is recorded by a gamma camera to detect the radioactivity. It provides useful visualisation of oesophageal function, particularly in the investigation of achalasia.

Physiological tests

Oesophageal manometry

A soft plastic multilumen tube connected to a pressure transducer system is passed orally or nasally and positioned at the required point in the stomach or oesophagus. Static measurements can be made at different positions, or the pressure profile of stomach, cardio-oesophageal junction and oesophagus can be obtained by recording during a wet swallow.

The upper oesophageal sphincter can also be assessed, determining the relationship of pharyngeal and oesophageal relaxation and contraction.

Ambulatory manometry is now available for investigation of infrequent oesophageal spasm. It is useful for assessment of motility disorders, dysphagia and the complications of anti-reflux surgery. However, it has low sensitivity for reflux. The technique is not widely available in most hospitals.

Twenty-four-hour pH monitoring

This is now the preferred method of pH assessment. Patients are assessed when they have been off all antacid or proton-pump inhibitor medication for 10 days. A twin pH probe is passed orally or nasally, the oesophageal transducer is positioned 5cm above the high-pressure zone in the lower oesphagus (as determined by manometry), and the gastric transducer is positioned in the stomach. The pH in both the oesophagus and the stomach is monitored for 24 hours. The patient can press an event marker when symptoms are experienced, and this can be correlated with pH recordings.

The procedure tends to be uncomfortable and requires patient compliance. It is not widely available in most hospitals.

Hiatus hernia

In this condition, the oesophageal hiatus in the diaphragm is enlarged, allowing part of the stomach to pass through into the chest.

There are three main types:
- ✦ type I (70–80%) sliding
- ✦ type II (8–10%) para-oesophageal
- ✦ type III mixed.

History

Take a general and oesophageal history.

Type I
- ✦ Often asymptomatic.
- ✦ May have symptoms of reflux oesophagitis, chronic blood loss or stricture.

Type II
◇ Mainly pressure symptoms when distended with gas or food.
◇ Pain, dyspnoea and tightness precipitated by food, bending and stooping.
◇ Pain sharp, beneath lower sternum and radiates to the back, often accompanied by a bloated sensation, anxiety, palpitations and dyspnoea.
◇ Pain often relieved by belching or vomiting.
◇ Symptoms of anaemia associated with ulcer within the hiatus hernia (Cameron's ulcer).
◇ Dysphagia in 20%.

Take a cardiac history to differentiate oesophageal symptoms from atypical angina.

Examination
◇ Perform a general examination.
◇ Examine for anaemia.
◇ Examine the chest for evidence of effusions or infection and examine the supraclavicular fossae for evidence of lymph node spread.
◇ Examine the abdomen for epigastric masses or evidence of liver enlargement.

There may be no abnormalities on examination, which makes the diagnosis of hiatus hernia more likely. Perform a cardiovascular examination if indicated by the history.

Investigations
◇ A CXR may show soft tissue mass or fluid level behind the heart.
◇ Oesophago-gastro-duodenoscopy shows reduced distance from incisors to GOJ, and the J-manoeuvre in the stomach may show the hernia.
◇ Barium swallow is usually diagnostic in cases not detected by OGD.
◇ Iron deficiency anaemia may be shown by FBC.
◇ Cardiovascular investigations are needed as indicated by atypical chest pain.

Treatment
Symptoms of reflux oesophagitis can be controlled medically with proton-pump inhibitors (PPI).

If symptoms are severe enough to merit intervention and the patient is a good operative risk, surgery can be considered.
◇ For type I, reduction and anti-reflux surgery (open or laparoscopic).
◇ For type II, repair of diaphragmatic defect with or without anti-reflux surgery. An infarcted or strangulated type II may need a thoracotomy or thoraco-abdominal surgery.

Follow-up
Most patients with oesophageal reflux secondary to hiatus hernia are treated by gastro-enterologists, who refer patients with uncontrolled or recurrent symptoms on medical therapy for surgery.

Patients with pressure symptoms in the chest may be referred directly to a surgeon. Investigations should be completed promptly, especially if a cardiac cause cannot be excluded on history and examination.

Post-operative follow-up
In routine cases patients are reviewed 4–6 weeks after surgery. Review the operation notes to determine whether there were any complications during the procedure. Early complications include wound infection and incisional hernia. Determine whether the operation has been successful in relieving the original symptoms.

Tight wrap

✧ Patients may complain of dysphagia or gas bloat as if the fundal wrap is too tight.

✧ This is usually mild and will resolve within three months with observation.

✧ Severe or persistent cases beyond three months require further investigation with barium swallow, OGD or oesophageal manometry.

✧ Treatment options include endoscopic balloon dilatation (often successful) or remedial surgery.

Slipped Nissen

The Nissen wrap either slips down the stomach, causing an hour-glass deformity and presenting as dysphagia and abdominal discomfort, or the wrap slips up between the crura into the chest, with accompanying dysphagia.

✧ Diagnosed by a barium meal.

✧ Requires prompt revision surgery.

Congenital diaphragmatic hernia

This condition is often diagnosed and treated shortly after birth. However, it may be asymptomatic and present later in life.

✧ Bochdalek hernia. There are persistent pleuroperitoneal canals. It presents in the neonatal period with respiratory distress.

✧ Morgagni's hernia. This parasternal hernia presents in adult life with episodes of pain and tenderness in the subcostal region and intermittent obstructive symptoms. Complete intestinal obstruction may intervene.

✧ Central tendon defect is associated with a defect in the pericardium. The intestine herniates into the pericardium.

History

Take a general oesophageal and gastrointestinal history. In particular, note any history of intermittent subcostal pain or dysphagia.

Examination

Perform a general examination. This is often found to be normal. There may be tenderness and/or fullness in the subcostal region.

Investigations

✧ Chest X-ray, posterior anterior view (CXR-PA) shows a round, gas-containing shadow to the right of the cardiac outline. Lateral CXR shows a gas-containing shadow behind the sternum.

✧ Barium swallow is usually diagnostic.

✧ On the right, ultrasound may be needed to differentiate diaphragmatic neoplasm (rare) from herniated liver parenchyma.

Treatment

Symptomatic patients are considered for surgical reduction and prosthetic mesh repair. Right-side abnormalities usually require no treatment, while left-sided and central hernias require surgical repair.

Follow-up

Follow-up should be at short intervals (1–4 weeks) until the diagnosis is made. Mild cases can be observed at gradually increasing intervals (1–6 months).

Post-operative follow-up

Determine if the operation has relieved the symptoms and detect any complications associated with abdominal and thoracic surgery.

Recurrence of symptoms may indicate recurrence of the hernia – investigate as for primary cases.

Traumatic diaphragmatic hernia

This hernia may present months or years after the event, e.g. seat-belt injury from a road traffic accident.

History

Take a general history. Symptoms tend to be related to the size of the herniated contents and to the onset of mechanical complications such as intestinal obstruction, strangulation, haemorrhage or progressive cardiorespiratory insufficiency.

Examination

Perform a general examination. Examine the chest for evidence of respiratory insufficiency, bowel sounds or infection.

Investigations

- ✧ CXR shows a space-occupying lesion. If spleen or omentum is herniated this appears solid.
- ✧ Barium swallow may confirm the diagnosis.
- ✧ Ultrasound scanning (USS) or CT can be helpful to determine chest contents.

Treatment

- ✧ If symptomatic, requires surgical repair through abdominal or thoracic approach.
- ✧ If asymptomatic, mildly symptomatic, or unfit for surgery, manage conservatively.

Follow-up

Severe cases need prompt investigation and treatment. Other cases can be managed with gradually lengthening follow-up (1–6 months), monitoring for the development of increasing symptoms and of deteriorating cardiorespiratory function.

Post-operative follow-up

Determine if the operation has relieved the symptoms and detect any complications of the thoracic and abdominal procedure.

Reflux oesophagitis

Reflux oesophagitis is caused by the abnormal retrograde movement of gastric contents into the oesophagus. Normal subjects have reflux, but this is harmless because the effect is short-lived, thanks to an effective oesophageal clearance mechanism. If the oesophageal clearance mechanism is overwhelmed, inflammation of the lower oesophageal mucosa occurs.

Oesophagitis may occur not just due to acid reflux but also because of bile salts, trypsin and lysolecithin, especially after partial gastrectomy.

Complications of reflux oesophagitis include chronic blood loss, deep ulceration with perioesophagitis, and the formation of strictures and webs.

The presence of columnar mucosal change indicates the development of a Barrett's oesophagus. Barrett's oesophagitis may lead to stricture, ulceration and the development of adenocarcinoma. Risk of developing cancer is relatively low (approximately 1% per annum), but is higher in those that develop mucosal dysplasia.

Library
Knowledge Spa
Royal Cornwall Hospital
Treliske
Truro. TR1 3HD

History

Symptoms include heartburn, regurgitation and dysphagia. Symptoms are aggravated by posture and are worse at night after large meals, bending or stooping. Dysphagia is intermittent. Persistent dysphagia usually suggests stricture formation.

Other presentations include odynophagia, waterbrash, atypical chest pain or asthma (due to aspiration).

Examination

◆ Perform a general examination (often normal).
◆ Examine for anaemia and weight loss.
◆ Examine the chest for signs of effusion or infection.
◆ Examine the abdomen for epigastric masses or liver enlargement.

Investigations

◆ Perform oesophago-gastro-duodenoscopy (OGD), and biopsy for histology.
◆ Barium swallow is good for demonstrating hiatus hernia.
◆ Perform 24-hour pH monitoring and manometry.
◆ A FBC may reveal anaemia.

Treatment

Uncomplicated disease

The patient should:
◆ lose weight
◆ avoid spicy foods
◆ raise the head of the bed.

If symptoms do not improve, prescribe antacids, proton-pump inhibitors and prokinetics (metoclopramide). Prokinetics are particularly useful for relief of nausea, fullness, regurgitation, belching and odynophagia. A full course of medical therapy lasts for three months, after which maintenance is continued indefinitely.

An alternative treatment is a proton-pump inhibitors (PPI), e.g. omeprazole, for eight weeks.

For neutral/alkali reflux in post-operative gastric surgery patients, a bile-salt binding agent such as cholestyramine is useful.

Complicated disease

If there is Barrett's with low-grade dysplasia, confirm the diagnosis with two endoscopic biopsies three months apart, after a course of PPI.

Confirmed cases may require anti-reflux surgery and acid-suppression therapy. This reverses columnar change in approximately 10%, but all cases need continued OGD surveillance.

High-grade dysplasia may represent carcinoma in situ and, if confirmed, is an indication for oesophageal resection. (Once resected, 30 to 40% are found to have invasive carcinoma in the histological specimen.)

Indications for surgical treatment

The following are indications for surgical treatment.
◆ Failure of medical therapy: persistent symptoms, intractable oesophagitis.
◆ Development of complications, stricture, Barrett's.
◆ Reflux associated with motility disorders or oesophageal chest pain.
◆ Reflux in children, persisting beyond the age of two.
◆ Reflux after upper abdominal surgery; acid or bile.

Surgical treatment

This consists of floppy Nissen fundoplication, which is usually laparoscopic.

The thoracic approach is preferred in patients with severe oesophagitis, stricture formation, perioesophagitis and oesophageal shortening.

Post-operative supercompetence and gas bloat occur in 20%, but with a properly constructed loose Nissen fundoplication, dysphagia is rarely encountered.

Follow-up

The majority of patients with oesophageal reflux are treated by gastroenterologists, who refer patients for surgery if they have uncontrolled or recurrent symptoms on medical therapy.

Different units have their own policies regarding Barrett's oesophagitis patients and whether regular endoscopy monitoring to detect malignant change is performed in all or just selected patients.

At present there is no conclusive evidence to suggest routine follow up of Barrett's is justified in any patient other than those with dysplastic change.

Post-operative follow-up

See hiatus hernia.

Persistent heartburn occurs in approximately 5–8%. It may be due to delayed gastric emptying because of unrecognised distal peptic ulcer disease, or disruption of the fundal wrap. Investigate with OGD, barium meal and oesophageal manometry.

Non-reflux oesophagitis

This may occur because of ingestion of corrosive substances; or it may be infective, drug induced or from radiation.

Specific disorders are Behçet's syndrome, Crohn's disease and scleroderma. All produce a mixture of strictures, motility disorders, hiatus hernias and occasional cancers.

The acute phases are treated as in-patients.

History

Take a general oesophageal history. Usually there will be a history suggestive of the underlying disorder and progressive dysphagia from liquids to solids.

Examination

✧ Perform a general and systemic examination.
✧ Look for other evidence of an underlying disorder.
✧ Examine hands, face, chest and abdomen.

Investigations

Assess by a combination of OGD, barium swallow, motility and pH studies. If Crohn's is suspected, a small bowel follow-through may be helpful.

Treatment

Mild cases are treated medically. More severe cases may be considered for surgery. They are those with:
✧ extensive persistent stricture
✧ need for frequent dilatations
✧ presence of high strictures or late bronchotracheo-oesophageal fistulas
✧ late oesophageal shortening with reflux oesophagitis
✧ severe dysplasia, carcinoma in situ or invasive carcinoma.

Extensive scarring may require total oesophagectomy and replacement with colon, isoperistaltic jejunum or stomach.

In some cases there is a frozen mediastinum – leave oesophagus and perform a bypass.

Follow-up
Follow-up is long term, as complications eventually develop in most cases. If symptoms are mild and stable, discharge with a plan to return if symptoms increase.

Post-operative follow-up
This is long-term follow-up. Initially, determine the success of the procedure and detect any complications associated with the abdominal and thoracic procedures.
- Monitor nutrition at regular intervals (weight, skin-fold thickness, routine blood tests). Dietary and vitamin supplements may be necessary.
- Monitor function of bypass with regular barium swallows.
- Endoscopic dilatation of strictures may be indicated.

Benign oesophageal strictures
All strictures need urgent OGD and multiple biopsies to exclude cancer.

History
Take a general oesophageal history. There may be a history of reflux oesophagitis or caustic fluid ingestion in the past. Generally dysphagia symptoms will be of slow onset and progressive from solids to fluids.

Examination
- Perform a general oesophageal examination.
- Look for evidence of weight loss, anaemia and sepsis.
- Examine the chest for respiratory and cardiovascular disease.
- Examine the abdomen for other gastrointestinal disease.
- Examination may be normal.

Investigations
Strictures are diagnosed by a combination of OGD and biopsies for histological examination. If surgery is considered, studies of oesophageal motility should be made.

A CT scan to detect scarring in the mediastinum can be performed to help in planning the procedure.

Treatment
Endoscopic dilatation
- An OGD is performed to visualise the stricture and Puestow's, Celestine tube or pneumatic guidewire guided dilatation is performed. Some centres prefer to perform this procedure under fluoroscopic guidance. Severe stenoses require 2–3 dilatation sessions every 1–2 weeks; each session consists of 3–4 dilator sequences consisting of a 6–8mm diameter increase. All patients should remain nil-by-mouth for some hours after dilatation and some centres routinely perform a CXR to exclude perforation before allowing the patient to eat. Complications include haemorrhage, perforation and septicaemia.
- An equally important aspect of the management of benign stricture is inhibition of acid reflux, usually with a PPI.

If bile reflux is a problem, revision surgery (Roux-en-Y gastric bypass) is usually necessary.

Subsequent treatment

Following a course of dilatation, 20–50% of patients remain symptom-free. Twenty per cent require frequent dilatation. In these cases surgery should be considered, or consider insertion of a self-expanding metal stent if unfit. Patients must remain on lifelong treatment if the stricture is not to recur.

Indications for surgery

✧ Young patients with reflux strictures.
✧ Frequent and increasingly difficult dilatations.
✧ Intractable/impassable stricture.
✧ Stricture associated with Barrett's oesophagus.

Surgery

Perform thoracotomy and intra-operative dilatation, then return to abdomen and perform Nissen's. If the oesophagus is too short, perform a Collis gastropexy.

Follow-up

Intervals should be short (1–2 weeks) until cancer is excluded.

If a course of dilatation is indicated, the patient should be reviewed in clinic 2–4 weeks after completion of the course to detect recurrent symptoms. Thereafter follow up intervals can be lengthened (1–6 months), and if the condition remains stable the patient may be discharged with advice to reconsult if the symptoms return. Patients are advised they must remain on lifelong anti-reflux treatment (PPI) if the stricture is not to recur.

Post-operative follow-up

Following surgery, the patient should be reviewed to determine whether the procedure has relieved the original symptoms and to detect complications. Complications include wound infection and incisional hernia. Thoracotomy complications include wound infection and pleural effusion. Patients are advised they must remain on lifelong anti-reflux treatment if the stricture is not to recur.

Motility disorders

Most motility disorders occur in young adulthood (occasionally children) to late middle age and can be classified as follows.
✧ Primary (achalasia, vigorous achalasia, diffuse oesophageal spasm, nutcracker oesophagus).
✧ Secondary
  ∝ neurological disorders (poliomyelitis, pseudobulbar palsy)
  ∝ myopathies (dermatomyositis)
  ∝ systemic disease (scleroderma).
✧ Parasitic infections (Chaga's disease).

Achalasia

Achalasia is the absence of peristaltic contractions within the oesophageal body and incomplete relaxation of the high-pressure zone (HPZ) of the lower oesophageal sphincter.

History

Take a general and oesophageal history. Symptoms include dysphagia, regurgitation and chest pain.
✧ Typically dysphagia is for solids and liquids, initially intermittent and aggravated by emotion, and it may be improved by sipping fluids or repeated swallowing and other manoeuvres, e.g. valsalva.

 ✧ Odynophagia may be prominent if dilatation is minimal.
 ✧ As dilatation increases, pain and dysphagia decreases and regurgitation increases –
   especially postural regurgitation of foamy, mucoid saliva.
 ✧ Halitosis and eructation of foul air may be described.

Advanced achalasia leads to massive dilatation of the oesophagus, causing severe dysphagia, weight loss, anaemia, respiratory complications due to aspiration; fever, sweating and breathlessness.

Examination
 ✧ Perform a general and oesophageal examination (may be normal).
 ✧ Look for evidence of weight loss, anaemia and sepsis.
 ✧ Halitosis may be noticed.
 ✧ Examine the chest for evidence of infection or effusion.
 ✧ Examine the abdomen for other gastrointestinal pathology.

Investigations
A CXR may show a convex shadow to the right of the vena cava and right atrium, with or without a fluid level within the shadow. The lungs should also be assessed for pneumonia.
   Barium swallow may show dilatation of the oesophagus and the characteristic rat's-tail appearance and absence of the gastric air bubble.
   An OGD should be performed to exclude peptic stricture and carcinoma of the oesophagus.
   In early or doubtful cases, oesophageal manometry may demonstrate no relaxation of the lower oesophageal sphincter with swallowing.

Treatment
In early achalasia, some patients benefit from long-acting nitrates (isosorbide). Endoscopic pneumatic balloon dilatation up to 90F can be helpful and can be repeated at regular intervals.
   Surgical myotomy (Heller's procedure) is indicated:
 ✧ in advanced disease with severe dilatation and oesophagitis
 ✧ in younger patients
 ✧ where there is co-existent pathology requiring surgical treatment, e.g. hiatus hernia, phrenic diverticulum
 ✧ with failure of dilatation
 ✧ on recurrence of symptoms.

Severe achalasia with a huge tortuous megaoesophagus may require subtotal oesophagectomy with gastric pull-through and cervical anastomosis.

Follow-up
Severe cases need prompt assessment and treatment within weeks. Mild cases may respond to nitrates and review at 2–3 monthly intervals to gauge response.
   Patients requiring frequent endoscopic dilatation are followed up in the endoscopic unit or have an open appointment for this treatment when required.

Post-operative follow-up
Patients are reviewed at 4–6 weeks. Early complications include wound infection, pleural effusion or other respiratory complications if a thoracotomy was performed.
   Recurrence of symptoms can be treated with further endoscopic dilatation if persistent.

Patients treated by oesophagectomy and pull-through procedures can experience complications of recurrent laryngeal palsy, gastric outlet obstruction, gastro-oesophageal reflux and dumping (*see* oesophageal cancer).

Vigorous achalasia

This combines features of achalasia and diffuse oesophageal spasm.

History

Take a general oesophageal history. Symptoms are similar to achalasia, but chest pain is more prominent. Patients may also present with dysphagia and regurgitation.

Examination

✧ Perform a general examination (which may be normal).
✧ Look for evidence of sepsis, weight loss and anaemia.
✧ Examine the chest for evidence of sepsis or cardiac disease.
✧ Examine the abdomen for evidence of gastrointestinal disease.

Investigations

A barium swallow/meal may show segmental spasm of the lower oesophagus with dilatation of the proximal half.

Manometry may show repetitive high-amplitude non-peristaltic contraction and failure of relaxation of lower oesophageal sphincter.

Treatment

✧ Long-acting nitrates may help mild cases.
✧ Endoscopic dilatation *does not help*.
✧ Surgery may be indicated for severe cases and requires a long myotomy.

Follow-up

Severe cases need prompt assessment and treatment within weeks. Mild cases may respond to nitrates and review at 2–3 monthly intervals to gauge response. Patients requiring frequent endoscopic dilatation are followed up in the endoscopic unit or have an open appointment for this treatment when required.

Post-operative follow-up

This is as for achalasia. Long-term follow-up is recommended, with a barium swallow performed six months post-operatively.

Chagas disease

Chagas disease is a result of infection by *Trypanosoma cruzi*, which infects the myenteric plexus of the oesophagus. It occurs mainly in Latin America and simulates achalasia, both radiologically and manometrically. Patients are usually in poor medical condition, so they are treated by endoscopic dilatation.

Diffuse oesophageal spasm

This condition involves hypertrophy of the muscular coats of the oesophagus, Wallerian degeneration of vagal fibres and sensitivity to cholinergic compounds.

History

✧ Take a general and oesophageal history.
✧ Typical symptoms are substernal midline chest pain (similar to angina pain, it radiates to back, neck and jaw).

✧ Symptoms include odynophagia and dysphagia, affecting equally solids and liquids.
✧ An emotional personality may be apparent.
✧ It is often diagnosed after normal coronary angiography.

Examination
✧ Perform a general examination (which is often normal).
✧ Look for evidence of weight loss and anaemia.
✧ Examine the chest for any respiratory or cardiovascular abnormalities.

Investigations
✧ Barium swallow shows corkscrew appearance.
✧ Provide OGD to exclude organic disease.
✧ Consider cardiology assessment if cardiac disease is suspected.
✧ Manometry shows simultaneous non-peristaltic repetitive contractions in response to swallowing; spontaneous contractions not related to swallowing; periods of normal peristalsis; and normal relaxation of HPZ.
✧ A radionuclide scan shows oscillatory movement of the isotope-labelled bolus and marked delay in transit time.

Treatment
Conservative treatment is with:
✧ long-acting nitrates and tranquillisers
✧ endoscopic pneumatic dilatation.

Surgery, e.g. thoracoscopic long myotomy, is indicated in fit patients in whom conservative therapy has failed.

Follow-up
Severe cases are investigated and treated promptly within weeks. Less severe cases can be assessed at longer intervals (1–2 months) to determine the effect of therapeutic agents. Assess the need for endoscopic dilatation, or in severe cases in fit patients, the need for surgery.

Post-operative follow-up
Assess for general complications, wound infection and chest complications. Some centres recommend a barium swallow at six months to assess the effect of surgery.

Recurrence may respond to further endoscopic balloon dilatation.

Motility disorders secondary to systemic disease
The most common systemic disorder causing oesophageal motility symptoms is systemic sclerosis (SS). Nearly all patients with SS and oesophageal involvement have symptoms of oesophageal reflux, often severe. Less common conditions are dermatomyositis, systemic lupus erythematosus (SLE) and rheumatoid arthritis (RA). Common defects consist of lower oesophageal sphincter incompetence and complete loss of peristaltic activity in the lower two-thirds.

History
✧ Take a general oesophageal history.
✧ Patients can present with symptoms of oesophagitis and dysphagia in association with symptoms of the underlying disorder.

Examination

Perform a general examination and look for evidence of an underlying disorder, e.g. Raynaud's phenomenon or rheumatoid joints.

Investigations

Investigations include barium swallow, OGD, manometry and pH studies.

Treatment

Treatment is mainly medical, using drugs which increase oesophageal motility (domperidone and metoclopramide are used but with inconsistent results). Treat reflux aggressively with standard medical regimes. Any peptic strictures are treated by endoscopic dilatation.

Follow-up

Follow-up is long term for treatment of the motility disorder and the underlying condition. Assess for development of strictures and diverticulae. Treat as appropriate with drugs and regular endoscopic dilatation.

Nutcracker oesophagus

This is symptomatic oesophageal peristalsis.

History

Take a general oesophageal history. The condition typically does not cause dysphagia. Instead, there are episodes of chest pain similar to both angina and reflux oesophagitis.

Examination

- ✧ Perform a general examination (which may be normal).
- ✧ Examine the chest for respiratory or cardiovascular disease.
- ✧ Examine for abdominal pathology.

Investigations

- ✧ Manometry shows normal peristaltic waves on swallowing, but primary waves of large amplitude (greater than 150 mmHg) in the distal oesophagus and of long duration (longer than 5.5 seconds).
- ✧ Perform 24-hour pH monitoring in all patients to diagnose reflux.
- ✧ Use OGD to detect oesophagitis.

Treatment

Treatment is medical. If there is reflux, treat with omeprazole, otherwise with long-acting nitrates or calcium antagonists.

Follow-up

- ✧ Intervals should be short (1–4 weeks) until cardiac disease is excluded and the diagnosis is achieved.
- ✧ Thereafter, follow-up can be at longer intervals to assess the effect of therapeutic agents.
- ✧ Discharge the patient once the condition has stabilised.

Pharyngo-oesophageal (Zenker's) diverticulum – pharyngeal pouch

This is a pulsion diverticulum that occurs through Killian's dehiscence of the posterior cricopharyngeus. It usually lies to the left side of the oesophagus and is caused by a motility defect (failure of relaxation of the cricopharyngeus). The pouch enlarges and pushes the oesophagus to one side, so food enters the pouch preferentially.

History
✧ Take a general oesophageal history.
✧ Spluttering and coughing with meals is typical.
✧ High dysphagia, progressing to regurgitation, constant throat irritation, gurgling noises during swallowing, chronic cough and recurrent aspiration pneumonias are also suggestive.
✧ Compression of the oesophagus causes the dysphagia and attacks of spluttering and coughing with each meal.
✧ Other symptoms include halitosis, hoarseness and anorexia.
✧ Regurgitated material is non-acid.

Examination
✧ Perform a general examination (which may be normal).
✧ Occasionally, a lump may be palpable in the left side of the neck.
✧ Gurgling may be detected on palpation of the left side of the neck at the level of the cricoid, performed after the patient is asked to swallow several gulps of air.
✧ Examine the chest for evidence of respiratory or cardiovascular disease.
✧ Examine for abdominal pathology.

Investigations
Investigations comprise:
✧ CXR for chest complications
✧ FBC for anaemia
✧ barium swallow and meal to exclude gross oesophageal motility disorder and hiatus hernia.

OGD is not necessary initially and carries a risk of perforation.

Treatment
Treatment is surgical. Relief of symptoms is commonly achieved by endoscopic division of the septum for elderly, unfit patients.

Follow-up
Severe cases should be investigated and treated promptly, within weeks. Less severe cases can be assessed at longer intervals.

Post-operative follow-up
Determine if operation has relieved the symptoms and assess for general post-operative complications.

Oesophageal cancer
Ninety-five per cent of cases of oesophageal cancer are either squamous cell or adeno-carcinomas. In the United Kingdom, adenocarcinomas of the lower third of the oesophagus predominate. Carcinoma of the gastric cardia that invades the lower oesophagus is a gastric cancer. Overall the five-year survival for oesophageal cancer is poor (10%).
   Risk factors include being male, aged between 30 and 80.
✧ High risk: smoking, excess alcohol intake, tylosis (type A), Plummer-Vinson syndrome.
✧ Intermediate risk: reflux, Barrett's, achalasia, ectopic gastric mucosa, previous radio-

therapy for Hodgkin's and non-Hodgkin's disease, previous squamous cell cancer of head and neck.

✧ Low risk: oesophageal diverticula, corrosive strictures, coeliac disease, scleroderma.

History

✧ Take a general oesophageal history.
✧ The typical history is of progressive dysphagia over a period of months.
✧ There may be symptoms associated with anaemia, caused by bleeding from the tumour, or there may be symptoms of bleeding.
✧ There may be a history of weight loss.

Examination

✧ Perform a general examination.
✧ Note signs of weight loss, sepsis, anaemia or palpable Virchow's node in the left supraclavicular fossa.
✧ Examine the chest for evidence of cardiovascular or respiratory disease.
✧ Examine for abdominal pathology, e.g. epigastric mass or liver metastases.

Investigations

✧ Urgent OGD and biopsy.
✧ Barium swallow may be useful if unable to do an OGD, as lesions longer than 5cm are associated with deeper invasion levels, irresectability and a worse prognosis.
✧ FBC to detect anaemia.
✧ Assess nutritional status (skin fold, haematological and biochemical indices – albumin, transferrin, haemoglobin (Hb), iron).

Staging

To establish the presence of inoperable mediastinal or subdiaphragmatic disease.
✧ Staging chest and abdominal CT scan.
✧ Endoscopic ultrasound (EUS) to stage the tumour and nodal status within the chest and abdomen.
✧ Bronchoscopy, if there is evidence of tracheo-bronchial invasion.
✧ Staging laparoscopy for lower oesophageal cancer, looking for peritoneal disease or liver metastases.
✧ Vocal cord paralysis (ENT examination) and phrenic nerve paralysis (ultrasound screening) may indicate mediastinal spread.

Treatment

Treatments include surgical resection, radiotherapy, stenting, laser or electrocoagulation and combined modality treatment; which treatment depends on stage and operative fitness, including nutritional state. Malnourished patients may require pre-operative nutrition.

Surgery

✧ The main objective is restoring the ability to swallow.
✧ Thirty to forty per cent of oesophageal tumours are resectable.
✧ Operative mortality is 5–10%.
✧ Surgical resection is the treatment of choice for tumours of the lower two-thirds, provided that:
  ∝ the patient is considered fit for major surgical intervention
  ∝ pre-operative staging tests indicate the tumour is resectable and there is no metastatic disease.

✧ Upper-third tumours are treated using either chemo-radiotherapy or pharyngo-laryngectomy.
✧ Malignant oesophagotracheal fistulas are treated by endoscopic insertion of a covered oesophageal stent.
✧ Other palliative options include laser or diathermy fulguration.

Follow-up

✧ Intervals are short until the diagnosis and staging are complete.
✧ Curative surgery is performed 4–6 weeks after neoadjuvant therapy.
✧ Palliation requires co-ordination between surgery and oncology.
✧ If symptoms are to be controlled with diathermy or laser fulguration, this treatment may need to be performed every 1–3 months to keep symptoms under control. Intubation or stenting may be considered as an alternative.
✧ After intubation, patients need to be reviewed regularly (1–3 monthly) to detect problems with the stent, e.g. blockage or displacement.

Post-operative follow-up

Long term follow-up will be required. Assess the patient to determine whether the operation has been a success in relieving the symptoms and completely removing the tumour.

Review the operation notes and the histology report. Assess for general complications of abdominal surgery and thoracotomy. More specific early complications include the following.

✧ Recurrent laryngeal nerve palsy may be caused during resection of the tumour. Patients may complain of a hoarse voice and a weak cough. If only one vocal cord is affected, the other side often compensates. The condition may be temporary and may improve over several months. If the paralysis is permanent, improvement in the voice can be achieved by referral to the ENT surgeons for teflon injection or a formal thyroplasty.
✧ Gastric outlet obstruction occurs if the stomach was mobilised and the vagus nerves cut without an adequate pyloroplasty. Investigate with a barium meal. Remedial surgery may be necessary in severe cases, but usually endoscopic dilatation is sufficient.
✧ Gastro-oesophageal reflux occurs if the stomach has been moved into the chest to establish continuity. Treatment is with PPI and prokinetic drugs such as cisapride, maxalon and erythromycin.

Dumping symptoms are common after oesophageal surgery but usually settle after 12 months with conservative treatment.

Late complications include anastomotic stricture, which can be treated with endoscopic balloon dilatation.

Evidence of recurrence that is untreatable will require palliation.

Stomach and duodenum

Richard Hardwick

FIVE

Introduction

A general surgical outpatient clinic will commonly have patients who have been sent up by their GP to discuss a laparoscopic cholecystectomy because an ultrasound scan has detected gallstones. However, there is a large overlap between biliary and gastroduodenal symptoms. It is vital that a careful history is taken to avoid inappropriate biliary surgery when the patient has a duodenal ulcer. More specialist upper gastrointestinal (GI) clinics will have large numbers of new and follow-up patients with very specific problems, some of which will be due to the disease process and some due to treatment they have received. New patients are usually seen by a consultant, but trainees should attend some of these consultations to learn how to take a rapid and focused history and formulate a management plan. Gastrointestinal surgeons should be just as competent at diagnosing and treating GI disease as are their gastroenterology colleagues. Clearly the two specialities bring their own unique skills and experience to bear on a patient's problem, but they should work closely together and refer freely between themselves as appropriate.

Assessment of gastric and duodenal disorders

Gastric and duodenal history

Pain

Pain is generally in the epigastric region and is caused by inflammation, ulceration, distension or tumour of the stomach.

Characteristics of pain due to peptic ulceration may vary according to the *site* of the ulcer.

- ✧ Gastric ulcer pain may be exacerbated by food and may be relieved by vomiting. Consequently, the patient is afraid to eat and loses weight.
- ✧ Duodenal ulcer pain is epigastric but may radiate through to the back. It is typically relieved by eating and may sometimes wake the patient at night.
- ✧ Pyloric stenosis: vomiting and weight loss are unusual and may suggest the development of pyloric stenosis. With the widespread use of acid-suppressing medication this is now a very rare complication in developed countries. Pain tends to be periodic, lasting 10–14 days every 3–4 months. Pain due to pyloric stenosis may cause abdominal distension, which is uncomfortable.
- ✧ Gastric carcinoma: pain due to cancer of the stomach is common and cannot reliably be distinguished from benign inflammation. Worryingly, patients with gastric cancer will usually report relief of their burning epigastric pain soon after starting a proton-pump inhibitor. This falsely reassures both patient and doctor that there is nothing sinister and delays the diagnostic endoscopy, which then is requested only when the pain returns or the patient loses weight.

Vomiting

Vomiting may be a feature of gastric ulcer disease with or without gastric outlet obstruction. Gastric outlet obstruction may also be caused by tumour. Patients report vomiting undigested food ingested several days before. Always take this symptom seriously and investigate it.

Water brash and heartburn

Water brash is caused by excess secretion of saliva. It tastes salty and is an indicator of oesophageal reflux. Heartburn is a much commoner symptom. It is often felt after meals, at night or when bending down. It can radiate into the neck and be very similar to cardiac chest pain. However, unlike the latter it is quickly relieved by antacids or acid suppression.

Dysphagia

This is primarily an oesophageal symptom but it may also indicate a gastric problem – carcinoma of the cardia obstructing the gastro-oesophageal junction. Always *investigate dysphagia urgently*.

Fatigue, malaise

These non-specific symptoms may indicate anaemia secondary to chronic blood loss from a peptic ulcer or tumour.

Drug history

The ingestion of certain medications, e.g. NSAIDs or steroids, may predispose to gastro-duodenal ulceration, or predispose to complications from ulceration, as, for example, does warfarin.

Past medical history

Previous peptic ulceration or gastric surgery may be relevant. A social history of smoking and excess alcohol ingestion is associated with peptic ulceration.

Gastric and duodenal examination

This will usually be entirely normal.

Look for the signs of advanced upper GI malignancy – weight loss, anaemia, an abdominal mass, ascites and lymphadenopathy. These are *signs of incurability* and it is sad that they are still used as 'alarm features' to guide GPs to refer patients for investigation.

Curable upper GI malignancy usually presents with *mild dyspepsia* only, and unless an endoscopy and biopsy is done then, the chance of cure is often lost.

Distension in the epigastrium and left hypochondrium may represent gastric distension secondary to gastric outlet obstruction. Auscultation in this region may reveal a succussion splash in response to rocking the abdomen. Surgical scars may indicate previous gastric surgery. Always look for the signs of liver disease, such as spider naevi, liver palms, hepatomegaly, jaundice and tremor.

Investigation of gastric and duodenal disorders

Laboratory investigations

✧ Haematology: routine indications, e.g. full blood count (FBC), may indicate anaemia; leucocytosis may suggest infection.
✧ Biochemistry: routine indications, e.g. abnormal liver function tests (LFT), may indicate liver metastases in malignancy. More specialised gastric acid secretion tests can be made.
✧ Immunology: for example, identification of serum antibodies to *Helicobacter pylori* (HP); parietal cell antibodies in pernicious anaemia.
✧ Cytology/histology: cytology of brushings or histology of biopsies taken at endoscopy.
✧ Urea breath test or faecal antigen test for *Helicobacter pylori*: patients *under the age of 55* (some would argue 45) who present with simple dyspepsia should be tested for HP and, when positive, undergo triple-therapy eradication treatment with a combination

of two antibiotics and a proton-pump inhibitor (clarythromycin, amoxicillin and omeprazole is one example). Serum antibody testing for HP is possible but will stay positive for many months after eradication and is less reliable than a urea breath test. Urea containing radio-labelled carbon is drunk by the patient. If HP is present in the stomach, the urease enzyme produced by it will split the urea into radio-labelled carbon dioxide (CO_2) and ammonia. The CO_2 is exhaled and can be detected. Faecal antigen testing using HP-specific antibodies is an alternative technique, but it is not as popular with patients and staff for obvious reasons. A gastric biopsy taken at endoscopy can also be tested using a test for *Campylobacter*-like organisms, the CLO test, which works on the same principle as the urea breath test, except that a colour change is induced by the urease rather than by CO_2.

Imaging techniques

Oesophago-gastro-duodenoscopy (OGD)

This should be the *first investigation* in all patients with gastroduodenal symptoms.
- ◇ The request form is usually an endoscopy request form. Include relevant history and request specific tests, e.g. antral biopsies for *Helicobacter*.
- ◇ The report will usually comment on the oesophagus, stomach and duodenum. Usually measurements will be given for the position of the oesophago-gastric junction (38–40cm), the presence of the Z-line (squamo-columnar junction) and, using the J-manoeuvre, the presence of a hiatus hernia. The first (D1) and second (D2) parts of the duodenum will be described. The site, size and character of any ulcers or other lesions will be described. If biopsies were taken, look for the histology report, which may also comment on the presence or absence of *Helicobacter pylori*. Recommendations for treatment are sometimes suggested.

The advantages of the procedure are that it allows *direct visualisation* of gastroduodenal lesions and enables biopsies to be taken for histological diagnosis. It can visualise oesophagitis, ulceration, varices etc. Certain therapeutic manoeuvres, e.g. injection of bleeding ulcers, can be performed.

Disadvantages are that it is an invasive procedure, and it is unable to diagnose early motility disorders. Some patients may find it unpleasant and are unable to swallow the scope. Complications include aspiration; or trauma to the oesophagus, stomach and duodenum that may cause bleeding, pain or occasionally perforation. This is particularly a risk in an unco-operative patient. Linitis plastica can be difficult to diagnose with OGD. Patients who are unable to swallow the scope may be offered a general anaesthetic.

CLO test for Helicobacter pylori

- ◇ Technique: this is often performed in conjunction with OGD. Endoscopic gastric biopsies are taken under direct vision from the gastric antrum. The tissue is placed in indicator medium, which detects the presence of urease activity by *H. pylori*. The presence of *H. pylori* results in an indicator colour change within a specified time-period, e.g. 60 minutes. Colour change after this time period is non-specific.
- ◇ Request form: write *request for CLO test* on the endoscopy request form. It is often performed as routine, even if not specifically requested.

The advantages are that it gives a quick result, enabling eradication therapy to be immediately prescribed. The disadvantages are that false negatives occur in 5–15%, so a negative result does not completely exclude the presence of *H. pylori*. PPI, bismuth and antibiotic use may interfere with the test and give a false negative result.

Alternative tests for H. pylori

H. pylori can also be detected, using immuno-histochemical stains, from gastric biopsies sent for histology.

Barium swallow/meal

This technique is used as a *second-line investigation* if OGD fails to provide a diagnosis. Indications for its use are:

✧ dysphagia in a frail person not suitable for OGD
✧ dysphagia when patient refuses OGD
✧ to exclude a pharyngeal pouch if there is concern prior to scoping.

An advantage of the technique is that it is useful in the investigation of dysphagia where endoscopy has not detected a mechanical cause and a motility disorder of the oesophagus or stomach is suspected. Double contrast (barium-air) barium meals are useful for the evaluation of suspected gastric cancer. Rigidity and absent peristalsis may occur at the site of a localised tumour, while linitis plastica produces an abrupt circumferential narrowing of the stomach lumen.

The disadvantages are that irradiation is used and simultaneous therapeutic procedures are not possible. Overall, it is not as sensitive as endoscopy for the detection of small lesions.

Ultrasound

The technique is mainly used non-invasively, with the ultrasound probe applied to the outside of the body after applying acoustic water-based gel. It often will be needed to exclude gallstones.

Its advantage is that it is a cheap, quick and safe way of imaging the liver, so it is useful for screening for liver metastases.

Endoluminal ultrasound (EUS)

This is a technique where a specialised probe is placed in the stomach to provide images of the stomach wall and adjacent lymph nodes. EUS can:

✧ help with diagnosis of gastric gastrointestinal stromal tumours (GIST)
✧ stage tumour
✧ obtain tissue (using EUS, fine-needle aspiration (FNA) and core biopsy).

Endoluminal ultrasound is good for determining intramural spread and lymph node involvement.

Combined laparoscopy and laparoscopic ultrasound is good for identifying transcoelomic spread and peritoneal seedlings, which can then be biopsied under direct vision. Laparoscopic ultrasound gives better images than external ultrasound of intra-abdominal organs, helping to detect smaller metastases, which can then be biopsied.

The disadvantage is that this is a limited application on its own. Confirmation of findings is needed by performing a computed tomography (CT) scan, so this tends to be preferred to ultrasound. Endoluminal ultrasound and laparoscopic ultrasound are not widely available.

CT scanning

The technique is used in gastric malignancy to demonstrate the extent of mural invasion; involvement of adjacent structures; and liver and lymph node involvement. Sometimes CT is used as a 'diagnostic fishing trip' when the clinician is worried that the patient has disseminated cancer but cannot find anything concrete on examination or blood tests.

An advantage is that invasion of the wall of the stomach is demonstrated as wall thickening (greater than 5mm). A thickness greater than 2cm generally correlates with spread beyond the stomach. Lymph node metastases can be detected in about 70% of cases. CT is good for detecting liver metastases.

Disadvantages include irradiation and a tendency to underestimate early peritoneal spread and lymph node metastases. It is not totally reliable in differentiating direct metastatic spread from reactive inflammation surrounding a tumour. Therefore it tends to understage tumours.

Barium meal

Barium meal is useful for defining the anatomy of a large hiatus hernia or seeing whether fluid empties from the stomach. In experienced hands it can be used to diagnose peptic ulcers and tumour, but it is inferior to endoscopy and should be reserved for specific cases.

Radioisotope techniques

The only test routinely used is a two-phase gastric emptying study. This is to investigate patients with suspected functional stomach problems (gastroparesis and gastric hurry).

Technetium-99m-HIDA scan

This scan is used to detect and quantify enterogastric reflux and afferent loop obstruction after gastrojejunostomy reconstructions.

In this technique, the patient is given an intravenous injection of technetium-99m-HIDA, which is secreted in the bile and concentrated in the gall bladder. The amount of radioactivity in the gall bladder is calculated and the gall bladder is stimulated to contract by administration of a milk meal. This expels the radioactivity into the duodenum. The passage of the radioactivity along the small bowel can be traced and the obstruction can be identified. Enterogastric reflux of radioactivity from the small bowel back into the stomach can be identified and quantified as a percentage of the total abdominal radioactivity.

Its advantages are that it provides quantitative assessment of the degree of enterogastric reflux and it can detect afferent loop obstruction in gastrojejunostomy reconstructions. Disadvantages include the use of radioactivity. It requires a functioning unobstructed biliary system.

Schilling test

This is a test used to assess the patient's ability to absorb vitamin B12. Radioactive vitamin B12 is given by mouth, and urine is collected for 24 hours.

A normal individual will excrete at least 10% of the original dose over 24 hours. A patient with pernicious anaemia will excrete less than 5%.

The advantage of this test is that it is a quantifiable measure of the ability of the gastro-intestinal tract to absorb vitamin B12. The disadvantages are that it does not localise the disease to stomach or terminal ileum and it uses radioactivity.

Laparoscopy

Laparoscopy is being increasingly used for the diagnosis and staging of tumours. The technique is performed in the operating theatre under general anaesthetic. A laparoscopic port is inserted under direct vision and CO_2 is insufflated to produce a pneumoperito-neum. It may be combined with intra-operative ultrasound using a special laparoscopic ultrasound probe. It also enables biopsy of focal lesions under direct vision. Laparoscopy is performed by a surgeon with a special interest.

The advantages are direct visualisation of abdominal pathology, and in gastric cancer it may establish irresectability without subjecting the patient to a full laparotomy. It enables direct biopsy of small lesions, e.g. peritoneal deposits, small liver lesions. Its disadvantage is that it is an invasive procedure requiring general anaesthetic.

Peptic ulcer disease
Chronic duodenal ulcer
Peak incidence occurs in the 25–50 age range. However, these ulcers are now *rare* in developed countries, due to effective treatment in the primary care setting.

History
- The patient typically presents with recurrent episodes of epigastric pain.
- Exacerbations are associated with stress, dietary/alcoholic overindulgence and smoking. Symptoms increase during fasting (night pain) and are decreased by food, especially milk or alkalis.
- Pain radiating through to the back is typical of posterior ulceration.
- Vomiting is uncommon unless associated with oedema/fibrosis around the ulcer causing pyloric obstruction.
- There may be a history of aspirin or non-steroidal anti-inflammatory drug (NSAID) ingestion. Often the patient is referred to surgery with a long history of H2-receptor antagonist (H2RA) or PPI treatment with relapses.

Examination
The patient may be overweight due to constant nibbling and there may be evidence of anaemia. On abdominal examination there may be diffuse epigastric tenderness. In cases with a degree of gastric outlet obstruction a succussion splash may be detected. Examination may otherwise be normal.

Chronic gastric ulcer
This is less common than duodenal ulcer. There are two distinct types.
- Type I is in the body of the stomach along the lesser curve. Type I may arise in normal mucosa or atrophic gastritis. These ulcers are not associated with hyperacidity, and in fact hypoacidity may be found. Hyperacidity tends to occur in the older age group.
- Type II is a pyloric channel ulcer (includes pre-pyloric). The natural history, acid secretory profile and therapeutic response are the same as for duodenal ulcers.

History
- Gastric ulcer patients may describe discomfort and fullness in the stomach.
- Eating increases the pain and is relieved by fasting – in fact patients may be afraid to eat, and they lose weight.
- These symptoms are the same as for gastric cancer, but cancer tends to be associated with more nausea and vomiting, and pain is more constant.

Examination
Examine for evidence of weight loss, anaemia and epigastric tenderness. A palpable epigastric mass suggests carcinoma of the stomach but may represent an inflammatory mass.

Investigations
- OGD and/or double contrast barium meal are used to investigate all dyspepsia patients.
- OGD combined with CLO testing of gastric antrum biopsies will establish *Helicobacter pylori* status.

OGD shows duodenal ulcer

✧ Diagnosis and biopsy of gastric antrum are needed to detect *H. pylori*.
✧ Two more biopsies are needed: one for the instant CLO test, one for histological examination.

If either is positive, the patient is started on *H. pylori*-eradication therapy and medical ulcer-healing therapy. OGD is repeated after medical therapy to check healing.

OGD shows gastric ulcer

Biopsy of the ulcer is mandatory to exclude gastric cancer; and also perform a biopsy of the antrum looking for *H. pylori* bacteria. If biopsy is benign, start on medical ulcer-healing therapy and *H. pylori* eradication, but repeat the endoscopy after 2–3 months of medical therapy. If the ulcer is not healed, repeat the biopsy. Failure to heal, even in the presence of negative biopsies, may be an indication for surgical therapy.

Medical treatment

The first step is to stop any medication such as NSAIDs that might cause ulceration, and to eradicate *H. pylori* infection. Thereafter use PPIs. A therapeutic course lasting 2–3 months heals 90%, with symptom relief achieved within 2–3 days.

✧ Resistant ulcers need a *double dose* of PPI. Only PPIs heal all resistant ulcers. Relapse is universal unless maintenance therapy is continued indefinitely.
✧ PPIs heal both duodenal and gastric ulcers. Problems of long-term PPI therapy are achlorhydria and hypergastrinaemia. There is evidence from rat studies of proliferation of gastric fundal endocrine cells and G-cells with the development of carcinoid tumours.
✧ Current triple-therapy regimes consist of a PPI, clarithromycin and metronidazole for 1–2 weeks. The PPI is continued for six weeks. Permanent healing rates are achieved in all patients in whom *H. pylori* infection is eradicated – approximately 90%. Patients undergo a urea breath test at 6–8 weeks to confirm eradication. If this fails, the original regime is tried.

Refractory ulcers

✧ A duodenal ulcer is considered refractory if there is no healing after eight weeks' therapy.
✧ A gastric ulcer is considered refractory if there is no healing after 12 weeks' therapy.

Perform an OGD to differentiate patients with a true refractory ulcer from those patients with persistent symptoms despite ulcer healing, which require investigation of alternative causes. If a refractory ulcer is present, successful *H. pylori* eradication should be confirmed by further biopsy for CLO test and histology. If *H. pylori* is still present, investigate its non-compliance with eradication therapy and, if indicated, prescribe another regime. If no *H. pylori* is detected, enquire regarding the presence of other ulcerogenic factors, e.g. smoking (measure urinary nicotine levels) or aspirin ingestion (measure blood salicylate levels).

True resistant ulcer

A true resistant ulcer fails to heal despite *H. pylori* eradication. A relapsed ulcer heals initially but then recurs.

✧ Perform an OGD and take multiple biopsies for evidence of neoplasia, infection or inflammation.
✧ Measure serum gastrin levels, and, if they are high, investigate for Zollinger-Ellison syndrome.

✧ Where no cause can be found, the ulcer can be termed an idiopathic refractory ulcer. Prolonged drug treatment and OGD surveillance, or surgery, is indicated to exclude undetected malignancy. Indications for surgical treatment of peptic ulcer disease are:

∝ failure to comply with maintenance
∝ ulcers resistant to *H. pylori* eradication therapy
∝ gastric ulcers that remain unhealed after three months treatment, irrespective of the biopsy findings
∝ complications associated with ulcers, e.g. pyloric obstruction, perforation, bleeding.

Always think: 'Could this be cancer?'

Follow-up
Follow up with medical therapy and follow-up OGD. Once the ulcer is healed and *H.pylori* eradicated, the patient can be discharged.

Post-operative follow-up
This is needed long term to detect complications, which include recurrent ulceration, dumping, diarrhoea and adverse nutritional consequences. However, remedial surgery for most chronic conditions is usually delayed for at least 18 months, as most symptoms improve.

Nutritional consequences of gastric surgery
Nutritional consequences are more common after gastrectomy, which results in:
✧ decreased food intake
✧ malabsorption of fat or nitrogen
✧ decreased small bowel transit time.

Iron deficiency anaemia
Iron deficiency is very common after vagotomy and drainage or gastric resections, especially in females. The incidence increases with time until it is 60–80% at 10–20 years. It is caused by altered handling of iron – the failure to reduce it to the ferric form for absorption. Iron absorption is unpredictable after gastrectomy, and close monitoring of the FBC is necessary for 1–2 years after surgery.

Macrocytic anaemia
This is caused by vitamin B12 deficiency. It invariably occurs after total gastrectomy due to loss of the intrinsic factor. After partial gastrectomy, diagnosis is by an abnormal Schilling test. Treat by three-monthly injections of cyanocobalamin, indefinitely. Partial gastrectomy and truncal vagotomy and drainage result in lower levels of vitamin B12 due to lack of an acid environment. The Schilling test is normal – treatment is with oral crystalline vitamin B12.

Bone disease
Bone disease may develop several years after gastric resection with duodenal exclusion; the duodenum is the major site of calcium absorption. Many females develop osteomalacia 10–20 years after gastrectomy. They may present with symptoms of generalised bone pain, weakness due to associated myopathy, and stress fractures. Investigations show a raised serum alkaline phosphatase and calcium, and areas of bone rarefaction on X-rays.

Calcium and alkaline phosphatase levels should be measured annually. After five years all patients should have a full assessment for metabolic bone disease. Treatment is with oral calcium and vitamin D. Post-menopausal women and all patients aged over 70 should take an oral calcium supplement, twice a day, for life.

Post-gastric surgery dumping and reactive hypoglycaemia
Dumping
This is rapid gastric emptying. Vasomotor symptoms occur within minutes of eating due to hypovolaemia (decreased cardiac output and peripheral resistance) caused by out-pouring of fluid into the bowel to dilute hyperosmolar gastric contents.

Treatment of mild or moderate dumping is to advise *small dry meals*, rich in protein and fat but low in carbohydrate. Methoxy pectin or bran can be added to the diet to slow gastric emptying. Dumping rarely has a surgical solution and should be managed conservatively. Time is usually the best healer, as symptoms will often settle down over 6–12 months.

Reactive hypoglycaemia
Symptoms of sweating and tremor due to hypoglycaemia occur 2–3 hours after a meal. Diagnosis is made by performing an in-patient extended glucose tolerance test. Following a meal this shows initial hyperglycaemia, provoking an exaggerated insulin release with increased plasma insulin and enteroglucagon levels. This results in the subsequent hypoglycaemia and occurrence of symptoms. Treatment is mainly dietary, with low carbohydrate-high protein meals. Ingesting fluids at the same time as solids should be avoided, to help reduce intestinal transit time.

Enterogastric reflux/reflux gastritis
Reflux of bile/pancreatic juice into the stomach causes a reflux erosive gastritis and bilious vomiting.

History
There is a history of epigastric pain, nausea and vomiting in the early postprandial period. It is a burning-type pain, aggravated by food and not relieved by antacids. Episodes culminate in the vomiting of bile-stained fluid 1–2 hours after a meal. Less commonly, vomiting occurs early in the morning after night pain. Iron deficiency anaemia develops.

Investigations
Diagnosis is confirmed by OGD which reveals gastritis and pooling of bile in the stomach.

Treatment
✧ Bile-salt binding agents such as cholestyramine, combined with Sulcralfate at night, are often effective.
✧ If medical therapy fails to control the symptoms, remedial surgery is indicated.
✧ Note that atrophic gastritis and intestinal metaplasia associated with enterogastric reflux has been implicated in the development of carcinoma and requires long-term follow-up with regular OGD assessment.

Extrinsic loop obstruction
This is a rare condition. It occurs after truncal vagotomy and gastroenterostomy. It usually affects the afferent loop and is predisposed to by the formation of antecolic anastomoses and long loops greater than 20cm.

Causes
Causes include internal herniation; kinking of the anastomosis; volvulus; stenosis;

jejunogastric intussusception; and development of gastric cancer in the stomach remnant. This operation is no longer performed, so the condition is relevant only to older patients who have had ulcer surgery in the 1960s and 70s.

History
✧ Usually, intermittent feelings of fullness and cramp-like pain and nausea occur within one hour of eating.
✧ The attack culminates in vomiting of copious amounts of bile-stained fluid, which relieves the symptoms.
✧ In acute cases there is no relief. It may be accompanied by development of acute pancreatitis, jaundice and necrosis with perforation.

Examination
During pain-free episodes examination may be normal. During attacks there may be upper abdominal distension and tenderness.

Investigations
Liver function tests may be abnormal and there may be a dilated small bowel loop on abdominal X-ray (AXR). Delayed emptying of the afferent loop may be demonstrated by 99Tcm-diethyl-IDA (EHIDA) scan. There may be failure of barium to enter the afferent loop during barium meal.

Treatment
Some cases are amenable to endoscopic pneumatic dilatation. Unresponsive cases require surgical correction.

Acute jejunogastric intussusception
There is severe epigastric pain and haematemesis and a palpable abdominal mass and high small bowel obstruction. Diagnosis is by AXR, which shows a soft-tissue mass surrounded by air. Treatment is by surgery.

Gastro-oesophageal reflux/oesophagitis
Mobilisation of the oesophagus during surgery may cause cardio-oesophageal incompetence. If associated with enterogastric reflux this may lead to a severe neutral/alkaline oesophagitis and stricture formation.

Post-gastric surgery diarrhoea
Three patterns of diarrhoea occur after gastric surgery:
✧ frequent loose motions
✧ intermittent episodes of short-lived diarrhoea
✧ severe intractable diarrhoea, which occurs in 2% after truncal vagotomy and, unlike dumping, is often precipitated by small meals.

Diarrhoea may be caused by malabsorption of bile salts and/or fatty acids; accelerated small bowel transit time; or bacterial overgrowth.

History
Determine the pattern of the diarrhoea and any precipitating or exacerbating factors. Estimate the severity of the symptoms.

Examination
Examine for anaemia, weight loss and dehydration.

Investigations

Investigations are usually delayed until simple treatments have failed to control the symptoms.

Investigations include faecal fat estimation, butter fat test, small bowel transit time and C14 glycocholate breath test for bacterial overgrowth.

Treatment

◆ Advise a diet low in animal fat. Intestinal sedatives (codeine phosphate, loperamide) and bile-salt binding agents (cholestyramine) usually give short-term relief.
◆ If symptoms are severe and fail to settle, consider remedial surgery, e.g. reversed small bowel segment – but results are poor.

Post-gastric surgery decreased appetite

A small stomach is created by extensive or total gastrectomy and it produces early satiety, which precludes adequate intake and can cause malnutrition. All patients should be warned accordingly. For many this symptom reduces with time but it rarely disappears completely.

History

Determine the average dietary intake and whether this is associated with weight loss.

Examination

Examine for evidence of anaemia and weight loss.

Investigation

Carry out FBC, urea and electrolytes (U&Es) and LFTs to estimate nutrition. Investigate serum iron, B12 and folate. Take contrast studies to examine the gastric remnant.

Treatment

◆ Mild cases are treated with small, frequent meals. There should be dietician input and high-calorie supplements.
◆ More severe cases may require elemental diets administered by Clinifeed tube.

Other complications after gastric surgery

Other complications after gastric surgery include the following.
◆ Gallstones.
◆ Bezoars – balls of undigested vegetable/fruit matter in the stomach remnant. There will be a history of nausea and vomiting; abdominal discomfort; halitosis; and early satiety. They lead to small bowel obstruction, severe gastritis and ulceration. Investigation is by OGD or barium meal. Medical treatment is with enzymatic cellulose. Small bezoars may be removed piecemeal endoscopically, but larger ones will need to be removed surgically. This may be possible with a laparoscopic approach.
◆ There is an *increased risk of carcinoma in the gastric remnant* at 15–20 years: OGD should be performed in any patient with new upper abdominal symptoms after any previous ulcer surgery. Some clinicians offer all patients who have had old-style gastric ulcer surgery surveillance endoscopy every 3–5 years, but this is controversial. They are undoubtedly at high risk of developing stump cancers in their gastric remnants.

Gastric volvulus

Usually a degree of gastric outlet obstruction develops, resulting in a big dilated stomach, which after a heavy meal is prone to twist.

History

Gastric volvulus can present in the outpatient with chronic symptoms of episodes of epigastric distress and vomiting; or acutely with severe epigastric pain, ineffectual retching with distension, tenderness and signs of shock.

Examination

Examination may be normal if performed between episodes, or there may be evidence of epigastric distension and tenderness with a succussion splash.

Investigations

An AXR may show abnormal gastric shadow. Barium meal may demonstrate an abnormal, big stomach but endoscopy is the investigation of choice.

Treatment

An acutely volved stomach may untwist if carefully decompressed with a nasogastric tube, or better, at endoscopy. It is does not, resuscitation and urgent surgery by an experienced upper GI surgeon will be necessary. A laparoscopic approach is often possible and offers many advantages to the frail elderly patient.

Follow-up

Follow up at short intervals until diagnosis is established.

Post-operative follow-up

This is as for gastrectomy and gastric ulcer surgery.

Gastritis
Types of gastritis

There are four main types of gastritis.

- ✧ Type A is an autoimmune condition. Circulating parietal cell antibodies cause pernicious anaemia with achlorhydria and absent intrinsic factor. The antrum is spared, so serum gastrin levels are high due to alkaline conditions. There is significant *increased risk of development of carcinoma*, usually of the diffuse type.
- ✧ Type B begins distally in the pyloric region due to *H. pylori* infection. Gastrin levels are normal. It is always present in duodenal ulceration.
- ✧ Lymphocytic gastritis involves infiltration of the gastric epithelium by T lymphocytes. OGD shows nodularity, erosions and enlarged mucosal folds.
- ✧ Erosive gastritis is caused by NSAIDs and alcohol.
- ✧ Other causes include reflux, stress, granulomatous (TB, Crohn's) gastritis, cystica polyposa, AIDS gastritis, eosinophilic gastritis, Ménétrier's disease, suppurative gastritis, and emphysematous gastritis.

History

Patients may complain of dyspepsia and abdominal pain. There may be a history of alcohol or NSAID ingestion.

Examination

Examination may be normal, or there may be evidence of anaemia, weight loss or an underlying disorder.

Investigations

Carry out OGD and biopsy for detection of dysplasia and *H. pylori*. Vitamin B12 and folate levels may be low. Perform a Schilling test if atrophic gastritis is suspected. Measure serum gastrin levels and carry out a FBC for lymphocyte and eosinophil levels.

Treatment
Treatment depends on diagnosis and the effect of symptoms and it should be given in combination with anti-ulcer therapy if indicated.
✧ Type A: vitamin B12 injection every three months.
✧ Type B: *H. pylori* eradication.
✧ Erosive gastritis: NSAID or alcohol withdrawal.
✧ Dysplasia: if mild to moderate, can be monitored by regular OGD surveillance. If there is severe dysplasia, gastric resection is indicated.

Follow-up
If gastritis is accompanied by dysplasia, surveillance by OGD is indicated. If dysplasia is severe, gastric resection is indicated.

Post-operative follow-up
✧ Review histology.
✧ Refer to oncology if indicated.
✧ Follow-up for complications is the same as for gastrectomy for peptic ulcer disease.
✧ Follow-up is usually long term.

Gastric polyps
Types of polyp
Adenomas and other benign tumours are rare. They account for 5% of benign gastric polyps. Many are found in the antrum. They may be single or multiple. Progression to cancer is possible. Adenomatous polyps *larger than 4cm* are associated with 11% malignant change over a four-year follow-up period.

The *majority* (75–95%) of gastric polyps are hyperplastic, which represents regeneration of the mucosa after mucosal damage. They are benign and have no malignant potential. The commonest polyps by far are fundic gland polyps, which are frequently seen in patients taking PPIs. They need surveillance only if large (1cm diameter or greater).

Polyps may also be associated with independent cancer elsewhere in the stomach (6.5%–25%). Gastrointestinal stromal tumours (GIST) most commonly arise in the stomach and are frequently polypoid. They are submucosal, may have both an intra-luminal and extra-luminal component and ulcerate causing haematemesis or anaemia.

History
Polyps are usually asymptomatic unless they are large and situated at the pylorus or cardia and are causing obstruction.

Examination
Examination is usually completely normal.

Treatment
✧ If polyps are small and found on endoscopy, then endoscopic removal is advisable for histological diagnosis.
✧ This is combined with multiple biopsies of the stomach with prophylactic anti-ulcer treatment.
✧ Since endoscopic resection is associated with 40% recurrence of polyps, endoscopic follow-up is essential.

Follow-up

Intervals should be short until the diagnosis is made and malignancy is excluded. After treatment, long-term follow-up with OGD surveillance is indicated to detect recurrence or malignant change.

Post-operative follow-up

Review histology to detect any evidence of malignancy.

Non-neoplastic gastric polyps

Regenerative polyps are inflammatory and associated with gastritis and peptic ulceration. All should be removed endoscopically for histology. Two per cent have areas of focal carcinoma, 4% dysplasia. Long-term follow-up with OGD surveillance is indicated.

Other polyps

Inflammatory fibroid polyps are found when eosinophilic gastritis occurs in the pyloric antrum and duodenum. It is caused by a gastrointestinal allergy.

Others include myoepithelial hamartomas; Peutz-Jeghers syndrome; and heterotopic pancreatic tissue in the antropyloric region.

Carcinoma of the stomach

Overall, five-year survival for carcinoma of the stomach remains depressingly low in the United Kingdom, at 5–10%. However, survival is dependent upon cancer stage at presentation and, to a lesser degree, on the radicality of resection. Early tumours with no or few involved nodes can be cured by D2 gastrectomy, so early detection is vital.

It is rarely seen before 40 years of age, except in patients with familial hereditary gastric cancer due to E-cadherin gene mutations. The incidence increases from the age of 55 years onwards and peaks in the sixth and seventh decades. The incidence of distal gastric cancer in the UK and other post-industrial societies has been falling for 30 years, but at the same time the incidence of proximal tumours in the gastric cardia, possibly due to gastrointestinal reflux, has been rising.

The male–female ratio is 2:1.

The aetiology of distal tumours includes *H. pylori* infection, spicy food, polycyclic hydrocarbons, high salt intake and tobacco smoking. For proximal tumours it is gastro-oesophageal reflux disease (GORD).

Risk factors are atrophic gastritis; pernicious anaemia; previous partial gastrectomy; adenomatous and regenerative polyps; familial polyposis; hypogammaglobulinaemia; blood group A; type III intestinal metaplasia; and severe dysplasia.

Dysplasia

Dysplasia can be a marker of gastric cancer.
- ⟡ Type A affects the metaplastic gastric epithelium and can lead to the development of the intestinal type of gastric cancer.
- ⟡ Type B arises in the non-metaplastic gastric epithelium and predisposes to diffuse or intermediate gastric cancers.

History

Most patients present with dyspepsia, and dysplasia is detected during routine investigation. Some cases are detected by screening.

Examination
A normal examination is a good sign. Look for evidence of malignancy such as epigastric mass and weight loss.

Investigations
✧   Diagnose by OGD and biopsy for histology.
✧   Dysplasia is graded into mild, moderate and severe (carcinoma in situ).

Treatment
✧   Mild to moderate dysplasia requires regular OGD surveillance.
✧   For severe dysplasia a second OGD and biopsy is mandatory within a few weeks. If severe dysplasia is confirmed, gastrectomy is advised.
✧   The histology of gastrectomy specimens shows that 40–50% have early invasive gastric cancer.

Follow-up is at short intervals initially, until neoplasia is excluded. Regular OGD surveillance to detect development of neoplasia and grade it is required.

Pathology of gastric cancer
The main classification of gastric cancers is into:
✧   intestinal type
✧   diffuse type.

Each is then classified into 'well differentiated', 'poorly differentiated' or 'undifferentiated'. The undifferentiated diffuse type is equivalent to linitis plastica.
    There are no reliable serum markers of gastric cancer.

Early gastric cancer
Cancer limited to the mucosa and submucosa, regardless of nodal status, if completely resected by gastrectomy has a five-year survival of 80%.
    Endoscopic appearance may be protruding, superficial or excavated. At the time of diagnosis, 10–15% of early gastric cancers have already spread to the lymph nodes.

Advanced gastric cancer
The tumour involves the muscularis propria. Advanced gastric cancer represents 95% of gastric cancer diagnosed in the UK. Most have lymph node spread as well as peritoneal and liver spread.

Staging of gastric cancer
This involves the TNM system. It describes: (T) the depth of the tumour's penetration into the stomach wall, (N) the involvement of local or distant lymph nodes and (M) distant metastases.
    Measurements are T1–4, N0–3 and M0–1 where N1 = 1–6 positive nodes, N2 = 7–15 positive nodes and N3 = more than 15 positive nodes.
    Stage for stage, intestinal tumours have a better prognosis than diffuse tumours; well differentiated tumours do better than poorly differentiated ones; and distally located cancers do better than proximal ones.

Spread
Nodal spread to lymph nodes on the lesser and greater curves, the so-called D1 tier of nodes, is common (stations 1–6). The second tier of nodes, the D2 group, includes those along the left gastric artery, the coeliac trunk, the common hepatic artery and the splenic

artery (stations 7–12a). Involved nodes beyond these locations are classified D3 and imply incurability.

Para-aortic nodal disease, peritoneal metastases and spread to the liver or lungs are incurable. Para-oesophageal nodes, if positive, usually count as distant metastases unless the tumour is located in the gastric cardia, in which case they are counted as regional D1 nodes and cure is still achievable if all the disease is resected (an R0 resection).

History

Early disease is often asymptomatic, or presents with mild dyspepsia which responds to acid suppression. Symptoms of malaise, early satiety, postprandial fullness, loss of appetite and weight loss usually indicate advanced disease.

Cardia lesions may present with dysphagia; middle and pyloric tumours may present with vomiting after meals. Advanced cases may present with haematemesis and melaena.

The most common presentation *is recent onset dyspepsia in someone over the age of 55.* Therefore all patients in this age group should have an urgent OGD before starting ulcer treatment. Younger patients should also be scoped if they have unexplained symptoms or persistent symptoms despite treatment. All patients with 'alarm symptoms' such as anaemia or weight loss should undergo urgent upper GI endoscopy (*see* NICE Guidance on Dyspepsia).

Examination

✧ No abnormal findings is a good sign.
✧ Anaemia often presents at diagnosis.
✧ Signs of weight loss, an epigastric mass and an enlarged left supraclavicular lymph node indicate late disease.
✧ Jaundice, hepatomegaly or ascites indicate incurable disease.

Investigations

✧ OGD and multiple biopsies and brush cytology.
✧ CT of chest and abdomen.
✧ EUS for local staging of proximal tumours involving the cardia.
✧ Staging laparoscopy to exclude peritoneal and small liver metastases.
✧ PET-CT can be useful to help determine the nature of distant lesions seen on CT if this is likely to radically change management (i.e. an adrenal metastasis).

Treatment

Treatment takes place in the setting of a multidisciplinary team.

Curative surgery

This should be performed in a high volume centre by a surgeon with appropriate training who does this type of surgery frequently and who works as part of a multidisciplinary team that can provide all aspects of specialist care 24 hours a day, 365 days of the year. The aim of surgery should be to obtain a complete resection of the primary tumour (R0); an adequate resection of regional lymph nodes (a minimum of 15 nodes for TNM staging by D1 or D2 resection); and to provide patients with the best possible quality of life. Open and close rates (failure of staging) and peri-operative mortality should both be less than 5%. Patients with locally advanced disease should be considered for neoadjuvant chemotherapy prior to resection.

Palliative treatment

Gastrectomy with palliative intent is rarely indicated. Incurable distal tumours causing outlet obstruction can be palliated by laparoscopic gastric bypass or endoscopic duodenal stenting. Cardia tumours can usually be stented, and tumours of the gastric body may be palliated by chemotherapy.

Chemotherapy

Cisplatin-based regimens can be used to shrink tumours prior to resection, increasing the chance of an R0 resection, or as palliative therapy for patients with incurable disease. Randomised controlled trials of palliative chemotherapy have shown a doubling of survival from three to six months and improved quality of life.

Radiotherapy

Radiotherapy can be useful for palliation to reduce bleeding from an incurable tumour. It is occasionally used as part of an adjuvant regimen of chemo-radiation post resection, but it is poorly tolerated and is not routine in the UK.

Follow-up

Make a baseline CT scan at three months and again at one year. There should be further CTs if there is any deterioration in clinical status. Perform examination and bloods three times in the first year, twice in the second year and annually thereafter for five years, then discharge. All total gastrectomy patients need B12 injections every three months.

Post-operative follow-up

Check histology to confirm complete excision and correct resection level. Arrange oncology referral if appropriate. Follow up for complications of gastric surgery as previously described.

Other tumours

- ✧ Other tumours include leiomyoma (benign) and leiomyosarcoma (malignant).
- ✧ Submucosal and intramuscular tumours occur in the upper and middle third of the stomach.
- ✧ Ulceration and/or bleeding is a common presentation.
- ✧ They are treated by wedge resection if small or partial gastrectomy if large.

Gastric lymphomas (2–5%)

These are mainly *B-cell non-Hodgkin's lymphomas* arising in the mucosa-associated lymphoid tissue (MALT), or *extra-nodal marginal zone B-cell lymphomas* according to the WHO classification. They are slow growing, remain localised until late and are less aggressive than non-Hodgkin's. They infiltrate the wall, producing mucosal thickening, and may present with ulceration and bleeding. Lymph node spread occurs late and tends to remain in regional lymph nodes.

History

- ✧ There are the usual dyspeptic symptoms, but nausea, vomiting and weight loss are more common. Diarrhoea is often present.
- ✧ Some patients will present as emergencies with perforation or haematemesis.
- ✧ Pain, fever and anorexia may also be features.

Examination

A palpable epigastric mass may be present in 20% of patients and does not indicate inoperability. However, hepatomegaly and/or splenomegaly suggest a diffuse process with a worse prognosis, as does general lymphadenopathy.

Investigations
✧ Faecal occult blood tests are positive in 50%.
✧ Erythrocyte sedimentation rate (ESR) is usually grossly elevated.
✧ Diagnosis is by OGD with cobblestone mucosal appearance and rugal hypertrophy, multiple tumour nodules.
✧ Biopsies for histology are taken but may be negative in a large proportion of cases due to the *submucosal location* of the tumour. Therefore, in the presence of a typical appearance a negative histology result does not rule out the diagnosis. Repeat.
✧ OGD and deeper biopsies may be indicated.
✧ Endoscopic ultrasound is useful.

Staging
✧ Ann Arbor or TNM for gastric lymphoma.
✧ CT scan of the chest and abdomen is performed to detect spread.
✧ Bone marrow aspirate and biopsy may demonstrate diffuse disease.
✧ Laparoscopy is useful for stage III and IV and distinction between primary gastric lymphoma and advanced primary nodal disease.

Treatment
Low-grade MALT lymphoma
If associated with *H. pylori* infection, this should be eradicated with triple therapy, as many tumours will regress. If this fails, chemotherapy with cyclophosphamide, doxorubicin, vincristine and prednisone (CHOP) regimen, with or without rituximab, is indicated. Surgery is not indicated.

High-grade MALT lymphoma or diffuse B-cell lymphoma
This is also treated with chemotherapy. Surgical resection is reserved for treatment failures. Survival rates of greater than 90% can be expected with this approach.

Follow-up
There should be regular OGD review and follow-up by haematologists.

Gastric carcinoids
These tumours are associated with atrophic gastritis (type A) and chronic hypergastri-naemia of pernicious anaemia. The incidence in pernicious anaemia patients is 2–9%. More recently, fundal enterochromaffin tumours in Zollinger-Ellison patients have been treated with omeprazole. The tumours produce gastrin, somatostatin, serotonin and vasoactive invasive peptide. They are generally *slow growing* and *indolent* but can metastasise if they exhibit abnormal cytology and are larger than 2cm.

History
✧ Rarely symptomatic.
✧ Usually diagnosed on endoscopy in investigation for dyspepsia.
✧ Other presentations include abdominal pain or evidence of gastrointestinal bleeding.
✧ The carcinoid syndrome can be produced by gastric carcinoids, but this is usually endocrinologically silent unless associated with liver metastases. Typically, gastric carcinoid produces bright red geographical flushing.

Examination
Examination may be normal, but examine for evidence of tumour and spread. Epigastric mass and liver enlargement are late signs.

Investigations
OGD with biopsy is usually diagnostic. Investigate for carcinoid syndrome if suspected.

Treatment
Treat with local resection (or endoscopic) followed by endoscopic surveillance.

Larger tumours require surgical excision, which may be possible laparoscopically. Resection of the gastric antrum reduces the gastrin drive to the remainder of the stomach.

Follow-up
Follow up at short intervals until diagnosis and treatment is performed. Tumours treated by endoscopic resection require long-term endoscopic follow-up to detect recurrence. Irresectable lesions require oncology referral for chemotherapy and, if necessary, treatment of the carcinoid syndrome.

Post-operative follow-up
Check histology for resection. There may be complications of gastrectomy, as previously described.

The small intestine and vermiform appendix
Alastair Windsor

SIX

Introduction
The basic functions of the small bowel are digestion and assimilation. Most chronic disorders of the small bowel tend to be managed by gastroenterologists with referral to surgeons if surgery is indicated. However, some knowledge of these disorders is necessary for the surgeon, especially in the case of small bowel inflammatory conditions such as Crohn's, small bowel tumours, and in the investigation of weight loss and diarrhoea, which may be referred to the surgical clinic.

Assessment of small bowel disorders
Small bowel history
Take a general gastrointestinal history. There are no symptoms which exclusively indicate small bowel disease, but small bowel disorders should be considered in patients presenting with intermittent, colicky central abdominal pain. These symptoms may be accompanied by diarrhoea, stool that are difficult to flush away and weight loss. Patients may also complain of symptoms typical of anaemia. Intermittent small bowel obstruction secondary to adhesions is very common after any abdominal surgery, so an enquiry about previous operations is important. Patients may complain of regular vomiting 1–2 hours after meals.

Small bowel examination
Perform a general examination. Examine for anaemia and weight loss. Examine the mouth and pharynx for ulcers. Abdominal examination may reveal distension, scars from previous surgery, tenderness or a mass. Rectal examination, sigmoidoscopy and biopsy if indicated complete the examination.

Laboratory investigations
Full blood count (FBC) may reveal anaemia due to gastrointestinal (GI) bleeding or chronic disease. Abnormal white cell count (WCC) may indicate infection or lymphoma. Raised erythrocyte sedimentation rate (ESR) and C-reactive protein (CRP) may indicate active inflammatory bowel disease.

Biochemistry
- Urinalysis: raised urinary levels of 5-hydroxyindoleacetic acid (5-HIAA) may indicate carcinoid syndrome.
- Serum biochemistry: routine indications. Abnormalities of serum albumin, transferrin, urea and electrolytes, including calcium, may occur in small bowel disease.
- Liver function tests (LFT): abnormal LFTs may be associated with inflammatory bowel disease.
- Blood sugar tests: may reveal diabetes mellitus.
- Estimation of faecal fat: from a 3–5 day collection on a standard diet containing 80–100 g of fat. Normal excretion is less than 6.0 g/day (18 mmol triglyceride). This is a non-invasive screening test for malabsorption.

Microbiology
Stool cultures are useful in various small bowel infections, e.g. *Yersinia*.

Cytology/histology – jejunal mucosal biopsy

The Crosby suction capsule is at the end of a fine-bore catheter. The patient swallows the capsule and time is allowed for the capsule to be propelled into the jejunum, which is confirmed by plain abdominal X-ray (AXR). The capsule is opened and suction applied via the catheter. The capsule is then closed, taking a jejunal mucosa biopsy, and the capsule is removed. The tissue is sent for histology.

This method is used for diagnosis of coeliac disease, Whipple's, parasites and amyloid. It is a random biopsy of jejunal tissue, not performed under direct vision. This technique has largely been replaced by endoscopy and biopsy of the second part of the duodenum, under direct vision.

Imaging techniques

AXR plain

An X-ray may identify dilated small bowel loops in obstruction, or thickened bowel loops in inflammatory disorders.

Small bowel follow-through (SBFT)

The patient drinks radiological contrast. The path of the contrast through the stomach and small bowel is followed at regular intervals by repeated X-rays. It is easier to perform than small bowel enema but provides less detail of the small bowel due to dilution of contrast, the time taken to empty from the stomach and overlapping bowel loops.

Small bowel enema (SBE)

Contrast medium is instilled through a Bilbao-Dotter tube directly into the upper jejunum. It has a high diagnostic yield for small bowel tumours, Crohn's, occult GI bleeding and malabsorption. Malabsorption shows flocculation and segmentation of barium, thickening of mucosal folds and dilatation of intestinal loops. There may be difficulty swallowing the tube and passing the tube through the pylorus.

Small bowel magnetic resonance imaging (MRI)

MRI is performed with small bowel contrast using water or locust bean gum. Although currently not universally used, the technique is increasingly being shown to be very accurate at imaging the small bowel. Most of the work has been done in Crohn's disease. Its ability to indicate areas of inflammation may allow differentiation between fibro-stenotic and inflammatory strictures.

Selective splanchnic angiography

An angiography catheter is passed, using the Seldinger technique, through the femoral artery, and the catheter is manipulated through the aorta into the visceral arteries (coeliac, superior mesenteric artery (SMA), inferior mesenteric artery (IMA). Radiological contrast is injected. Certain appearances are characteristic of certain lesions, e.g. intraluminal bleeding, tumour or stenoses/occlusions of the coeliac, or mesenteric arteries indicating mesenteric ischaemia.

The technique allows identification of obscure GI bleeding not identified by oesophago-gastro-duodenoscopy (OGD) or colonoscopy. It is diagnostic for angiodysplastic lesions during active bleeding and may be useful for diagnosis of mesenteric ischaemia. It is an invasive technique that can have complications associated with arterial puncture, e.g. haemorrhage, haematoma, false aneurysm; and with the use of radiological contrast, e.g. allergic reactions, renal failure.

Contrast CT

The patient drinks, or has instilled through a nasogastric tube, a special radiological contrast solution (E-Z-CAT®) to opacify the intestine. The patient is then passed through the CT body scanner. The scan is useful for detecting thickening of the bowel wall and the presence of enterocolic and enterovesical fistulas. It provides detailed information about the small and large bowel, but it is expensive and time-consuming and it uses ionising radiation.

Ultrasound scan

An ultrasound probe is passed over the abdomen using aqueous gel as a coupling medium. Images of the underlying organs are formed from the differential amount of ultrasound reflected from different organs. Using the Doppler Effect and colour coding, blood flow can be imaged in major arterial and venous vessels. It is useful for detecting fluid-filled loops of small bowel, detecting peristalsis, estimating bowel wall thickness, detecting intra-abdominal fluid and detecting blood flow in major vessels.

Visualisation of the small bowel
Small bowel enteroscopy

A long endoscope is inserted into the duodenum, a balloon is inflated, and gut peristalsis carries the scope to the caecum, as confirmed by X-ray screening. Inspection is made as the instrument is withdrawn. It may be useful to visualise obscure bleeding but is not widely available.

Capsule endoscopy (CE)

The PillCam video capsule contains a miniaturised camera, a light source and a wireless circuit for acquisition and transmission of signals. The patient swallows a capsule and the device is passively propelled through the gastrointestinal tract by peristalsis. Images are transmitted to a data recorder and then downloaded to be reviewed on a monitor. The capsule is passed in the patient's stool usually in 24–48 hours. Currently, best evidence for its use includes evaluation of patients with obscure bleeding, inflammatory bowel diseases, suspected small bowel tumours, hereditary polyposis syndromes and complicated coeliac disease. It cannot be used in patients with motility disorders or mechanical obstruction.

Radioisotope techniques
Isotope scintigraphy

Isotope scintigraphy involves intravenous administration of a radio-labelled compound or autologous cells. It may be useful to show occult GI bleeding, suspected intra-abdominal localised inflammation/abscess, inflamed Crohn's and intestinal transit time, and also for evaluation of bilioenteric anastomoses. However, it requires radioactivity and it poorly localises bleeding points or abscesses in the abdomen.

Small bowel transit time

This is shown by external scintigraphy after administration of isotope-labelled meals or by breath tests. For meals the detection of caecal radioactivity is used as the end-point for the estimation of small bowel transit time (includes gastric emptying time as well). Breath tests are a simpler way of obtaining similar information.

White cell scan

Indium 111-labelled autologous leucocytes are injected intravenously and settle in areas of abscess/inflammation. An abdominal scintiscan is performed at 2, 6, 20 and 24 hours. The scan can be used to detect the extent and severity of inflammatory bowel disease.

Tests of small bowel function
Breath tests
Breath tests are used in the detection of bacterial overgrowth, the demonstration of carbohydrate malabsorption and the assessment of small bowel transit time.

Bacterial overgrowth
The 14C-glycocholate breath test can show bacterial overgrowth in the small intestine. Bacteria deconjugate the compound, which is absorbed into the bloodstream and exhaled. It can also be positive in the presence of ileal disease, and in this circumstance 14C-D-xylose is more reliable.

Carbohydrate malabsorption
Ingestion of 14C-lactose is the conventional test for lactose intolerance, i.e. brush-border lactase deficiency.

Hydrogen breath test for small bowel transit time and bacterial overgrowth
The hydrogen (H_2) breath test is supplanting other tests for small bowel transit time. Repeated measurements of H_2O in end-expiratory air are taken after a drink of lactulose or a meal of mashed potato and beans. When the meal reaches the caecum bacterial fermentation occurs, resulting in increased breath H_2.

The test includes gastric emptying time. If the meal is radio-labelled with technetium-99m (^{99m}Tc), both gastric emptying and small bowel transit times can be calculated from the one investigation.

Tests of intestinal permeability
51Cr-labelled EDTA is given orally. It is not absorbed in a healthy person. Urinary estimation is performed and if EDTA is detected this indicates abnormal intestinal permeability. It may be useful in the diagnosis of obscure cases of Crohn's, but it is not widely available.

Ileal malabsorption
The Schilling test shows the ability of the ileum to absorb vitamin B12.

The SeHCAT test assesses the ileal absorptive capacity for bile salts.

Investigation of specific small bowel abnormalities
Investigation of intestinal bleeding
Causes may be Meckel's diverticulum, polyps and tumours – especially smooth muscle neoplasms and vascular malformations.

Tests
OGD and SBE are usually negative. The use of radio-labelled red cells is suitable for intermittent bleeding, but not for active rapid bleeding. For rapid bleeding, it is best to use angiography and embolisation.

Investigation of suspected malabsorption
Malabsorption is either due to small bowel disease, bacterial overgrowth or pancreatic exocrine insufficiency.

Tests
✧ The first test is for abnormal faecal fat excretion (greater than 6.0 g/day).
✧ For the second test give SBE. If it is normal, perform a mucosal biopsy, and if this is

normal perform pancreatic function tests. If the small bowel enema is abnormal, a mucosal biopsy can be performed, or proceed directly to the Schilling test and follow with tests for bacterial overgrowth.

Syndromes resulting from disease or surgery on the gastrointestinal tract

These syndromes include bacterial overgrowth (stagnant loop syndrome), short gut syndrome and protein-losing enteropathy.

Bacterial overgrowth

The causes of bacterial overgrowth fall into two groups.

◇ Excessive entry of bacteria into the small intestine, caused by achlorhydria, gastrojejunostomy, partial/total gastrectomy, enterocolic fistulas, cholangitis or loss of ileocaecal valve following right hemicolectomy.

◇ Intestinal stasis, caused by Crohn's disease (stenosis), TB (stenosis), small bowel diverticulosis, afferent loop stasis, entero-enteric anastomosis and other intestinal bypass procedures, subacute obstruction or blind loops. Also diabetes mellitus, radiation enteritis, scleroderma and amyloidosis.

History

There may be asthenia, nausea and vomiting, excessive borborygmi or weight loss. Diarrhoea is frequent and watery. Less common is steatorrhoea.

Examination

Look for glossitis, stomatitis, anaemia, hypoproteinaemia with peripheral oedema, tetany, osteomalacia and rickets.

Investigation

Carry out 14C-glycocholate or 14C-D-xylose breath tests.

Treatment

Treatment is of the underlying condition. Surgery is not indicated because there is widespread disease. Treat with intermittent courses of antibiotics. Neomycin or metronidazole for 10–14 days may give symptomatic improvement for several months. Fresh unpasteurised yoghurt or lactobacillus preparations should be given with and after antibiotics to inhibit recolonisation.

Follow-up

Follow up long term at regular intervals, depending on the clinical condition.

Short gut syndrome

The causes of short gut syndrome include operations requiring extensive small bowel resection, Crohn's, mesenteric infarction, radiation enteritis, midgut volvulus, multiple fistulas and small bowel tumours.

A small bowel that is less than 2 m long has a diminished work capacity and those with less than 100cm require parenteral nutrition for life. Those with borderline length may benefit from enteral feeding and/or additional intravenous fluids. Ileal resections are less well tolerated than jejunal resections, largely because active transport sites for bile salts and vitamin B12 are localised in the ileum. Efforts should be made to try to retain a portion of the terminal ileum and the ileocaecal valve if possible.

Consequences of short gut syndrome

Short gut syndrome has a number of consequences.

✧ Malabsorption and malnutrition (also gastric hypersecretion – transient).
✧ Gallstone formation, mainly cholesterol stones due to decreased bile salts.
✧ Hepatic disease: fatty liver, onset of liver failure after jejunoileal bypass. If there is a history, up to six months post-operatively, of flu-like illness, anorexia, nausea and vomiting, weight loss and decreased serum albumin, it is an indication to restore intestinal continuity.
✧ Impaired renal function and stone formation: diarrhoea and loss of electrolyte-rich fluid leading principally to hyponatraemia. There may be metabolic acidosis and formation of urinary calculi. Increased aldosterone leads to chronic hypokalaemia causing muscle weakness, anorexia and cardiac arrythmias.
✧ Metabolic bone disease: hypocalcaemia and hypomagnesaemia are common. Treat with 1-alpha-hydroxy-cholecalciferol.

History

Take a general small bowel history. Enquire about the causes of short bowel syndrome and the consequences of it (*see* above).

Examination

Perform a general examination. Look for evidence of anaemia and weight loss. Examine for evidence of the consequences of short gut syndrome.

Treatment

Support the patient until adaptation occurs – up to six months post-operatively. Give parenteral nutrition in the immediate stage of 3–6 weeks' transition to an oral diet. If one metre of small bowel remains, a normal diet may be achieved. However, these patients may require long-term enteral feed with polymeric or elemental formula diets and, on occasion, additional intravenous fluid (saline). Supplements of calcium, magnesium and vitamin C are needed, and in cases of ileal resection, Vitamin B12 injections are needed every three months for life.

Follow-up

Follow-up is long term at regular intervals determined by the clinical condition. There are the following possible complications.

✧ High output states: sodium and water can be lost in significant amounts. A combination of oral fluid restriction, loperamide and, on rare occasions, infusion/subcutaneous injection of long-acting somatostatin may be needed.
✧ Steatorrhoea: the cause is excess fat in the diet. Treat by substituting fat with medium chain triglycerides which do not require the presence of bile salts for digestion.

Long-term treatments include combined hepatic and small bowel transplant or techniques such as reversed antiperistaltic small bowel segment to decrease the diarrhoea. If the patient is young and symptoms are not improving, transplantation may be considered.

Protein-losing enteropathy

The causes of protein-losing enteropathy include coeliac disease, Whipple's disease, bacterial overgrowth and inflammatory bowel disease (IBD).

History/examination

Usually the clinical picture is dominated by the underlying condition, but the loss of protein leads to hypoproteinaemia with secondary water and salt retention. Albumin and immunoglobulin A (IgA) are depleted more than other larger proteins.

Investigation
Albumin labelled with iodine-131 or chromium-52 is injected intravenously and levels are monitored for two weeks. A plasma die-away curve is plotted and faecal radioactivity is measured. Daily enteric losses are calculated and excessive loss can be detected.

Treatment
Treatment is with albumin infusions or surgery of the underlying condition. A high-calorie, high-protein diet is needed.

Follow-up
Follow-up is long term, at regular intervals determined by the clinical condition.

Vascular anomalies, hamartomatous lesions and vasculitic/connective tissue disease (CTD) of gastrointestinal tract
Bleeding into the small intestine may be part of systemic vasculitic and connective tissue disorders. The conditions in which intestinal involvement is common are polyarteritis, Henoch-Schönlein purpura, pseudoxanthoma elasticum and Ehlers-Danlos syndrome.

Angiodysplasia
Angiodysplasia consists of clusters of arteriolar, venular and capillary vessels in the mucosa and submucosa of the gastrointestinal tract, so it is not visible or palpable from the outside. Rupture of the mucosal component causes bleeding. It commonly occurs in the right colon but also occurs in the stomach and small intestine.

History
There is increased incidence in patients suffering from aortic valve disease and chronic lung disease. Colonic lesions are commonest between ages 50–55, small bowel lesions between ages 30–35. There is episodic or chronic occult GI bleeding over the years. It may present as iron deficiency anaemia, overt melaena or acute haemorrhage.

Examination
Perform a general examination. Examine for signs of weight loss and anaemia. Examine for general features of connective tissue disease. Abdominal examination may be normal but rectal examination may reveal melaena.

Investigation
Use OGD and colonoscopy to locate or exclude these sites as the source of bleeding. Colonic angiodysplasia is well visualised by colonoscopy as cherry red lesions similar to a spider naevus. If the small bowel is suspected as the source, options include radionuclide scan using ^{99m}Tc, Sc or 99mT-labelled red cells. Selective mesenteric angiography is useful to demonstrate abnormal vessel patterns, even in the absence of active bleeding.

Treatment
Treatment is conservative, as blood vessels are involved. Endoscopy and diathermy are especially useful in colonic lesions. Laparotomy with peroperative endoscopy can be used to transilluminate the bowel and localise the lesion for excision.

Follow-up

Intervals should be short or the patient should be admitted for investigation until the source of bleeding is identified. One this has been treated, follow up at regular intervals (1–6 months) until further episodes are excluded.

Other causes of small bowel bleeding

Other causes of small bowel bleeding include the following.

✧ Phlebectasia: a meshwork of dilated veins in the submucosa frequently occurs in the oesophagus, mid-small bowel and rectum, but they are a rare cause of bleeding.

✧ Haemangiomas (vascular malformations) occur in the small and large intestine. Treatment is by either surgical excision or selective embolisation.

✧ Hereditary haemorrhagic telangiectasia – Peutz-Jeghers syndrome – causes bleeding from polyps in the bowel. There is a risk of malignancy, so all polyps larger than 2cm should be removed.

✧ Polyarteritis: systemic necrotising vasculitis with fibrinoid necrosis affecting blood vessels of several organs including the gut. Weakened vessels lead to aneurysm formation. They rupture, bleed and thrombose.

Inflammatory bowel disease (IBD)
Crohn's disease

Crohn's disease most commonly affects the terminal ileum, colon and rectum, stomach and duodenum, and oesophagus, in that order.

A chronic granulomatous disease, it is a segmental condition with areas of involvement strongly demarcated from the contiguous normal bowel. Oedema, sloughing and linear ulceration lead to the formation of pseudopolyps and mucosa bridges. Ulcers are typically deep, penetrate into the muscle layers (fissuring) and account for the tendency to localised perforation, adhesions and fistula formation.

History

Crohn's may present in a variety of ways and variable presentation often delays diagnosis. It is commonest in the third decade of life, with abdominal pain that varies from discomfort to severe and colicky. It is often associated with diarrhoea and weight loss. There is early satiety or a sense of fullness. Abdominal distension occurs during bouts of abdominal pain. Colonic rectal bleeding may present.

✧ Pseudoappendicitis syndrome shows acute abdominal pain. Remove the appendix if caecum appears normal. Only one in eight cases of acute terminal ileitis are due to Crohn's. Always review the histology.

✧ Small bowel obstruction is usually partial or subacute. It is more commonly due to adhesions or stricture. Early operation is advisable. Intermittent self-limiting episodes invariably have gross bacterial overgrowth which may cause malabsorption.

✧ Abscess results from localised perforation or lymph node mass. It presents with local signs and increased catabolism, weight loss, fever and anorexia. It is commonest in the right iliac fossa. The abscess may track through to the pelvis and under the inguinal ligament to the anterior compartment of the thigh. Free perforation causing peritonitis is rare.

✧ A perianal fistula may present before intestinal disease. An enterocutaneous fistula is classified as high or low output. Spontaneous closure with parenteral nutrition is usually only possible with low-output fistulas.

✧ Diarrhoea is present in 70–80%. It is colonic, associated with mucus and blood. The small bowel is associated, with protein-losing enteropathy and/or steatorrhoea due to bacterial overgrowth or bile salt malabsorption.

Examination

Perform a general examination. Examine for evidence of anaemia and weight loss and other systemic features of Crohn's such as clubbing, proximal myopathy, easy bruising, and, in toxic cases, raised temperature, tachycardia and oedema. Abdominal examination may be normal or there may be evidence of a mass, particularly in the right side of the abdomen. Examine the anus for fissures, fleshy skin tags and sinuses.

Investigations

These should be a combination of luminal investigation (usually endoscopic) with appropriate histology, in association with raised inflammatory markers (CRP, ESR and white cell count). In addition, a number of serological markers such as anti-*Saccharomyces cerevisiae* antibodies (ASCA), antineutrophil cytoplasmic antibody (ANCA) and OMP-C may provide additional information about disease severity. Demonstration of diseased segments can be made by contrast radiology and/or MRI, showing narrowing of lumen, nodularity of mucosal pattern, irregularity and deep ulcers or fistulas. The string sign may be seen. Fistulas and sinuses are shown by injection of contrast +/– CT scans.

Treatment

The management of Crohn's disease is dependent on the assessment of the disease location and its severity. The therapeutic goals are to induce a clinical remission, to maintain that remission and to prevent post-operative relapse.

Mild to moderate disease

The initial choice is 5-aminosalicylate (5-ASA), although there is little evidence to support its efficacy. Budesonide seems to be as effective as prednisolone, with a reduction in adverse effects. Metronidazole and ciprofloxacin regimens can give similar results to 5-ASA, particularly in Crohn's ileocolitis and in perianal disease.

Moderate to severe disease

Steroids provide rapid remission but their use should be short and sharp to prevent side effects. There is no role for steroids in maintenance of remission. Introduction of immunosupression such as Azathioprine or Methotrexate will allow long-term control of the disease.

Severe Crohn's disease

Patients are admitted into the hospital. They require standard resuscitation and then are treated with intravenous medication. Options include steroids, cyclosporine and biological therapy such as infliximab.

Dietary manipulations

Evidence exists to support the use of an exclusive enteral diet in the management of mild to moderate disease. This provides an equivalent, if slower, remission rate to that of oral steroids. Compliance may be a problem.

Surgery

Common indications for surgery include:
- intestinal obstruction
- abscess formation
- fistula formation
- failure of medical treatment for limited disease
- need to raise an ileostomy to defunction diseased bowel
- nutritional failure

✧ small bowel perforation (rare)
✧ acute severe haemorrhage (rare).

Procedures are small bowel resection, strictureplasty and ileostomy.

Post-operative follow-up
Review with histology to confirm diagnosis and exclude other diagnoses, e.g. small bowel lymphoma. Examine for any post-operative complications, including anastomotic leakage resulting in fistula formation or intra-abdominal abscess. Long-term follow-up is indicated to continue medical management in an attempt to reduce post-operative recurrence.

Complications of surgical treatment in Crohn's disease
The incidence of post-operative complications is 10–15%.
✧ Acute complications include anastomotic leakage, fistula formation, intra-abdominal abscess and haemorrhage.
✧ Late complications are short bowel syndrome, urinary lithiasis, cholelithiasis, gastric hypersecretion and peptic ulcer disease.

Recurrence after resection for small bowel resection is 30% at five years. Medical treatment may influence the recurrence rate.
  Short gut syndrome treatment options include home parenteral nutrition, small bowel transplant or small bowel and hepatic transplantation.

Ileostomy care
Patients require adequate salt and water intake, as they typically lose 500 to 600 mls of fluid and 40–50 mmols Na+ each day via the ileostomy.
  Local complications of terminal ileostomies – stenosis, prolapse – may require revision surgery.
✧ Peristomal irritation occurs in 20–40% but responds to regular cleaning and use of skin barriers like Stomahesive or Comfeel.
✧ Para-ileostomy hernia in 5% leads to ill-fitting of appliance and leakage, and it may cause internal strangulation. It may require surgical re-siting, but it tends to recur so reserve this for the severe cases.
✧ Ileostomy diarrhoea: the causes include proximal stoma, partial obstruction, internal abscess formation and recurrence of Crohn's. Investigations include AXR, small bowel enema (through stoma) and endoscopic examination through the stoma.
✧ Treatment of high output ileostomy (*see* short bowel syndrome).

Tumours of the small intestine
These are rare – fewer than 10% of all GI neoplasms.

Benign tumours
Most are detected as incidental findings at post-mortem. They include tubular and villous adenomas, lipomas, haemangiomas and neurogenic tumours. Adenomas may also occur in association with familial polyposis coli, Gardner's syndrome (intestinal polyps and epidermoid cysts), and Turcot's syndrome (intestinal polyps and brain tumours). In addition to the known risk of colonic carcinoma, these patients are liable to develop carcinoma of the duodenum and biliary tract. In the non-familial group, villous adenomas are prone to malignant change.

History

May present acutely as intussusception, or chronic bleeding causing iron deficiency anaemia, or occasionally overt haemorrhage. Most are asymptomatic. Take a general small bowel history. Enquire regarding the symptoms of anaemia, family history or history relating to the rare causes outlined above.

Examination

Perform a general examination. Depending on the mode of presentation the examination may be normal or there may be signs of anaemia and an abdominal mass. Rectal examination may reveal melaena.

Investigations

Faecal occult blood test (FOB) may be positive for blood. Make OGD to exclude other causes of GI bleeding and to diagnose duodenal tumours. SBE may demonstrate lesions further down the small bowel. Use an ultrasound scan (USS) to detect lesions and examine the liver to exclude metastases.

Treatment and follow-up

Treatment is by surgical resection. Follow-up is at short intervals until diagnosis is obtained and malignant tumours are excluded.

Post-operative follow-up

Review the histology to confirm the benign nature of the tumour and ensure complete excision. Detect complications related to laparotomy and small bowel resection. Discharge once asymptomatic. Long-term follow-up is needed for Gardner's and Turcot's syndromes.

Polyposis and duodenal tumours

Peutz-Jeghers syndrome

Background

Peutz-Jeghers syndrome is an inherited autosomal dominant polyposis syndrome. Multiple hamartomatous polyps develop throughout the stomach and the small and large bowel. Patients usually have speckled pigmentation around the oral and buccal mucosa.

History

The polyps eventually produce symptoms such as obstruction or anaemia secondary to chronic bleeding. Malignant change may occur in the polyps.

Investigation

Investigate with contrast radiology, endoscopy and capsule endoscopy.

Treatment

Surgery for small bowel polyps is indicated if the patient becomes symptomatic or the polyps exceed 1.5cm in diameter. On-table enteroscopy with endoscopic snare resection is the intervention of choice for small bowel polyps, as endoscopy can control colonic, gastric and duodenal polyps.

Duodenal tumours

Background

Duodenal neoplasms are rare. They are most common in the first part of the duodenum. The risk of malignancy increases as they become more distal.

History

Presentation is most commonly with gastrointestinal haemorrhage. Adenomas are the most common tumours. Presentation may be with obstructive symptoms or an abdominal mass.

Investigation

Investigate with endoscopy and cross-sectional imaging.

Treatment

If the lesion is resectable, pancreaticoduodenectomy is the procedure of choice. More commonly, however, radical resection is contraindicated due to local invasion or meta-static disease, and then palliation only is appropriate. This may involve biliary stenting or surgical bypass if there is biliary obstruction, or a surgical gastrojejunostomy for duodenal obstruction.

Duodenal disease in familial adenomatous polyposis

Background

Familial adenomatous polyposis (FAP) was previously known as familial polyposis coli, the change in name reflecting the recognition of extracolonic polyps and cancers. Adenomas tend to be noted in the duodenum approximately 15 years after colonic polyps occur.

Investigation

Investigate with regular endoscopy and biopsy. The severity of duodenal polyposis can be quantified using a staging system developed by Spigelman and colleagues, which relies on clinical and histological assessment of the duodenum to provide a four-stage scoring system.

Natural history

Polyposis is associated with a high frequency of duodenal or periampullary cancer with estimates of between 1 and 12%. These cancers are the commonest cause of death in polyposis.

Treatment

Treatment is endoscopic surveillance with therapeutic options such as mucosal resection and argon beam coagulation. Duodenectomy or pancreaticoduodenectomy is needed for more advanced polyps and/or cancer.

Malignant small bowel tumours

These are rare and present late. They are adenocarcinoma (40%), carcinoid tumours (30%), lymphoma (25%) and smooth muscle tumours (5%). Of the adenocarcinomas, 40% are duodenal, 40% jejunal and 20% ileal. Most duodenal carcinomas are found in the periampullary region and in the third part of the duodenum. They spread to regional lymph nodes, the liver and the peritoneal cavity.

Carcinoma in Crohn's disease has a particularly poor prognosis. It occurs in the 40–50 year age-group. It is more common in males (3:1) and affects the ileum in 75% of cases.

History

They mainly occur in the over-60 age group. They present with epigastric or periumbilical discomfort or pain. Pain is usually postprandial and colicky. There may be nausea and vomiting and weight loss; GI bleeding; and intestinal obstruction or intussusception.

Duodenal carcinoma presents with obstructive jaundice.

Examination

Perform a general examination. Examine for evidence of anaemia or jaundice. The abdominal examination may be normal, or there may be a mass or evidence of small bowel obstruction. The liver may be enlarged due to metastases.

Investigations

Malignant tumours are diagnosed by OGD for the duodenum and by small bowel enema for jejunal and ileal lesions.

Treatment

Treatment is by surgical resection. Small intestine adenocarcinomas do not respond to chemotherapy or radiotherapy.

Follow-up

Intervals should be short (1–4 weeks) until diagnosis is obtained.

Post-operative follow-up

This should be long term, looking for signs of recurrence. Five year survival is 20–45%, but better for duodenal tumours.

Carcinoid tumours

Classification

Carcinoid tumours are classified into three groups.
- ❖ Foregut – stomach, duodenum, pancreas, biliary tract and bronchus.
- ❖ Midgut – jejunum, ileum and right colon.
- ❖ Hindgut – left colon and rectum (do not secrete active peptides).

Foregut and midgut tumours may secrete almost any gut hormones and serotonin.

Tumours smaller than 1.0cm are rarely malignant; those 1.0–1.9cm may be malignant; those greater than 2.0cm are invariably invasive and metastasise. Invasion occurs into the bowel wall, mesentery and parietal peritoneum and adjacent organs. There is spread to lymph nodes and the liver and less frequently to lungs and bones.

The commonest sites for tumours are the appendix, jejunoilium and rectum, in that order.

History

The commonest age group is 45–55 years. Duodenal carcinoids present with vomiting or bizarre endocrine syndrome. Jejunoileal carcinoids present with diarrhoea or intestinal obstruction and/or a palpable abdominal mass. Appendix tumours present usually as acute appendicitis. The presence of symptoms of the carcinoid syndrome indicates advanced disease with extensive hepatic involvement.

Examination

Perform a general examination. Examine for presence of a tumour and metastases, e.g. enlarged liver. Examine for carcinoid syndrome (see below).

Investigations

Carry out OGD, SBE and USS of the abdomen and liver. Measure urinary levels of 5-hydroxytryptamine (5-HT) (*see* below).

Treatment

Treatment by resection of the tumour, with wide margins of healthy tissue, regional lymph nodes and associated mesentery is standard. External beam radiotherapy for inoperable tumours has given disappointing results. Resectable hepatic deposits can be treated by surgical resection. Debulking of the tumour may help distressing symptoms.

Follow-up

Follow-up is at short intervals (1–4 weeks) until diagnosis is obtained.

Post-operative follow-up

This should be long term to detect recurrence or onset of carcinoid syndrome. Many patients survive long periods despite the presence of residual or metastatic disease. There is 60% five-year survival.

Carcinoid syndrome

Carcinoid syndrome is rare, affecting 10% of carcinoid tumours. It indicates advanced disease with extensive hepatic involvement. Inappropriate secretion of 5-HT and other vasoactive substances is responsible for the symptoms.

History

Patients may describe several types of flushing syndromes – cutaneous flushing affecting the upper part of the body and accompanied by sweating, itching, oedema, palpitations and hypotension. Patients may also complain of intestinal colic and diarrhoea, broncho-spasm and hypoproteinaemia and oedema. Other presentations include cardiac lesions, tricuspid insufficiency or pulmonary stenosis, photosensitive dermatitis, neurological signs, peptic ulceration and arthralgia.

Examination

Perform a general examination. Examine for evidence of flushing and/or dermatitis and oedema. Examine the chest for presence of cardiac lesions and bronchospasm. Examine the abdomen for evidence of a tumour and/or metastases or an enlarged liver. Perform a neurological examination.

Investigations

Look at urinary levels of the metabolite 5-hydroxyindole acetic acid (5-HIAA). Take a USS of the liver and perform investigations for a carcinoid tumour as described above.

Treatment

Carry out surgical resection/debulking covered by antiserotonin therapy with cyprohep-tadine and parachlorophenylalanine. Also use selective arterial embolisation (cover with antibiotics and methylprednisolone).

Chemotherapy uses cyclophosphamide, Adriamycin and 5FU, which are given intravenously or by infusion into the hepatic artery using implantable reservoirs. Use somatostatin and antiserotonin drugs.

Follow-up

Follow-up is long term at regular intervals determined by the clinical condition.

Primary gut lymphomas

Characteristically, primary gut lymphomas of the small bowel are seldom diagnosed pre-operatively and at operation may be confused with Crohn's disease. When gut lymphoma is diagnosed, one of the first tasks is to determine the type of lymphoma and whether this primarily affects the bowel or whether the bowel is involved as part of a systemic lymphoma.

Criteria for diagnosis of primary gut lymphomas

✧ No palpable superficial lymphadenopathy.
✧ No mediastinal lymph nodes on CT or CXR.
✧ Normal white cell count, normal bone marrow.
✧ Patients present with GI symptoms.
✧ Bowel lesions predominate at laparotomy and only regional lymph nodes (LN) are involved.
✧ Liver and spleen are not involved.

Primary gut lymphoma is rare. Predisposing conditions include immunoproliferative small intestine disease (IPSID), ulcerative colitis, Crohn's disease, AIDS and other immunodeficiency states.

Site

Primary gut lymphoma arises in the following sites: duodenum 8%, jejunum 33%, ileum 59%, more than one site 32%.

Type of lymphoma

Hodgkin's lymphoma accounts for less than 1% of gut lymphomas. Non-Hodgkin's lymphoma accounts for the vast majority – mostly B-cell lymphoma (mucosa-associated lymphoid tissue (MALT) lymphomas).

Histological grading

Polymorphic B-cell lymphomas stay localised. They are classified into high grade and low grade and they metastasise late. There are many different types. Centrocytic lymphomas are characterised by wide and extensive mucosal involvement and are therefore not controlled by surgery – treatment is by chemotherapy. T-cell lymphomas also occur. There are many types, differentiated into high grade and low grade.

Staging

This is modified Ann Arbor.
✧ Stage I: disease confined to one extralymphatic site.
✧ Stage II: localised involvement of one organ site and involvement of a group of regional lymph nodes on one side of diaphragm.
  ∝ II1 – regional adjacent lymph node involvement.
  ∝ II2 – regional but non-confluent lymph node involvement
✧ Stage III: localised involvement of organ or site plus involvement of lymph node.
✧ Stage IV: diffuse disseminated disease with involvement of more than one organ and lymph node enlargement.

History

Lymphomas occur at any age except infancy. There is a peak in the sixth decade and a small peak in the first to third decades. They often present as an emergency with intestinal obstruction, haemorrhage or perforation. Chronic symptoms are malaise, abdominal pain, weight loss, diarrhoea/steatorrhoea and anaemia (may be normochromic). There may be a previous history of coeliac disease, previously controlled, with symptoms returning usually in the fifth to seventh decade.

Examination
Perform a general examination. Examination may be normal or there may be evidence of weight loss and anaemia. Examine all lymph node sites and examine the abdomen for hepatosplenomegaly. An abdominal mass may be present.

Investigations
Look for ESR increase and hypoproteinaemia. Take a FBC to detect raised WCC. Most cases are diagnosed on SBE, USS or CT. Occasionally laparoscopy and biopsy provides the diagnosis. IPSID abnormal alpha chain is diagnosed by immunohistochemistry of tumour sections.

Treatment
- For the acute, disease treatment is by resection of disease with post-operative chemotherapy.
- Elective surgery is followed by chemotherapy/radiotherapy for stage I and stage II. Chemotherapy alone is used for more advanced disease.

Follow-up
Follow-up is at short intervals until diagnosis is obtained (1–4 weeks).

Post-operative follow-up
Review with histology and liaise with oncologists. Complete the grading and staging procedure. Detect early complications related to laparotomy and small bowel resection.

Gastrointestinal stromal tumours
Background
These were previously known as leiomyoma and leiomyosarcoma.

History
In the 60–70 age group, with a long history of bleeding, abdominal pain, anaemia and weight loss. Repeated episodes of melaena (or haematemesis). They are 60% gastric, 40% small bowel, rare elsewhere.

Examination
There is a palpable mass in one-third of patients.

Investigations
Use cross sectional imaging, such as CT or MRI.

Treatment
Treat with surgical excision for local disease. Non-resectable or metastatic disease responds to tyrosine kinase inhibitors.

Post-operative follow-up
Review with histology to confirm diagnosis and that there is adequate resection. Thereafter follow up long term to detect recurrence.

Chronic infective/inflammatory conditions of the small bowel
Yersinia
Yersinia is one of the most common and clinically important infections. In the acute phase the differential diagnosis includes *Salmonella* and *Campylobacter*, which also may become chronic infections.

History/examination
The acute condition is self-limiting. The chronic disease in children may simulate Crohn's disease. There is a swollen terminal ileum and colon exhibiting ulcerated, nodular and cobblestone change.

Investigations
It is diagnosed by recovery of the organism from stool. It also causes a pseudoappendicitis syndrome in older children and adults. SBE may exhibit typical Crohn's type changes. At operation the terminal ileum and lymph nodes are inflamed and oedematous. Send lymph nodes for culture.

Treatment
Yersinia usually resolves and never progresses to Crohn's.

Intestinal tuberculosis (TB)
There are four macroscopic forms: hypertrophic, ulcerative, fibrotic and ulcerofibrotic.
✦ Hypertrophic shows thickening of the terminal ileum and colon. There is recent subacute obstruction, pain and vomiting.
✦ Ulcerative affects the terminal ileum: there are deep ulcers which may reach serosa and perforate. There is subacute obstruction and pain, vomiting and constipation.
✦ Fibrotic is in the terminal ileum, caecum and ascending colon. There is shortening and narrowing of segments.
✦ Ulcerofibrotic is a combination of ulcerative and fibrotic subtypes.

History
Take a general small bowel history. It mainly occurs in children and young adults – 25% have co-existing pulmonary disease and give a history of chronic ill health, malaise, anorexia, fever, night-sweats, dyspepsia and weight loss.

Examination
Perform a general examination. Examine for evidence of weight loss and general debility. Examine lymph node fields and the chest for evidence of systemic TB. Examine the abdomen for abdominal masses or intestinal obstruction (may be normal).

Investigations
Mantoux test may be negative. Try to culture TB from gastric washing, faeces and peritoneal fluid and lymph node biopsy. AXR may show extensive calcification. Barium studies have the above changes according to the type of intestinal TB, but the changes may be indistinguishable from Crohn's. Laparoscopy and sampling of peritoneal fluid may be required for diagnosis.

Treatment
In the absence of obstruction or perforation give chemotherapy for 12 months.
    Surgery (e.g. right hemicolectomy) is needed for complications and failure of medical therapy.

Follow-up

Follow up at regular intervals, e.g. three-monthly during the first eighteen months, to detect obstruction, perforation or intra-abdominal abscess formation. Discharge when the patient has finished chemotherapy and remains asymptomatic.

Actinomycosis

Actinomycosis is rare – diagnosis usually follows perforated appendix.

History/examination

The patient presents some weeks after appendicectomy with abscess and sinus formation and fixed indurated mass in the right iliac fossa. It may progress to abscesses in the liver.

Investigations

Do a FBC; microbiology of pus; and a USS of mass and liver.

Treatment

Treatment is prolonged therapy with penicillin and lincomycin.

Follow-up

Follow up at regular intervals until the patient is off all treatment and asymptomatic.

AIDS, opportunistic small bowel infection and HIV-1 enteropathy

Small bowel infections are extremely common in AIDS. They are mostly due to opportunistic ulceration with protozoa, bacteria, viruses and fungi. In some 30% no pathogen is identified – this is AIDS enteropathy.

History/examination

There is diarrhoea, weight loss and abdominal pain.

Investigations

Investigate with sigmoidoscopy and stool cultures.

Treatment

For bacterial infection, treat with antibiotics. Otherwise give symptomatic treatment with loperamide.

Follow-up

Follow up in conjunction with a specialist AIDS clinic. Make regular stool cultures and sigmoidoscopy until asymptomatic then discharge to a specialist AIDS clinic.

Radiation-induced bowel disease

Symptoms are encountered in most patients during the first few weeks of radiotherapy – they include anorexia, nausea and vomiting and central nervous system (CNS) effects and they should settle.

In true radiation-induced disease the interval may be from two months to two years after radiotherapy.

History/examination

There is vague abdominal discomfort, diarrhoea, mild rectal bleeding and passage of mucus. Intestinal obstruction may be acute, subacute or recurrent.

Investigations

Investigations include SBE, barium enema, malabsorption studies, flexible sigmoidoscopy and colonoscopy.

Treatment

Treatment should be conservative whenever possible, including correction of nutritional deficiencies. Use Lomotil, Salazopyrin and steroids. Give Predsol enemas for radiation proctitis; antibiotics for bacterial overgrowth; and bile-salt binding agents for ileal disease. Dietary management includes elemental diets. If there is extensive disease it requires intermittent or indefinite total parenteral nutrition (TPN).

Surgical resection is used in localised disease. Protect anastomoses with a stoma. For fistulas and extensive disease carry out a complete bypass and exclusion of the diseased segment – these procedures can be safer than resection.

Follow-up

Follow-up is long term at regular intervals until the patient is asymptomatic or symptoms are well controlled.

Appendicitis follow-up
Objectives

The main objectives of the follow-up visit after surgery are the detection of post-operative complications and the exclusion of underlying pathology such as inflammatory bowel disease or tumours of the appendix. Always ensure that you have read the histology report before you see the patient. Complications include:

✧ chronic wound infection
✧ abscess/mass in right iliac fossa (RIF)
✧ faecal fistula
✧ intraperitoneal abscess formation – solitary (pelvic/subphrenic) or multiple small loop abscesses
✧ recurrent intestinal obstruction – late complication secondary to adhesions
✧ pylephlebitis (portal pyaemia).

Superficial chronic wound infection that has not responded to antibiotics may indicate a stitch sinus, which can be treated by exploration of the wound either in the clinic or as a day-case. It is a local anaesthetic procedure and the residual stitch material is removed.

Deeper chronic wound infection, or the presence of a mass or faecal fistula, may indicate the presence of an underlying condition such as Crohn's, a tumour or chronic infective inflammatory conditions.

Inflammatory bowel disease

The histology report may describe changes suggestive of Crohn's disease. In this situation a full assessment for Crohn's is required, including SBE (*see* Crohn's section).

Tumours of the appendix

This includes carcinoids, adenocarcinoma, mucinous neoplasm and lymphoma. Assess according to the relevant section.

Carcinoid

Carcinoid usually occurs at the tip. There is invasion of muscularis mucosa in 30% but nodal and distal metastases are rare. Appendicectomy is usually curative but assess as described in the section on carcinoid.

Adenocarcinoma

Adenocarcinoma is rare. It may present as acute appendicitis or intestinal obstruction. The correct treatment is right hemicolectomy.

Mucinous neoplasm

This is a simple mucocele where there is obstruction but no infection. The lesion may calcify.

Chronic appendicitis

There is some controversy as to whether this condition exists, but removal of the appendix appears to be gaining in popularity when combined with a diagnostic laparoscopy and is successful in relieving the symptoms in a number of patients.

History

There are episodes of recurrent right iliac fossa pain. They may be severe and debilitating. Pain is often colicky in nature but the patient appears otherwise well. Take a full gastro-intestinal and gynaecological history. In particular, enquire about bowel habits. Consider irritable bowel syndrome – ask regarding symptoms in other body systems suggestive of this, e.g. intermittent dysphagia.

Examination

Perform a general examination. This is usually normal. Examine for abdominal masses and tenderness. Perform a rectal examination and arrange for a gynaecological examination.

Investigations

Carry out routine biochemistry and haematology plus investigations to exclude inflammatory bowel disease and gynaecological disease in females. The main finding in chronic appendicitis may be that a barium enema is normal but the appendix does not fill because the appendix is often long fibrotic and contains faecoliths.

Diagnostic laparoscopy combined with appendicectomy is an alternative to invasive radiological investigations.

Treatment

Give conservative treatment; or laparoscopic appendicectomy if other pathology has been excluded.

Follow-up

Follow up at regular intervals as determined by the severity and effect of the symptoms, until serious causes are excluded. Then either provide treatment for the specific disorder; discharge with advice; or proceed to laparoscopic appendicectomy.

Post-operative follow-up

Review with histology. If it is normal, discharge with advice and reassurance.

Meckel's diverticulum

Meckel's diverticulum arises from the antimesenteric border of the ileum, within 90cm of the ileocaecal valve. It is a true diverticulum, i.e. it contains all three layers of bowel wall. There is ectopic tissue (gastric, pancreatic, duodenal, colonic) in 50–70% of cases. Ulceration of ectopic gastric mucosa may cause copious rectal bleeding.

History

Take a general small bowel history. Most are asymptomatic. However, the patient may complain of symptoms similar to peptic ulceration but in a different abdominal site; intestinal colic; or intermittent GI bleeding or melaena. Unexplained anaemia may be another presentation. It may present acutely as acute appendicitis or perforation.

Examination

Perform a general examination. Examine for evidence of anaemia and abdominal tenderness. Occasionally there may be an inflammatory mass to palpate but examination is often normal.

Investigations

Ectopic gastric mucosa can be identified by ^{99m}Tc scan.

Treatment

If there is an uninflamed Meckel's at laparotomy with a wide base and normal to palpation – leave it. If there is a narrow neck, or it is nodular, chronically inflamed or has faecoliths – excise. Symptomatic Meckel's require excision.

Follow-up

This should be at short intervals until diagnosis is obtained and other causes excluded.

Post-operative follow-up

Review with histology and ensure that all ectopic mucosa has been excised. Check for post-operative complications associated with laparotomy and small bowel resection. Discharge the patient once they are recovered and asymptomatic.

The spleen and lymph nodes

Neville Jamieson

SEVEN

The spleen

The spleen has important haematological and immunological functions. However, the main involvement of the surgeon is to remove the spleen. One of the commonest indications for removal of the spleen is trauma, which seldom presents to the outpatient department. However, patients return to the surgical clinic following splenectomy and it is important to have an appreciation of the implications of the long-term management of the asplenic patient. In particular, trauma patients are young, fit individuals who had an otherwise healthy spleen removed, so no other clinical specialities (e.g. haematology) will have been involved. Splenectomy is also performed as an intentional part of resection for other pathologies, e.g. carcinoma of the stomach. In this instance, as well as managing the primary condition the effects of splenectomy must also be considered. The spleen may also be removed during operations on the pancreas or, less commonly, as part of the treatment of portal hypertension.

In other situations the patient will be referred from another speciality for consideration of splenectomy because the spleen itself is diseased or involved in a disease process, or because it is adversely affecting haematological function.

In the commonest diseases to affect the spleen, enlargement occurs (splenomegaly) and a common result of this enlargement is that the spleen becomes overactive (hypersplenism). The commonest clinical features of a diseased spleen are splenomegaly and an abnormal blood film result. Key to understanding these disease processes and the effects of splenectomy is an understanding of the normal function of the spleen and the effect of an overactive or underactive spleen.

Haematological function

The spleen removes fragmented, damaged or senescent red blood cells (culling). It removes mature red blood cells (target cells – high membrane to intracellular haemoglobin). It removes intra-erythrocytic inclusions (pitting), e.g. Howell-Jolly bodies (nuclear remnants), siderotic granules (haemosiderin) and Heinz bodies (aggregates of denatured haemoglobin (Hb)). It removes irregular-shaped red blood cells (acanthocytes, irregular crenated cells and target forms). All of these appear in the bloodstream after splenectomy. Within its volume is a large number of sequestered platelets.

Following splenectomy there is a transient thrombocytosis. There is no haemopoiesis after foetal life unless the bone marrow becomes diseased, e.g. myelofibrosis.

There is storage of iron and factor VIII.

Immunological function

The spleen is involved in antibody production and cell-mediated responses. It is important for phagocytosis and the maturation of lymphoid cells, and it is significant in lymphopoiesis.

Clinical manifestations of splenic disorders

Most common splenic disorders cause pathological destruction or pooling of blood elements. Splenic enlargement, as occurs with venous thrombosis and congestion, causes entrapment and pooling resulting in destruction of normal cells.

Hypersplenism

Hypersplenism is splenomegaly plus decreased numbers of circulating blood elements (anaemia, leucopenia and/or thrombocytopenia). This is different from 'work hypertrophy', where the spleen enlarges due to constant exposure of the spleen's phagocytic mechanism to abnormal cells. Hypersplenism leads to a decreased number of normal cells. If the bone marrow cannot compensate, the patient becomes anaemic.

Splenomegaly

Causes of splenomegaly include the following.
- Infections:
  - acute (mononucleosis, septicaemia)
  - subacute (bacterial endocarditis, tuberculosis (TB), brucellosis)
  - chronic (fungal diseases, syphilis, bacterial endocarditis).
- Congestive in a setting of portal hypertension due to:
  - cirrhosis of all causes
  - prehepatic portal hypertension
  - posthepatic
  - segmental portal hypertension usually due to splenic vein occlusion as a result of inflammation (post severe pancreatitis) or tumour.
- Haematological:
  - haemolytic disorders
  - myeloproliferative (myeloid metaplasia, essential thrombocythaemia)
  - miscellaneous (megaloblastic anaemia).
- Malignant:
  - haematological (acute or chronic leukaemias, lymphomas)
  - intrinsic malignancies (primary – lymphosarcoma, plasmacytoma, fibrosarcoma; secondary – carcinoma, melanoma; benign – hamartoma).
- Inflammatory or granulomatous: Felty's, systemic lupus erythematosus (SLE), rheumatoid arthritis.
- Storage: Gaucher's, Wilson's.
- Miscellaneous: cysts, parasitic and non-parasitic. Other causes, e.g. amyloid, hyperthyroidism.

Hyposplenism

The causes of hyposplenism include the following.
- Splenectomy.
- Splenic agenesis.
- Atrophy: coeliac disease, dermatitis herpetiformis, sickle cell anaemia, thrombo-cytopenia, SLE.

Assessment of splenic disorders

The main purpose of the assessment is to determine whether the spleen is enlarged because of a primary disorder or because it is involved in a generalised disease process. Therefore, assessment may also involve a haematological investigation, investigation of hepatobiliary disease and portal hypertension (ultrasound and oesophago-gastro-duodenoscopy (OGD)) and investigation of the causes of lymphadenopathy (lymph node biopsy).

Splenic history

The patient may be asymptomatic with regard to the spleen; or be referred from another speciality with the diagnosis already made; or be referred from the GP because of detection of an abdominal mass. Occasionally if the spleen is very large the patient may complain of a heaviness in the left subcostal region, especially on exercise. The patient may complain of weakness, tiredness or lethargy due to anaemia or may complain of haemorrhage or the appearance of skin purpura or ecchymoses related to other haematological abnormalities.

Further questioning is directed at differentiating the common causes of splenomegaly as outlined above. Remember to ask about other diseases, family history, drug history and travel abroad.

Splenic examination

Perform a general examination looking for any of the causes of splenic enlargement. Look for evidence of haematological abnormalities, e.g. purpura, ecchymosis, lymphadenopathy, signs of liver disease and portal hypertension. Examine the abdomen. Differentiate splenic from renal enlargement and other abdominal masses, e.g. stomach, colon. Features of an enlarged spleen are that the examining hand cannot get above it; there is a notched anterior border; it enlarges towards the right iliac fossa; and there is usually an absence of bowel gas in front of it (unlike the kidney). With a renal mass the kidney moves downwards on respiration and organ shapes are different. Examine for liver enlargement and the presence of ascites. Rarely, auscultation may reveal a rub when there is a splenic infarct.

Investigation of splenic disorders
Laboratory investigations
Haematology

Full blood count and blood film provide information on the number of blood cells circulating and the presence of abnormal cell types (as described above).
- Hypersplenism results in anaemia, leucopenia and/or thrombocytopenia.
- Hyposplenism results in abnormal red blood cells (Burr cells, target cells, pitted cells); red cell inclusions (Howell-Jolly bodies, siderotic granules); abnormal platelet morphology; thrombocytosis; and leucocytosis (neutrophilia, lymphocytosis, monocytosis).

Tests of clotting, haemolysis and bone marrow aspiration/biopsy are part of the haematology work-up. Refer if initial blood results indicate a possible haematological disorder.

Biochemistry

Liver function tests (which include a clotting profile) may indicate underlying liver disease.

Immunology

Look at autoantibodies as a cause of haemolytic anaemia. Investigate rheumatoid arthritis, Felty's syndrome and SLE.

Lymph node biopsy

Investigation of lymphadenopathy associated with splenomegaly.

Imaging techniques
Abdominal X-ray (AXR)

AXR may show an enlarged soft-tissue shadow or calcification in the spleen, which may represent old infarcts, hydatid cyst or TB.

Ultrasound scan (USS)

This is the first-line investigation for differentiating splenic from renal enlargement. It is good for detecting all forms or splenic enlargement, e.g. splenic cysts. It can also detect other disease processes, e.g. portal hypertension, ascites, liver enlargement.

Computed tomography (CT) scan

This may give better visualisation of the spleen than USS, especially in the presence of ascites or obesity. It is particularly useful for the detection of intra-abdominal lympha-denopathy. However, it is expensive and involves the use of radiation.

Magnetic resonance imaging (MRI) scan

MRI may give better visualisation of the spleen and additional definition of tissues, but it is expensive and time-consuming, with limited availability.

Radioisotopes

Technetium-99m-labelled colloid can be injected into the patient and scanned by a gamma camera to detect the position and size of the spleen or to detect accessory spleens. Some of the patient's own red blood cells are heat damaged and then labelled with 51Cr; or platelets are labelled with indium-111; and they are reinjected. Scans with a gamma camera are performed after hours or days to provide information about the sequestration of these elements in the spleen. The method provides quantifiable information on the activity of the spleen. It uses radioactivity, albeit in small doses, and is becoming less common.

Indications for splenectomy
Definite indications for splenectomy

These include the following.
- Neoplasms of spleen (primary, lymphomas, benign).
- Splenic abscess (not small septic emboli).
- Echinococcal cysts.
- Splenic vein thrombosis with segmental portal hypertension and resulting gastric varices.
- Splenic artery aneurysm (asymptomatic splenic artery aneurysm less than 1.5cm diameter can be observed – rupture is common during pregnancy).
- En bloc resection of adjacent neoplasm.
- Non-salvageable splenic injury.

Splenectomy is desirable

Indications include the following.
- Hereditary spherocytosis.
- Idiopathic thrombocytopenia purpura.
- Autoimmune haemolytic anaemia, genetic defects of red cells, e.g. pyruvate kinase deficiency.
- Gastro-oesophageal devascularisation procedures for oesophageal varices.

Splenectomy is debatable

The necessity for splenectomy is debatable for the following.
- Small splenic cyst – may be observed if less than 5cm diameter.
- Small pseudocyst.
- Thalassaemia syndromes.
- Lymphoma and specific cytopenia or pancytopenia.
- Thrombotic thrombocytopenia purpura.
- Myeloproliferative disorders.

Pre-operative preparation

Check full blood count (FBC), clotting and liver enzymes. Platelet transfusion may be needed intra-operatively to correct thrombocytopenia (platelets are not usually given until the spleen has been devascularised, as otherwise they will simply disappear into the spleen and be ineffective – discuss with haematology).

If thrombocytopenia is due to immune disease, do not give platelet infusion. Give human immunoglobulin (IgG) to increase platelets. Correct coagulopathies with fresh frozen plasma or cryoprecipitate.

Post-operative follow-up

Following splenectomy, patients are reviewed six weeks after leaving hospital. They are at specific risk of sepsis due to capsulated bacteria and they require appropriate prophylaxis. Ideally, *Haemophilus influenzae* type b (HIB), Meningovax and Pneumovax vaccinations should be given prior to surgery, but if not given pre-operatively they may be given post-splenectomy once the patient is stable. Patients should also receive long-term low-dose antibiotic prohylaxis (usually with penicillin/amoxycillin or erythromycin in sensitive patients); be advised to have annual flu vaccinations; and take advice about additional prophylaxis if travelling to malarial areas. They should be advised to seek early medical advice should they become unwell. Most hospitals will now have a written protocol and patient advice sheet.

Early complications

Early complications include bleeding and left subphrenic collection. Immediately follow-ing splenectomy, thrombocytosis is common, with an increased risk of thrombotic events. The platelet count should be monitored daily and will usually rise for a number of days before falling back to normal values. In addition to standard thrombo-embolic prohylaxis, if the platelet count increases to more than 1000×10^9/dl give an anti-platelet agent such as low-dose aspirin or an alternative (Persantin, clopidogrel).

Necrosis of the greater curve of the stomach due to poor surgical technique is a rare complication that may lead to subphrenic abscess and/or fistula.

Trauma to the tail of the pancreas leads to subphrenic fluid collections, abscess or pancreatic fistula. Diagnose by USS or CT scan and treat by percutaneous drainage under imaging.

Late complications

Late complications include migrating thrombophlebitis or deep-venous thrombosis (DVT) caused by thrombocytosis. It needs long-term anticoagulant therapy. Recurrence of presenting symptoms may mean retained accessory spleen. Image with radio-labelled nuclear scan and plan curative surgical resection.

Remember to educate the patient regarding overwhelming post-splenectomy infection (OPSI) and meningococcal, pneumococcal and *H. influenzae* vaccination. Make sure they have an advice sheet. Consider the possibility of a MedicAlert® bracelet.

Postsplenectomy sepsis

Increased risk and incidence is related to the indication for splenectomy. Trauma has a low risk with an incidence of 1–2%; thalassaemia has an incidence of 25%. Strep pneumonia is responsible for over half of all septic episodes, *Escherichia coli, H.influenzae* and *Neisseria meningitidis* for most of the rest. The mechanism responsible is thought to be impaired filtration, decreased phagocytosis, decreased immunoglobulin M (IgM) levels and loss of the opsonic tetrapeptide, tuftsin.

Overwhelming post-splenectomy infection (OPSI)

This life-threatening disorder is a constant threat in patients who have a splenectomy. Constant vigilance on the part of the patient and the surgeon is required if effective treatment is to be started in time.

History/examination

It is an insidious viral-like illness leading to high fevers, nausea and vomiting, dehydration, hypotension and collapse.

Investigation

Investiage with gram stain of peripheral blood smears.

Treatment

Admit the patient for intravenous antibiotics and fluids.

* Prognosis: mortality is 50–80%. Often a post-mortem shows bilateral adrenal haemorrhage.
* Prevention: the pneumococcal vaccine covers 90% of pneumococcal variants but leaves 10% uncovered. Vaccination should precede splenectomy by 10–14 days. Not all patients convert, but those who do should have elevated pneumococcal antibodies for 42 months. However, no form of prophylaxis is completely effective, so close surveillance is necessary with specific patient education to seek medical attention at the first signs of infection. The key to successful management is aggressive treatment and awareness of the risk of OPSI.

Specific disorders of the spleen
Splenic infarction

Apart from sickle cell, splenic infarction most commonly occurs with congestive disease, chronic myeloid leukaemia (CML) and myelosclerosis, but it can also occur as a result of arterial emboli (rare) or as a complication of severe acute pancreatitis.

History

Take a general splenic history. There may be sudden-onset left-sided abdominal and loin pain. Infarction causes a capsular reaction, irritating the left hemidiaphragm and leading to left basal pleurisy with or without rub and pain to the left shoulder. Pain may be worse on inspiration.

Examination

Perform a general examination. The patient may be in pain. Examine the chest for signs of a left basal rub or effusion. There may be tenderness in the left side of the abdomen and loin.

Investigations

USS may be useful to exclude other pathologies. CT scan with contrast is diagnostic.

Treatment

Give appropriate analgesia. Splenectomy is reserved for severe cases or diagnostic confusion.

Follow-up

Monitor for development of hyposplenism, but management of the underlying condition will usually take precedence. Discharge if stable after follow-up and when the underlying condition resolves.

Post-operative follow-up
As for splenectomy.

Splenic abscess
A splenic abscess is a complication of severe sepsis, bacterial endocarditis, leukaemia, diabetes or prematurity. Multiple abscesses are often fatal.

History
Take a general splenic history. It may be non-specific with fever, pain and possibly left upper quadrant (LUQ) tenderness.

Examination
Perform a general examination. Splenomegaly occurs in less than 50%.

Investigations
Chest X-ray (CXR) shows left pleural effusion and USS shows immobile diaphragm.

Treatment
Treat with USS percutaneous drainage or splenectomy. A rupture is fatal.

Follow-up
If the patient recovers from the acute episode, monitor for development of hyposplenism. Discharge when stable.

Post-operative follow-up
As for splenectomy.

Splenic cysts
Most splenic cysts are post-traumatic. True cysts are rare. They include haemangioma, lymphangioma, parasitic, epidermoid and dermoid. They may occasionally rupture or become infected.

History
The history is mostly size-related, but they are usually asymptomatic.

Examination
There is a mass in the LUQ.

Investigation
USS can identify cysts. Use CT scan with contrast if doubts exist.

Treatment
If cysts are small and asymptomatic, observe or treat with laparoscopic deroofing. Splenectomy is advised for large or symptomatic cysts or any complications.

Follow-up
Monitor for development of complications or enlargement. Discharge when stable.

Post-operative follow-up
As for splenectomy.

Splenic vein thrombosis

Splenic vein thrombosis follows acute pancreatitis or may arise in chronic pancreatitis or a pancreatic tumour. Isolated splenic vein thrombosis (without portal vein thrombosis) results in splenomegaly and segmental portal hypertension (predominantly gastric varices – oesophageal varices are present but are less prominent). Portal venous pressure is normal. Varices are often missed on endoscopy.

History/examination

It may present with massive gastrointestinal (GI) haemorrhage. Splenic vein thrombosis should be suspected in cases of GI bleeding with a history of previous pancreatitis.

Investigations

Carry out endoscopy, Duplex USS and selective visceral angiography. MRI is better.

Treatment

The condition is cured by splenectomy.

Post-operative follow-up

As for splenectomy.

Splenosis

There is a need to differentiate between splenosis and accessory spleens. Accessory spleens are found at the hilum of the spleen and omentum; number fewer than 10; and have hilar vessels with normal splenic architecture. Implantation splenosis tends to number more than 20; there is a history of trauma; they are scattered over the peritoneum; and do not have a co-ordinated circulation.

Treatment

Neither condition needs therapy unless it is causing recurrent disease.

Gaucher's disease

Gaucher's is a hereditary lipid storage disease.

Clinical

There is hypersplenism and massive splenomegaly.

Treatment

Splenectomy is needed for the symptoms and complications of hypersplenism.

Disorders affecting the spleen and lymph nodes

Disorders affecting both the spleen and the lymph nodes can be considered in three main groups.
- Immunological reactivity: non-specific, granulomatous (caseating, non-caseating).
- Neoplasia (mainly non-Hodgkin's and Hodgkin's lymphoma).
- Primary haematological disorders: myeloid leukaemia, myelosclerosis and polycythaemia rubra vera (PRV).

History

Take a general splenic history. Ask questions regarding each of the causes of splenomegaly. Ask about foreign travel. If there is a history of prior pancreatitis or abdominal pain, exclude a splenic vein thrombosis. If there is pruritus, exclude PRV and other myeloproliferative disorders.

Examination

Perform a general examination. A left upper quadrant mass with a spleen auscultation may reveal a rub. With a renal mass the kidney moves downwards on respiration, organ shapes are different and there is usually colonic resonance in front of the kidney. Search for lymphadenopathy, including posterior pharynx. Look for the stigmata of chronic liver disease. Look for purpura or bruising.

Investigations

- ✧ Take peripheral blood film and bone marrow.
- ✧ Take FBC and serology to investigate infective causes. Mononucleosis shows atypical lymphocytes on blood film, positive Paul Bunnell test and raised Epstein-Barr virus titre.
- ✧ If there is a positive history for travel, perform blood smears for malaria or bone marrow tests for Leishman-Donovan bodies.
- ✧ If the patient is an immigrant, test for TB.
- ✧ Ultrasound scan or CT.
- ✧ Splenic vessels: Duplex, dynamic CT or selective angiography.
- ✧ Splenic function: injection of labelled platelets.

Disorders of the lymph nodes

Palpable lymph nodes should be considered diseased until proven otherwise. Always remember that in addition to haematological disorders and infection, a lymph node may be the first sign of metastatic carcinoma at a yet undetermined site. This is particularly important in the neck, where node biopsy should not be performed without an appropriate ENT examination, as such a biopsy may preclude potentially curative ENT surgical excision and block dissection of diseased lymph nodes.

Localised lymphadenopathy

Acute infections usually subside.
- ✧ Chronic infections:
    - ∝ lymphadenopathy without signs of inflammation may be cat scratch fever
    - ∝ single tender node: primary bovine TB
    - ∝ chronically enlarged lymph nodes matted together: syphilis, leprosy, fungal infection, lymphogranuloma venereum.
- ✧ Occipital: chronic scalp infection.
- ✧ Posterior auricular: rubella.
- ✧ Anterior auricular: bacterial infection of eyelids or conjunctiva.
- ✧ Axillary: distal upper limb infection, occasionally lymphoma or Hodgkin's.
- ✧ Neck: most common site for lymphomas.
- ✧ Painless epitrochlear: childhood viral illnesses, secondary syphilis or TB.
- ✧ Mediastinal hilar: not noticeably enlarged with bacterial pneumonia, mainly TB (unilateral hilar lymphadenopathy). Infectious mononucleosis may cause mediastinal lymphadenopathy for several months. Most common cause of persistent mediastinal lymphadenopathy is malignant disease and sarcoidosis.
- ✧ Intra-abdominal or retro-peritoneal: lymphadenopathy is not commonly inflammatory.

Generalised lymphadenopathy

Noticeable lymph node enlargement in more than one drainage site is most commonly viral, e.g. mononucleosis, viral hepatitis, influenza, cytomegalovirus, rubella and also has other causes such as syphilis, TB, salmonella and toxoplasmosis. But malignant causes should always be excluded.

Malignant conditions of lymph nodes

Metastatic carcinomas rarely produce a generalised lymphadenopathy – they present more often as a group of nodes adjacent to the primary tumour site. Hodgkin's and non-Hodgkin's lymphomas commonly present with superficial lymph node enlargement.

Hodgkin's lymphoma

Hodgkin's is found mostly in men, presenting with a group of painlessly enlarged anterior cervical lymph nodes. Axillary is the first site in 20%, mediastinal or inguinal in 15%.

History

There will be a history of fevers, pruritus, malaise, weight loss, anorexia and sweats. The absence of systemic symptoms is signified by adding 'A' to the stage; the presence of systemic symptoms is signified by adding 'B' to the stage.

Examination

Examination reveals painless enlarged lymph nodes. Hepatosplenomegaly appears late.

Investigation

Investigation is by lymph node biopsy (excisional) and bone marrow aspirate. A team approach is essential. Staging laparotomy has now been replaced by high-quality cross-sectional imaging.

Staging

Classification is for stages I-IV. Staging depends on the history and examination findings; CXR and AXR; and CT chest, abdomen.

Treatment

Treatment depends on the Hodgkin's stage:
- Hodgkin's I and II: wide field radiotherapy
- IIIA: radiotherapy and/or chemotherapy
- IIIB and IV: multiagent chemotherapy.

Follow-up

Follow-up is under a haematologist/oncologist.

Non-Hodgkin's lymphoma

This may present with painless enlargement of one or more superficial lymph nodes. Extranodal disease may be present.

Biopsy is now assessed with multiple immuno stains to accurately define cellular type and direct treatment.

Staging

Staging depends on results of node biopsy, bone marrow biopsy, and cross-sectional imaging.

Treatment

Localised disease is commonly still managed with radiotherapy. More advanced disease is managed with various chemotherapy regimes including monoclonal antilymphocyte preparations such as rituximab.

Tumours of the peritoneum

Tumours of the peritoneum are mainly secondary, including pseudomyxoma peritonei. Primary methothelioma may occur, but is rare.

Pseudomyxoma peritonei

The peritoneum is filled with yellow-brown mucoid substances caused by the presence of a well-differentiated pseudomucinous cystadenoma/carcinoma. The most common primary is the ovary; then the appendix, uterus, bowel and urachus. The primary tumour is often slow growing and rarely metastasises or invades adjacent viscera.

History
Patients complain of increasing abdominal distension or present acutely with abdominal pain, peritonitis or intestinal obstruction.

Examination
Perform a general examination. The main finding is abdominal distension.

Investigations
Perform a diagnostic peritoneal tap and biopsy.

Treatment
Treatment is by aggressive surgical evacuation and resection of the primary tumour. This is followed by systemic chemotherapy including cisplatin. Radiotherapy is ineffective.

Prognosis is guarded but long-term survival can occur. One useful prognostic factor appears to be the number of cells in the mucus. There is poor correlation between histology of the primary and survival. Management following diagnosis is usually in a regional or supra-regional specialist centre.

Follow-up
Follow-up is long term to detect deterioration and provide symptomatic support.

Peritoneal mesothelioma

Peritoneal mesotheliomas carry a poor prognosis of 8–12 months. There are two main types: diffuse malignant (the majority) and fibrotic benign (rare, and can be cured by surgical excision). Among the malignant tumours the only treatable lesions are the stage I tumours that are confined to one hemithorax or to the peritoneum.

History
Peritoneal mesothelioma presents with anorexia, ascites and intestinal obstruction. There is fever and weight loss.

Investigations
Perform paracentesis and laparoscopy and peritoneal biopsy.

Treatment
Treatment for stage I is surgical resection, radiotherapy and chemotherapy (systemic and intraperitoneal).

Follow-up
Follow-up is long term to detect deterioration and provide symptomatic support.

Desmoid tumours (of abdominal wall)

These are slow-growing well-circumscribed hard tumours that involve fascial and muscle layers. They recur after local excision (10–20%). They may be associated with Gardner's syndrome.

Treatment

Treatment is surgical, by wide local excision.

Follow-up

Follow-up is long term to detect recurrence, or discharge with advice to GP to continue follow-up.

Liver, biliary system and pancreas

Satyajit Bhattacharya and Adrian O'Sullivan

EIGHT

Introduction

In this chapter, disorders of the liver, pancreas, biliary system and spleen are considered separately. However, it is important to appreciate that these systems are closely inter-related and may present with similar clinical features. For example, a patient may be jaundiced due to a primary liver disorder such as cirrhosis, due to a biliary problem such as choledocholithiasis, or due to obstruction of the extrahepatic bile duct by a pancreatic neoplasm. Conversely, each of these conditions can in turn, if not corrected, eventually cause secondary biliary cirrhosis. When a patient presents with jaundice, one of the main tasks is to determine what the primary disorder is and then determine the effect this has had on the function of the liver, pancreatic and biliary systems.

Assessment of liver disorders

Liver disease

The main clinical features of liver disease are jaundice and signs of liver failure. As the assessment and management of liver disease is complex, it is useful to have an initial overview of the consultation objectives.

Objectives

Confirm that the symptoms and signs of liver disease are present.
1. Determine the cause through history, examination, urine and blood tests, imaging and histology.
2. Detect the clinical consequences of liver disease through history, examination, urine and blood tests (Child score (*see* later)), imaging and endoscopy:
   - encephalopathy
   - ascites
   - portal hypertension
     - hypersplenism
     - gastrointestinal bleeding – varices (oesophageal, gastric or rectal)
     - ascites
   - jaundice
   - clotting abnormalities
   - hepatorenal failure.
3. Treat the underlying cause of the liver disease, which may lead to improvement in the clinical consequences of liver disease.
4. Treat the clinical consequences:
   - measures to reduce encephalopathy
   - treat ascites
   - treat the consequences of portal hypertension
     - hypersplenism: splenectomy if surgery for portal shunt considered
     - varices: Sengstaken tube, vasoactive drugs, injection sclerotherapy or fibrin glue, transjugular intrahepatic portosystemic shunt (TIPS), surgery
     - ascites: medical, tap ascites, peritoneovenous shunt
   - jaundice: symptomatic, or relieve obstruction if present
   - clotting abnormalities: correct with vitamin K or fresh frozen plasma
   - hepatorenal failure: treat underlying liver condition, provide renal support.

Liver history

Start with a general gastrointestinal history. When responses indicate a possible liver problem, a more detailed liver history is required. This includes questions about general symptoms, aetiological factors and symptoms related to the clinical consequences of liver disease.

General symptoms that may indicate liver disease include jaundice, fatigue, malaise, headache, myalgia, arthralgia and fever. To determine the aetiology of the liver disease ask about excessive or chronic alcohol ingestion, the ingestion of drugs (therapeutic or recreational), occupation, pets, foreign travel, contact with jaundiced individuals, family history of jaundice or liver problems, recent anaesthetics, surgery or blood transfusions, sexual contacts and ingestion of raw shellfish or wild mushrooms.

The clinical consequences of liver disease include:

✦ encephalopathy – a range of reversible neuropsychiatric states ranging from confusion and forgetfulness to coma
✦ ascites – the presence of intra-abdominal fluid
✦ portal hypertension (varices) – which may be asymptomatic or may present with haematemesis (vomiting of bright red blood) or melaena
✦ jaundice – patients may simply report that they have turned yellow. Enquire about pale stools, dark urine and pruritus. Determine if the jaundice is painless or associated with right upper quadrant or epigastric abdominal pain
✦ clotting abnormalities – spontaneous bleeds, easily bruised
✦ hepatorenal failure – increasing lethargy, nausea, oedema.

Liver examination

Perform a general examination and once again look for general signs of liver disease, aetiological signs and signs of clinical consequences. Liver disease commonly presents with jaundice. However, other signs may also be present: palmar erythema, finger clubbing, leuconychia, bruising, asterixis, spider naevi, gynaecomastia, muscle wasting, scratch marks, ascites, caput medusae, hepatosplenomegaly, testicular atrophy and loss of axillary and pubic hair. Hepatomegaly may be real or apparent (pushed down by over-inflated lung) and enlargement may be focal or generalised, smooth or irregular. Liver tenderness may be elicited by palpation or percussion through the rib cage. Auscultation over the liver may reveal a friction rub (tumour, abscess) or a systolic bruit.

Aetiology may be indicated by the smell of alcohol, tattoos or evidence of drug injections (e.g. antecubital fossa).

The following are signs of clinical consequences.

✦ Encephalopathy: poor scores on cognitive function tests, inability to draw a star, liver flap, decreased consciousness level.
✦ Peripheral neuropathy may indicate the effect of liver failure on the nervous system.
✦ Ascites: abdominal distension, eversion of umbilicus, flank dullness, shifting dullness.
✦ Portal hypertension: dilated periumbilical veins (late), anaemia, ascites, splenomegaly, hepatosplenomegaly.
✦ Jaundice: yellow conjunctiva, pale stool on rectal examination, dark urine.
✦ Clotting abnormalities: evidence of bruising.
✦ Hepatorenal failure: oedema, decreased urine output, uraemia.

Investigation of liver disorders
Laboratory investigations
Urinalysis
✧ The technique is dipstick urinalysis. A variety of dipsticks can test for a number of substances in a fresh specimen of urine, including conjugated bilirubin. Generally the presence of conjugated bilirubin indicates obstructive jaundice, although some other conditions associated with excess bilirubin production also result in some bilirubin in the urine.
✧ There is no request form.
✧ The results are sticks that are compared to a reference chart.
✧ The advantage is it is a quick and easy method that can be performed in the clinic.
✧ The disadvantage is that limited information is available.

Blood tests
Blood tests form an integral part of the diagnosis of liver disorders. The commonest tests are described under the department that analyses the samples.

Biochemistry
Release of integral membrane enzymes
Minor increases of alanine transaminase (ALT) or serum glutamic pyruvic transaminase (SGPT), and aspartate aminotransferase (AST) or serum glutamic oxaloacetic transaminase (SGOT) occur in cholestasis and chronic liver disease. Major increases are associated with acute hepatitis or with liver cell necrosis of any cause.

Alkaline phosphatase (ALP) from the liver, biliary tract, bone, intestine, kidney and placenta can be differentiated by immunoassay. Cholestasis and obstructive jaundice are associated with an increased alkaline phosphatase.

Gamma-glutamyl-transpeptidase (gamma GT) is particularly raised in alcoholic liver disease and obstructive jaundice from any cause. Secondary tumour deposits cause a rise in alkaline phosphatase and gamma GT and a small rise in bilirubin. These can vary depending on the burden of underlying disease.

Serum markers of liver disease
✧ Serum protein changes: hypoalbuminaemia often occurs in liver disease. An altered albumin/globulin ratio may occur in the presence of a normal albumin, e.g. increased immunoglobulin (IgG) in cirrhosis and chronic active hepatitis. Primary biliary cirrhosis is associated with increased immunoglobulin M (IgM) and antimitochondrial antibody.
✧ Marker proteins: alpha-foetoprotein (AFP) is the most commonly used tumour marker for hepatocellular carcinoma. It may also be raised in pregnancy, germ cell tumours, and chronic liver disease. Abnormal prothrombin antigen (APT) is increased in 90% of primary hepatocellular carcinoma (greater than 300 ng/ml indicates primary hepatocellular carcinoma). There are small increases in other disorders. Levels decrease or are eliminated after curative resection or chemotherapy. There is little correlation between APT and AFP. Human chorionic gonadotropin (beta-hCG) and carcinoembryonic antigen (CEA) are also useful liver tumour markers.
✧ Urea and electrolytes may indicate electrolyte abnormalities, particularly hyponatraemia and hypoglycaemia. Evidence of raised urea and creatinine levels may indicate impaired renal function associated with liver disease (hepatorenal syndrome).

Haematology
✧ Full blood count (FBC) may reveal anaemia of chronic disease or indicate blood loss from gastrointestinal (GI) bleeding. Other abnormalities of the blood cells may be

detected, such as haemolytic anaemia, leukaemia and lymphoma. Thromocytopenia may suggest hypersplenism.
✧ Clotting tests: clotting, in particular the international normalised ratio (INR), may be abnormal in liver disease due to the defective production of clotting factors.

Immunology

Hepatitis serology is routine screening in liver disease, for hepatitis A, B and C.

There is also screening for autoimmune disease and primary biliary cirrhosis (anti-mitochondrial antibody).

Imaging techniques
Ultrasound scanning (USS)

Ultrasound uses high-frequency sound waves that enter the tissues and are reflected in different amounts from structures of different compositions. The reflected waves are detected and used to construct representative images of the underlying insonated tissues. Acoustic water-based gel is applied and an ultrasound probe manipulated over the abdomen by the sonographer.
✧ The request form is from radiology/ultrasound (check if your department uses the same or different forms).
✧ Results are in a written report compiled by the radiologist or sonographer, with a selection of ultrasound photographs.
✧ USS is a very good non-invasive technique for visualising the liver parenchyma. It can detect small (1cm) focal lesions, including liver cysts and abscesses, and primary and secondary liver tumours. Liver cirrhosis is suggested by areas of increased and irregular attenuation. The intrahepatic and extrahepatic bile ducts and the gall bladder are well visualised, and dilatation and stones can be detected. Using colour Duplex, blood flow in the portal vein can be identified and the diameter can be measured, giving an estimation of the presence of portal hypertension. Ultrasound-guided biopsy can be performed.
✧ The disadvantages are that accuracy is dependent on the experience of the operator; it is less reliable in fat or gaseous patients; and it is *less reliable* than computed tomography (CT) for defining lesions such as haemangiomas, but it can be used to follow these lesions once CT has established the diagnosis.

CT scan

In this technique X-rays are used to obtain multiple cross-sectional slices of the patient, which are then reconstructed by a computer to produce the images. Intravenous contrast to outline the vessels and focal lesions within the liver can also be given, and multiple scans can be performed to give non-contrast, arterial, venous and delayed phases of scanning. Oral contrast agents can be given to outline the stomach and duodenum. Modern multi-slice spiral CT scans can be performed quickly (15–30 seconds) using 5mm cuts, giving more detail and allowing sophisticated reconstructions. *See also* CT angioportography and lipiodol CT.
✧ The request form is from radiology or use a specific CT request form.
✧ Results are in a report written by the radiologist and a selection of still CT images.
✧ When used with contrast, CT is more sensitive than USS at determining the nature of lesions within the liver, especially differentiating between small tumours, cysts or abscesses. CT-guided biopsies can be performed. It is invaluable in planning liver resection surgery.
✧ Disadvantages are that it is expensive and time-consuming; it uses ionising radiation; and certain lesions such as hepatic adenomas or focal nodular hyperplasia may be difficult to differentiate on CT.

Liver scintiscan

A liver scintiscan uses isotopes technetium-99m, gallium-67 citrate or indium-113. The isotopes are injected intravenously and concentrated in liver lesions. Excess uptake is detected by a gamma camera.

❖ The radioisotopes request form is usually in the medical physics department.
❖ The results are as a written report and selection of images.
❖ The advantages are that technetium-99m is taken up by the reticuloendothelium system and can detect lesions larger than 2cm in about 66% of cases; gallium-67 citrate is concentrated in neoplastic lesions and abscesses; indium-113 is concentrated in haemangiomas.
❖ The disadvantage is that it uses radioactivity. Other techniques usually provide the same information.

Magnetic resonance imaging (MRI)

MRI detects minute quantities of energy released by hydrogen ions when they are forced to change direction by a strong magnetic field. The patient passes through the scanner, which is quite claustrophobic and noisy.

❖ There is a specialised MRI request form.
❖ The advantages are that it provides detailed information regarding liver parenchymatous disease, especially certain types of cirrhosis, e.g. haemochromatosis, Wilson's and primary biliary cirrhosis; MR cholangiopancreatography (MRCP) is very useful for non-invasive imaging of the biliary tree; MRI is very useful as an adjunct to other imaging modalities to further characterise liver lesions; and recent advances include liver-specific MRI constrast agents.
❖ The disadvantages are that it is expensive and time-consuming; and patients may find the experience unpleasant.

Angiography/venography; hepatic wedge pressure and venography; portography techniques

These invasive techniques to visualise the hepatic vasculature are being less commonly used.

Portography

This involves puncture of the spleen percutaneously through an intercostal space and the injection of contrast to outline the splenic and portal vein and enable the measurement of portal venous pressure. A transhepatic route may also be used.

Hepatic wedge pressure and venography

A catheter is passed from the brachial vein or internal jugular vein through the superior vena cava into the hepatic veins as far as possible, and the wedge pressure is measured. Under certain circumstances this is representative of the portal venous pressure. Injection of contrast can demonstrate the presence of thrombus or occlusion, e.g. in Budd-Chiari syndrome.

Angiography/venography

The coeliac and superior mesenteric arteries are selectively catheterised. The arterial supply of the liver can be visualised and the venous phase can demonstrate the portal system. Selective angiography can be combined with CT scanning for the technique – CT angioportography. Contrast is delivered into the splenic artery or SMA and enhances the liver via the portal venous blood. Liver tumours are supplied almost exclusively by hepatic artery blood and are therefore visualised as non-enhancing lesions. Another variation is lipiodol CT. Iodised poppy-seed oil, injected via angiography of the hepatic artery, is retained for long periods by hepatocellular carcinoma, causing dense enhancement of these lesions on subsequent CT scan (two weeks later).

✦ The request form is from radiology, but these are specialised investigations. Contacting a radiologist directly to discuss the indications is recommended.

✦ Results are a written report by the radiologist and a selection of images.

✦ The advantages are that the methods provide direct measurements and images of the portal system; and selective arteriography is useful in planning resection of liver tumours.

✦ The disadvantages are that the procedures are invasive and associated with complications; much of this information can be obtained by less invasive means, e.g. Duplex ultrasound, MRI angiography, spiral CT.

Liver needle biopsy

This is usually performed as an in-patient procedure (or as an outpatient/day-case procedure in selected patients) as the patient requires strict bed rest and frequent observation after the procedure.

Indications for liver biopsy include alcoholic liver disease, cholestatic jaundice without dilatation of the bile ducts on ultrasound, unexplained hepatomegaly, drug-induced liver disease and unexplained focal lesions of the liver (after consultation with a liver surgeon). The procedure is only performed when the INR is normal and the platelet count exceeds 60 000/ml.

Usually a Tru-cut needle is preferred. The patient is placed supine with the right arm abducted. A lateral intercostal approach is used, or if a focal mass is apparent this is approached directly (better performed under ultrasound control). The liver dullness is percussed and marked. Local anaesthetic is infiltrated and a small incision is made in the skin. The patient is instructed to cease breathing in expiration and the needle is inserted, the sample is taken and the needle is removed. The patient resumes respiration and the sample is placed whole into fixation fluid. The patient remains in bed with frequent observations of pulse and blood pressure.

✦ The procedure requires admission to hospital as an in-patient or a day-case. Determine the exact arrangements for request forms in your hospital. The sample is sent for histology.

✦ Results are as a written report from the histopathologist.

✦ The advantage is that it provides a core of tissue for histological diagnosis.

✦ The disadvantages are complications, including haemorrhage, intrahepatic haematoma, pleurisy, arteriovenous fistulae and biliary peritonitis. If there is any suspicion of a pnemothorax, an urgent chest X-ray is obtained and a chest drain is placed.

Laparoscopy

This operation is being increasingly used for the assessment of a number of disorders such as jaundice, chronic liver disease, ascites of unknown origin and the staging of primary and secondary hepatic and pancreaticobiliary tumours. A general anaesthetic is required. The laparoscope is inserted using an open technique through an infraumbilical approach. Further ports may be inserted if necessary. The technique can be combined with intra-operative liver biopsy, ultrasound and cholangiography.

✦ There is no request form. It is usually performed as an in-patient procedure.

✦ The results are a written or printed operation note recording the main intra-operative findings, and a histology report if any biopsies were taken.

✦ The advantages are direct visualisation of lesions, enabling accurate characterisation and biopsy. After biopsy haemostasis can be confirmed. In experienced hands, ultrasound applied directly to the liver is more sensitive at detecting abnormalities.

✦ The disadvantages are that it requires a general anaesthetic and is an invasive procedure that is expensive and time-consuming. Risks and benefits must be carefully balanced.

The clinical consequences of liver disease
Assessment of hepatic dysfunction
Certain management options depend on an objective assessment of the degree of liver impairment. One such assessment is Pugh's modification of Child's scoring for hepatic dysfunction (Table 8.1). A worse prognosis is associated with a higher score.

TABLE 8.1 Pugh's modification of Child's score for hepatic dysfunction.

	1	2	3
Encephalopathy	None	1–2	3–4
Ascites	Absent	Slight	Moderate
Albumin g/l	35	28–35	<28
Prothrombin time (sec prolonged)	<3	4–10	>10
Bilirubin (micromol/l)	<34	35–51	>51

Grade A (good) = 5–6, Grade B (moderate) = 7–9, Grade C (poor) = 10+

Hepatic encephalopathy
A spectrum of syndromes exists:
✧ acute (fulminant) liver failure
✧ cirrhotic patients with a precipitant
✧ chronic portal-systemic encephalopathy.

Grades are from I to IV, ranging from mild confusion, to drowsiness, to somnolent-but-rousable, to coma.

Causes are acute liver failure from any cause and exacerbation of chronic disease by precipitants such as GI haemorrhage, infection, drugs, hypokalaemic alkalosis, diuretic therapy, sedation, sepsis and portosystemic surgical shunting.

History
There may be a history of chronic liver disease and symptoms of intellectual impairment. There may also be a history of recent GI haemorrhage, diuretic therapy or other causes of encephalopathy.

Examination
Examination shows a decreased level of consciousness and abnormalities on cognitive testing – apraxia, hyperactive stretch reflexes.

Treatment
Withdraw the underlying cause (e.g. sedatives), stop haemorrhage and give phosphate enema to treat infection. The effect of GI haemorrhage is reduced by purgation with magnesium sulphate. Bacterial production of protein metabolites within the bowel is reduced using neomycin, metronidazole and lactulose. Ensure a protein-restricted diet.

For chronic treatment, decrease protein diet, but not less than 40 g. Severe encephalopathy after insertion of surgical shunts is treated by radiological blocking of the shunt.

Follow-up
Follow-up is long term at regular intervals (1–3 months) with frequent assessment for the presence of subclinical encephalopathy.

Portal hypertension

Obstruction to portal venous flow results in increased pressure in the splanchnic venous circulation. Normal portal pressure is 5–10 mmHg with a portal flow in the region of 1.5 l/min. Portal hypertension occurs if the pressure in the portal venous system exceeds 20 cm of saline or 12 mmHg.

Causes of obstruction include the following.

✧ Extrahepatic compression of the portal vein, or thrombosis of portal, mesenteric or splenic veins. Twenty five per cent of patients with portal hypertension will have an extrahepatic block, and a proportion of these will have underlying liver disease or polycythaemia. Chronic pancreaticobiliary disease or pancreatic neoplasm may precipitate portal vein thrombosis.

✧ Compression of portal venous radicles within the liver, by disease. Most commonly this obstruction is sinusoidal and results from cirrhosis of the liver. In cirrhosis, portal hypertension is due to both obstruction and increased splanchnic blood flow secondary to elevated levels of vasodilators, e.g. glucagon, and decreased sensitivity to vasoconstrictors. Pre-sinusoidal obstruction can develop in schistosomiasis.

✧ Obstruction to venous outflow from the liver, usually due to thrombosis of the hepatic veins. Causes of thrombosis include the contraceptive pill, ingestion of Bush teas, congenital diaphragm of the vena cava or congestive right heart failure. These patients rarely present with bleeding but have intractable ascites, painful hepatomegaly and rapidly deteriorating liver function.

Obstruction of portal venous flow results in enlargement of portosystemic communications and a risk of bleeding from oesophageal and gastric varices. Bleeding from varices usually occurs when the portal hypertension exceeds 30 cm saline. However, only 50% of varices ever bleed and only 15–40% of patients with chronic liver disease develop portal hypertension.

Clinical features of portal hypertension

Three clinical syndromes can be attributed to portal hypertension: hypersplenism, gastrointestinal bleeding and ascites.

Objectives

Detect portal hypertension, determine the cause, detect the syndromes associated with it, treat portal hypertension and its effects.

Hypersplenism (an overactive spleen)

Portal hypertension causes the spleen to enlarge (splenomegaly). Enlargement of the spleen causes increased sequestration of blood elements, enough to result in haemolytic anaemia, leucopenia and thrombocytopenia. These seldom cause major symptoms but may debilitate. After portal decompression, hypersplenism may remain. Therefore, pancytopenia in patients requiring portal decompression may be an indication for incorporating splenectomy as part of the procedure.

Gastrointestinal haemorrhage

The main causes of haemorrhage are oesophageal varices and gastric fundal varices. Colonic and rectal varices are detectable but seldom cause haemorrhage. After diagnosis of varices, 30% of patients bleed within two years – then a smaller proportion bleed each year after that. Increased risk of bleeding is associated with the following endoscopic characteristics: size graded from I (small) up to III, cherry-red spots, overlying varices, red whale markings and blue varices (as opposed to white). Grade I varices may be reversible with improvement of the liver condition. Other grades do not regress.

History

The patient may present with symptoms and signs of anaemia, massive haematemesis, a herald bleed (a mouthful of bright red blood) or melaena.

Examination

There may be stigmata of chronic liver disease.

Investigations

The primary investigation is endoscopy, performed by an operator experienced in dealing with variceal haemorrhage. FBC may reveal anaemia; clotting screen may detect a raised INR. Liver function tests (LFT) may be abnormal. Blood urea may be raised.

Treatment

The initial management of acute variceal bleeding is resuscitation and institution of measures to stop encephalopathy. Treatment to stop the bleeding may consist of drug therapy such as somatostatin to lower transhepatic venous gradient or of other vasoactive drugs such as terlipressin. Pentagastrin induces contraction of the lower oesophageal sphincter, as does metaclopramide.

Use balloon tamponade followed by endoscopy and sclerotherapy, banding or fibrin glue. If these measures fail to arrest the bleeding, a transjugular intrahepatic porto-systemic shunt (TIPS) procedure should be considered. Surgery can be an option, but the procedure carries a significant mortality in the acute setting. After the bleeding has stopped, management is aimed at preventing recurrent bleeding by treating the under-lying liver condition, treating the varices and reducing the portal hypertension. This is co-ordinated from the OPD.

Endoscopic sclerotherapy

Sclerotherapy (using ethanolamine oleate, 3% tetradecyl sulphate or absolute alcohol) is repeated at three-weekly intervals until all the varices are obliterated.

Complications of sclerotherapy

There may be oesophageal ulceration, perforation, stricture, acute respiratory distress syndrome (ARDS), mediastinitis, bacteraemia (10%), anaphylaxis (especially with ethanolamine), pneumatosis intestinalis, pneumoperitoneum and portal vein thrombosis (36% – therefore use with caution in good-risk Child's A patients who may later require a shunt operation or liver transplant).

Recurrence of oesophageal varices after initial obliteration by sclerotherapy occurs in about 60% of patients. Failed sclerotherapy is managed by oesophageal transection or shunt procedure.

Endoscopic banding

Using rubber band treatment to ensnare the varices is producing results as effective as sclerotherapy.

TIPS can be considered in persistent bleeding for suitable patients (without extrahepatic venous thrombosis). Access is obtained by cannulating the internal jugular and then the middle hepatic vein. A needle is then passed from the hepatic venous system to the portal venous system, which is then replaced by a wire and subsequently an expanding metal stent.

Complications of TIPS include haemorrhage, stent dislodgement or occlusion, infection and shunt encephalopathy.

Surgical treatment

Indications include patients who continue to bleed or have recurrent bleeding. Bleeding often downgrades a patient from Child's A/B to C. Portosystemic shunting in the emergency carries a prohibitive mortality, and oesphageal transection is performed instead.

In the elective situation two groups of patients are considered for surgery.
- Bleeding arrested and good liver function (Child's A/good B). Since there is no effective method for prevention of further bleeding, portosystemic shunting or oesophageal transection with devascularisation (Sugiura procedure) should be considered.
- End-stage liver disease (Child's C) controlled by sclerotherapy – consider for transplantation. For patients considered for hepatic transplantation, surgery should be avoided but TIPS has been successfully employed to achieve portal decompression and avoid further bleeding.

Liver transplant should be considered in all patients with variceal bleeding and good liver function but with poor quality of life.

Follow-up

Review at three-weekly intervals until all the varices are obliterated. Look for other signs of liver dysfunction and syndromes associated with portal hypertension. Detect complications of sclerotherapy. Estimate the Child score and formulate a plan for definitive management. Follow-up endoscopy every 6–12 months is recommended. Beta blockade should be considered. If rebleeding occurs after successful obliteration of varices, a shunt procedure or oesophageal transection procedure should be considered. Consider liver transplantation for suitable candidates.

Ascites

Ascites is clinically detectable when volume exceeds one litre.

Causes of ascites include:
- infection – TB, peritonitis
- inflammation – Crohn's, starch peritonitis
- hypoproteinaemia – nephrotic syndrome, liver disease, protein-losing enteropathy
- lymphatic obstruction – TB, filariasis, lymphoma, metastatic carcinoma, Milroy's disease, rupture/damage of abdominal lymphatics
- increased lymph flow/pressure – cirrhosis, congestive cardiac failure, constrictive pericarditis, Budd-Chiari syndrome
- neoplasms – primary and secondary tumours of the peritoneal cavity
- chronic pancreatitis – pancreatic ascites (caused by disruption of the pancreatic duct).

Intractable ascites is seen in advanced chronic liver disease, Budd-Chiari and peritoneal carcinomatosis. These patients cease to respond to diuretic therapy and develop pre-renal azotaemia. Pericardial effusions occur in 60% of alcoholic cirrhotics.

Differential diagnosis

This includes large ovarian cysts, pancreatic pseudocysts, mesenteric cysts, hydramnios and acute gastric dilatation.

Objectives

Diagnose the cause, treat the underlying disorder, treat ascites.

History

Take a general liver history. Patients may report increasing abdominal girth and fullness.

They may also complain of leg swelling or difficulty breathing due to splinting of the diaphragm. Ask about symptoms associated with each of the causes outlined above.

Examination
Perform a general examination. Early signs include dullness in the flanks. Shifting dullness and a fluid thrill may be elicited. Later, ascites may produce a tense, distended abdomen with grossly elevated intra-abdominal pressure, causing venous congestion and lower limb oedema. Respiratory distress may occur due to splinting of the diaphragm. Umbilical hernias are not uncommon. Look for signs associated with each of the causes outlined above.

Investigations
Use ultrasound to confirm presence of ascites.

Carry out diagnostic paracentesis – take off 20–50 ml and send samples of fluid for biochemistry, cytology, culture and sensitivity, and TB culture.

Determine serum/ascitic fluid albumin ratio. Gradients less than 11 g/litre are present in patients without portal hypertension. Gradients greater than 11 g/litre are associated with portal hypertension. This ratio helps to distinguish high-protein transudates in patients with portal hypertension from true exudates (e.g. TB and peritoneal carcinomatosis).

Laparoscopy is useful for uncertain cases, for inflammatory cases and for performing a peritoneal biopsy. Ascitic fluid can be described as serous, pseudochylous, bloodstained (often malignant) and myxomatous. Chylous ascites has a milky appearance and a high fat content on analysis. When chylous ascites arises spontaneously, it can indicate lymphatic obstruction by lymphoma or nodal deposits from carcinoma.

Treatment
Restrict sodium. Give spironolactone diuretic – loop diuretics increase the risk of encephalopathy, especially in the presence of subclinical renal impairment. The aim is for gradual loss of fluid of about 3 kg/week.

If this fails or patients become oliguric, other treatments apply.
- Therapeutic paracentesis with intravenous 5% albumin infused over two hours with 50 mg of frusemide and 250 ml of 20% mannitol over 20–30 minutes. If diuresis is not established, peritoneovenous shunting is indicated.
- Peritoneovenous shunting is effective in decreasing hospital stay; increasing muscle mass; and providing adequate long-term control on patients with ascites and good liver function (Child's A and B). It is ineffective and increases mortality in patients with advanced disease. Contraindications to peritoneovenous shunting include encephalopathy, uncorrectable bleeding diathesis, renal failure due to primary renal disease, recent variceal haemorrhage and cardiac failure. There have been reports of the successful use of the long saphenous vein as a saphenoperitoneal shunt. This avoids the cost and foreign body complications of an artificial shunt.

Follow-up
Follow-up is long term at regular intervals (1–3 months) to detect complications, which include blockage of the shunt and the development of disseminated intravascular coagulation (most commonly occurs just after shunt insertion).

Renal disease and hepatorenal failure
Hepatorenal syndrome is characterised by the development of renal failure in patients with severe liver disease without underlying renal disease. Diagnosis is dependent on a low glomerular filtration rate; absence of shock; ongoing sepsis; fluid loss or haemorrhage;

no improvement despite adequate plasma volume and diuretic withdrawal; proteinuria less than 500 mg/day; and no evidence of renal tract obstruction.

There are two types. Type 1 is rapidly progressive, of less than two weeks' duration and doubling of the initial creatinine, with a mortality of 80% at two weeks. Type 2 satisfies the criteria for diagnosis but is not rapidly progressive. It does not usually respond to dialysis. Best treatment is to improve underlying liver function.

Jaundice

Jaundice is recognised when serum bilirubin exceeds 40 umol/l. Mechanisms include excess bilirubin production, impaired uptake by the hepatocyte, failure of conjugation, impaired secretion of conjugated bilirubin into bile canaliculi, and impairment of bile flow subsequent to the secretion by the hepatocytes (cholestatic or obstructive). Causes include haemolysis, liver disease, adverse drug reactions and biliary tract obstruction (intrahepatic or extrahepatic). Table 8.2 shows types of jaundice.

TABLE 8.2 Types of jaundice.

TYPE	MECHANISM
Hepatocellular	Defective secretion of conjugated bilirubin into the bile canaliculi
Cholestatic intrahepatic/extrahepatic	Impairment of bile flow subsequent to the above secretory step
Haemolytic	Excess bilirubin production
Benign congenital hyperbilirubinaemia	Defective bilirubin uptake, conjugation or secretory defect

Hepatocellular jaundice

✥ The acute form is seen in viral hepatitis, liver cell necrosis and acute alcoholic hepatitis.
✥ The chronic form is seen in chronic active hepatitis, cirrhosis–alcoholic, cryptogenic, primary biliary. It is characterised by increased transaminases on the LFTs. If alcoholic, gamma-glutamyl-transpeptidase (gamma GT) is also raised.

Cholestatic jaundice

✥ Intrahepatic is functional (drugs, hepatitis) or organic (obstruction of intrahepatic biliary tree).
✥ Extrahepatic examples are duct stones and pancreaticobiliary cancer. It is characterised by:
  ∝ conjugated hyperbilirubinaemia
  ∝ increased alkaline phosphatase, gamma GT and 5-nucleotidase (5-nucleotidase is the most reliable, as it is not influenced by bone disease and not induced by alcohol)
  ∝ minor or no elevation of transaminases
  ∝ bilirubin in the urine
  ∝ elevation of serum cholesterol and bile acid levels.

Haemolytic jaundice

Unconjugated hyperbilirubinaemia results from haemolysis. Unconjugated bilirubin is not water soluble and is therefore carried in the blood bound to albumin. Increased unconjugated bilirubin leads to increased production of conjugated bilirubin and this leads eventually to increased urobilinogen and urobilin in urine. Therefore prolonged and recurrent haemolysis may produce a cholestatic component. Causes of haemolysis include abnormalities of red cells or increased red-cell destruction.

Assessment of the jaundiced patient
Objectives
Diagnose jaundice, diagnose the underlying cause, treat jaundice, treat the complications of jaundice, treat the underlying cause.

History
Take a general liver history. Enquire regarding drug intake (legal and illicit), injection with hypodermic needles (legal and illicit), alcohol abuse, anaesthetics, transfusion of blood and blood products, contact with jaundiced individuals, family history, sexual contacts, travel to hepatitis-endemic areas and ingestion of raw shellfish and wild mushrooms. Ask about the colour of urine, stools, itching and previous surgical procedures.

Examination
Perform a general examination. Is the patient jaundiced and has the patient any evidence of parenchymatous liver disease? Look for evidence of jaundice, e.g. yellow sclera. Examine for palmar erythema, spider naevi, bruising, splenomegaly, hepatomegaly or decreased liver size, fluid retention (ascites and oedema), muscle wasting, finger clubbing, white nails, enlargement of parotid gland, gynaecomastia and testicular atrophy. Scratch marks are commonly seen. Look for inco-ordination; neurological signs including hyper-reflexia and apraxia; altered sleep rhythm; confusion; flapping tremor; stupor; and foetor hepaticus.

Is there any evidence of malignancy, such as recent weight loss, enlarged left-sided supraclavicular lymph nodes, enlarged nodular liver, palpable gall bladder (Courvoisier's sign), palpable intra-abdominal mass (epigastric, iliac fossae) rapidly arising ascites or rectal neoplasm on rectal examination.

Investigations
Is the jaundice cholestatic? Cholestatic jaundice is characterised by dark and frothy urine and pale stools. There is bilirubin in urine. Serum alkaline phosphatase and gamma GT are elevated. There are slightly increased transaminases, usually less than 400 IU/ml (this amount virtually excludes significant hepatocellular damage). Check hepatitis A, B and C status in all jaundiced patients.

Is there dilatation of the biliary tree? Ultrasound is good at differentiating intrahepatic and extrahepatic jaundice, identifying stones and demonstrating the level of obstruction. Further investigation of the nature of the obstruction involves cross-sectional imaging (CT or MRI) and a cholangiogram (MRCP, endoscopic retrograde cholangiopancreatography (ERCP) or percutaneous transhepatic cholangiography (PTC)).

Intrahepatic cholestasis requires further investigation with liver biopsy for histology and serum autoantibody screen (antimitochondrial, anti-smooth muscle and immuno-globulin titres).

Liver biopsy can be performed (if clotting is normal) as a day-case or in-patient under USS guidance, or during diagnostic laparoscopy. If liver biopsy suggests bile duct obstruction despite a non-dilated duct, visualisation of the biliary tract is best achieved by ERCP.

Treatment
For the surgeon this consists of:
✧ treating the specific cause of the jaundice
✧ treating the general effects of jaundice prior to any radiological/surgical intervention.

General management of jaundice

Pre-operative management aims to minimise the incidence of complications associated with prolonged or severe cholestasis, which include infection (cholangitis, septicaemia, wound infections), disorders of the clotting mechanism, renal failure, liver failure and fluid and electrolyte abnormalities. Delayed wound healing is more associated with malignancy than jaundice alone.

Correct disorders of nutrition

Oral dietary supplements are preferred to intravenous supplements to control gut bacteria. Some centres advocate the oral administration of bile salts, and more recently lactulose, to reduce the intestinal absorption of endotoxins for the intestinal microflora and thus minimise the incidence of renal failure following surgical intervention. There are suggestions that probiotics may help modulate intestinal microflora. Hypokalaemia is frequent and should be corrected.

Prevention of infective complications

Prophylactic antibiotics are given to cover high-risk patients: all jaundiced patients, patients with rigors and pyrexia, patients undergoing emergency biliary procedures/operations, elderly patients, and patients with common bile duct stones or secondary biliary interventions.

Correct disorders of coagulation

When prolonged prothrombin time secondary to vitamin K deficiency (give intravenous injections of 10 mg vitamin K until deficit is corrected). Poor prognosis is associated with poor response, therefore give FFP just prior to surgery. Severely jaundiced patients need careful monitoring of fibrinogen levels, fibrin degradation products and platelet counts to rule out disseminated intravascular coagulopathy DIC.

Prevention of renal failure

The patient should be well hydrated. Administer intravenous fluids, e.g. 12–24 hours prior to surgery infuse 5% dextrose intravenously, then give mannitol at induction of anaesthesia.

Prevention of hepatic encephalopathy

Particularly consider this in patients with prolonged bile duct obstruction and those with pre-existing hepatocellular disease such as cirrhosis or chronic active hepatitis.

Stenting

If jaundice is severe (serum bilirubin greater than 150 umol/l); the patient is very distressed with pruritus; there are signs of cholangitis; there is going to be an undue delay in getting to surgery; or there are signs of impending liver failure; then a period of decompression is indicated by insertion of a biliary stent via ERCP. PTC can be performed if ERCP fails, and it is more likely to be needed in obstruction at the hilum.

Hepatomegaly

A patient may be referred to the surgical clinic with an enlarged liver, or hepatomegaly may be discovered on routine abdominal examination. Generally a liver that is palpable below the costal margin is thought to be enlarged, but this is not always the case. Determine the following features.

❖   Is the liver truly enlarged? True enlargement is suggested by liver dullness extending from the fifth intercostal space to a point below the costal margin. Apparent enlargement may occur when a liver is pushed down by a hyperexpanded lung, as occurs in chronic obstructive airways disease, and is suggested by lower level of liver dullness.

✧ Is the enlargement focal or generalised? Localised swellings are caused by conditions such as Riedel's lobe, hydatid cyst, amoebic abscess and primary carcinoma.

✧ Is generalised enlargement smooth or irregular? Causes of smooth enlargement include congestive cardiac failure, cirrhosis, reticuloses, Budd-Chiari and storage diseases. Irregular enlargement is associated with metastatic liver tumours, macronodular cirrhosis, primary liver tumours and polycystic disease.

✧ Is jaundice present? Smooth enlargement associated with jaundice includes viral hepatitis, biliary-tract obstruction and cholangitis. Irregular enlargement associated with jaundice occurs with macronodular cirrhosis and multiple metastases.

Objectives

Identify the cause, identify treatable causes, treat the cause.

History

Take a general hepatobiliary history. If jaundice is present take a general jaundice history. Establish whether there has been previous treatment for malignancy. If not, are there symptoms in other systems to suggest malignancy?

Examination

Determine whether true liver enlargement exists. Determine whether this is localised or generalised, smooth or irregular. Determine whether jaundice is present. Perform a general examination looking for causes of liver enlargement and evidence of liver impairment.

Investigations

Carry out urinalysis, liver function tests, FBC and clotting studies. Ultrasound is often diagnostic and answers the above questions in more detail. Liver biopsy may be indicated in cirrhosis and tumours (after consultation with a liver surgeon).

Treatment

Treat according to the specific condition diagnosed.

Follow-up

Intervals should be short until diagnosis is established and malignancy excluded: 1–2 weeks.

Liver cirrhosis

Cirrhosis is the end result of liver cell death by whatever cause – alcoholic, metabolic or cholestatic. Three morphological types are described: micronodular (alcoholic, malnutrition); macronodular; and mixed. Cirrhosis has two major consequences: hepatocellular failure and portal hypertension.

Objectives

Diagnose cirrhosis, detect the underlying cause, detect major consequences, treat cirrhosis, treat the underlying cause, treat consequences.

History

Take a general liver history. Uncomplicated cirrhosis is often asymptomatic. Ask about the complications of cirrhosis, e.g. gastrointestinal haemorrhage (varices) or hepatocellular failure. Ask about possible underlying causes, e.g. alcohol, drugs, hepatitis, previous biliary disorders, metabolic disorders or autoimmune disorders.

Examination

Perform a general examination. Examine for palmar erythema or unexplained peripheral oedema, muscle wasting, ascites, jaundice or hepatic encephalopathy.

Prior to any surgical procedure in the presence of liver disease, assess the risk using a Child score.

Investigations

LFTs, USS and liver biopsy are usually diagnostic. Other useful investigations include FBC, clotting and serology for hepatitis A, B and C, autoimmune disease and primary biliary cirrhosis (antimitochondrial antibody). OGD to detect varices is performed if indicated.

Treatment

Treatment is mainly medical but is important to the surgeon if a patient with cirrhosis is to undergo a surgical procedure or requires surgical intervention for the consequences of cirrhosis, e.g. bleeding varices. Note that cirrhotic liver does not regenerate as normal liver does. There is no specific medical treatment for cirrhosis. Treatment is aimed at the underlying cause and at detecting and treating the consequences of cirrhosis, such as hepatocellular failure and portal hypertension (see relevant sections). Liver transplantation should be considered in patients heading towards end-stage liver failure, provided they meet the eligibility criteria.

Follow-up

Follow-up is long term for detection of hepatocellular failure and portal hypertension. There should be periodic (six-monthly) estimations of AFP and liver USS to detect the development of primary liver tumours in Child's A/B cirrhotics.

Alcoholic liver disease

Damage varies, from fatty infiltration to alcoholic hepatitis, hepatic fibrosis and cirrhosis.

Objectives

Diagnose alcoholic liver disease, assess the severity, treat the alcoholic liver disease, treat the underlying cause.

History

Take a general liver history. There may be general symptoms of liver disease and a history of high and/or prolonged alcohol ingestion. Enquire for symptoms suggesting the development of liver failure or portal hypertension. There may be associated symptoms of alcohol damage to other organs, chronic pancreatitis, cardiomyopathy, myopathy, peripheral neuropathy and neurological effects.

Examination

Perform a general examination. The commonest and earliest sign of liver disease is hepatomegaly, which may progress to a tender liver from fatty infiltration of the parenchyma and from jaundice. Examine for evidence of liver failure or portal hypertension.

Investigations

LFTs may show raised transaminases, FBC may indicate anaemia and there may be a leucocytosis indicating hepatitis. An elevated mean corpuscular volume (MCV) may be indicative, but can also be elevated in other conditions such as B12 and folate deficiency. Clotting abnormalities may be present. Liver biopsy is performed – early disease shows

fatty infiltration, later cases show the classic features of micronodular cirrhosis.
Raised gamma GT is suggestive of diagnosis.

Treatment

Abstinence from alcohol and psychiatric help may be necessary. Corticosteroids may be prescribed in alcoholic hepatitis. Liver transplant can be an option for synthetic failure or the complications of liver failure if six months abstinence is documented. Otherwise treatment is as for cirrhosis.

Follow-up

Follow-up is generally managed by a gastroenterologist with a liver interest with involvement of the surgeon if the patient is referred for treatment of co-existing disorders or being considered for transplant. If cirrhosis is present, follow-up is the same as for cirrhosis.

Cholestatic liver disease

This consists of impaired bile secretion/excretion leading to conjugated hyperbilirubinaemia and raised ductular enzymes.

The causes include excess alcohol ingestion, viral hepatitis and obstructive lesions of biliary tract, both intrahepatic and extrahepatic.

Primary biliary cirrhosis

Intrahepatic bile ducts are progressively destroyed by an immunological process. It is often asymptomatic for long periods, and it is diagnosed on abnormal liver function tests.

History

Take a general liver history. The patient may be asymptomatic or complain of itching, weight loss, malaise and icterus.

Examination

Perform a general examination. Examination may be normal in early disease but later the liver becomes enlarged and the development of portal hypertension leads to splenomegaly. Deposition of cholesterol in the tissue around the orbits and extensor surface of the large joints may be detected. In advanced disease, intrapulmonary shunting leads to finger clubbing. Malabsorption of fat-soluble vitamins may lead to osteoporosis.

Investigations

Test urea and electrolytes (U&E) to detect hyponatraemia. LFTs are abnormal with a raised alkaline phosphatase. Antimitochondrial antibodies are found in all patients. IgM and smooth muscle antibody is also elevated. Clotting may be abnormal. USS may not be diagnostic but it helps to exclude other causes such as extrahepatic biliary obstruction, and it may detect portal hypertension.

Treatment

There is no effective medical treatment. Treat symptoms with cholestyramine for itching and ursodeoxycholate for other symptoms, and this may improve the liver function tests. If there is no improvement, prednisolone may be effective in decreasing fatigue and itching and in causing an improvement in LFTs. Give a monthly injection of fat-soluble vitamins.

Surgical intervention is liver transplantation before the onset of hyponatraemia or significant osteoporosis. Indications for surgery include decreased quality of life or bilirubin greater than 100 mmol/l and/or portal hypertension.

Follow-up
Follow-up is long term, for life.

Metabolic liver disease
Metabolic liver disease can be classified into two main types:
⋄ disorders of mineral deposition
⋄ disorders associated with defective enzyme production or release.

Objectives
Diagnose metabolic liver disease, diagnose the underlying cause, treat cirrhosis, treat underlying cause, treat the complications of cirrhosis.

Haemochromatosis
Primary is genetic, autosomal recessive; secondary is acquired due to multiple blood transfusions and polycythaemia.

Primary haemochromatosis leads to progressive iron deposition in the liver, heart, pancreas, joints and endocrine glands, with sparing of the spleen, lymph nodes and bone marrow. Hepatic accumulation leads to cirrhosis with increased risk of hepatocellular carcinoma.

History
History of diabetes (75%) and increasing pigmentation ('brown diabetes').

Examination
There is dusky brown pigmentation of skin, buccal mucosa and conjunctiva; and cirrhosis. Also look for polyarthropathy, hypopituitarism and hypogonadism.

Investigations
Investigate with liver biopsy. There is excessive iron in the hepatocytes and Kupffer cells, with fibrosis or macronodular cirrhosis. Serum ferritin and transferrin saturation exceeds 55%.

Treatment
Treatment is by phlebotomy, decreasing dietary intake of iron, giving iron chelating agents and long-term follow-up.

Follow-up
Follow-up is long term. Monitor for development of hepatocellular carcinoma.

Wilson's disease
There is copper deposition in the liver, cornea, kidneys and central nervous system (CNS) (basal ganglia). Liver fibrosis and cirrhosis occurs at an early age.

History
Symptoms are similar to cirrhosis. Enquire about symptoms of liver failure and portal hypertension.

Examination
Look for Kayser-Fleischer rings of pigment in the cornea. Examine for evidence of cirrhosis liver failure and portal hypertension.

Investigations

Perform routine liver investigations: FBC, clotting, LFTs, USS liver biopsy. Copper studies show serum copper and serum caeruloplasmin are reduced and urinary copper levels are elevated in all young patients with chronic liver disease. There is low serum caeruloplasmin and aminoaciduria.

Treatment

Treatment is by chelation with penicillamine or tientine; avoid copper and zinc supplements. Liver transplant can be considered for end-stage liver disease.

Follow-up

Follow up long term for the treatment of copper storage and the consequences of cirrhosis.

Cystic fibrosis

Of cystic fibrosis patients, 25% have clinical and biochemical evidence of liver disease, including fatty change, focal biliary cirrhosis and portal fibrosis followed by multilobar biliary cirrhosis. They may develop intrahepatic and extrahepatic strictures. Prognosis is determined by the pulmonary disease rather than the liver disease, and as patients are living longer features of liver disease may become more common.

Treatment

Treatment is long term for the development of cirrhosis. Ursodeoxycholic acid alters bile flow and composition, leading to an increase in less toxic hydrophilic bile acids. Liver transplant either alone or in combination with lung transplantation can be considered for end-stage liver disease.

Alpha-1-antitrypsin deficiency

Lack of inhibition of neutrophil elastase leads to pulmonary and liver damage.

Treatment

There is no effective medical treatment. Plasma derived or synthetic α1-antitrypsin has been used to treat pulmonary disease. Surgical treatment is liver transplantation and is the second commonest indication for liver transplant in childhood.

Hereditary tyrosinaemia type 1

This is an autosomal recessive disorder resulting in the lack of the enzyme fumaryl acetoacetate hydrolase and leading to the accumulation of the toxic products of amino acid degradation in the kidney, liver and nervous tissues.

The acute form leads to liver failure in infancy and death in the first year of life.

In the chronic form there is renal tubular dysfunction, rickets, progressive liver disease and development of hepatocellular carcinoma (40%).

Treatment

Treatment is by hepatic transplantation.

Hepatic abscess

There are two main types: pyogenic and amoebic. All abscesses are more common in the right lobe and both types have a high incidence of right lower lung abnormalities (50%). Mortality is increased by multiple abscesses, hyperbilirubinaemia and co-morbid disease.

Objectives
Diagnose abscess, diagnose the cause, treat abscess.

Pyogenic abscess
The main aetiology is from bile duct-ascending cholangitis, caused by *Escherichia coli* and anaerobic organisms. Other causes include portal pyaemia, e.g. from complicated diverticular disease; septicaemia; direct extension from suppurating cholecystitis; penetrating peptic ulcer disease or devitalised liver from trauma. In the frail geriatric population, liver abscesses may be insidious and non-specific, caused by *Strep. milleri*. Pyogenic abscesses can be either pus, surrounded by a fibrous capsule or, if antibiotics are used early in the course, a solid abscess containing inflammatory cells, dying liver cells and fibrotic tissue, mimicking a neoplastic lesion.

Amoebic abscess
This spreads to the liver via the portal vein from the bowel. It tends to affect younger patients.

Hepatic candidiasis
This occurs in immuno-compromised patients and complicates systemic candidiasis. There is often combined hepatic and splenic involvement. It forms target lesions – a central mass of fungus surrounded by necrotic liver cells, detected by CT or USS. Needle biopsy is *not* performed. These lesions need open or laparoscopic wedge excision for diagnosis and treatment.

History
Pyogenic abscesses tend to present as a primary disorder with fever, rigors, profuse sweating, anorexia and vomiting – pain is a late symptom. Amoebic abscesses present with a low-grade fever but with more pain, which is aggravated by movement and coughing.

Examination
Hepatomegaly may be a feature and 50% will have diarrhoea. In right lobe disease the patient may exhibit bulging and pitting of the intercostal spaces.

Investigations
FBC may show anaemia and leucocytosis. LFTs usually show an abnormal alkaline phosphatase, and alanine transaminase may also be raised. The ESR is raised. Amoebic abscess is diagnosed by positive serological tests (serum complement fixation test), amoebic trophozoites in abscess fluid and a rapid response to anti-amoebics. USS and CT scan are performed and diagnostic aspiration under imaging control is performed if indicated. CXR may detect lung involvement. In pyogenic abscesses with no obvious source of sepsis in the gut or biliary tree, look for an occult focus of infection elsewhere (e.g. endocarditis, dental sepsis); do blood cultures before starting antibiotic therapy.

Treatment
Treat pyogenic abscess with aspiration or drainage under radiological control and appropriate antibiotics based on microbiological samples. Treat amoebic abscess with metronidazole. If there is no improvement and the cyst is single and unilocular, provide percutaneous drainage. Otherwise surgical drainage is indicated.

Follow-up
Treatment is mainly as an in-patient. After percutaneous or surgical drainage, monitor by

frequent USS until there is evidence of resolution, then discharge with advice to return if symptoms recur. Very occasionally a neoplasm may mimic an abscess.

Liver cysts

There are two main types: non-parasitic or parasitic.

Non-parasitic liver cysts

These may be developmental, traumatic, dermoid or associated with other disorders such as congenital hepatic fibrosis, hamartoma, Caroli's disease, choledochal cyst or polycystic disease (liver, kidneys). Non-parasitic cysts are usually detected in middle-aged females.

Objectives

Diagnose the cause, treat the cause.

History

Most are asymptomatic until large enough to press on other structures. They are often present with non-specific symptoms of vomiting, upper abdominal pain and occasionally diarrhoea. Torsion, rupture or haemorrhage into a cyst produces sudden-onset pain.

Examination

Most have a non-tender liver swelling. Jaundice is rare.

Investigations

Liver function tests are usually normal. USS is usually diagnostic, although CT can also be used. It is important to identify cystic neoplasms (e.g. biliary cystadenoma). If in doubt, do fine-needle aspiration of the cyst fluid under ultrasound guidance and send the fluid for cytology and CEA level (high levels suggest a mucinous neoplasm). Ultrasound is useful in detecting cysts in the kidneys, which develop before liver cysts in polycystic disease. Occasionally multiple cysts can be confused with metastases.

Treatment

Small asymptomatic cysts do not require treatment unless complications occur. Treatment is confined to single large cysts, which are treated by laparoscopic surgical deroofing. Polycystic liver disease treatment is confined to those patients who develop local symptoms or portal hypertension due to compression of the portal vein. Aspiration of cysts with instillation of fibrosing agents is almost never effective. Laparoscopic deroofing and liver resection have been advocated in specialised centres.

Follow-up

Intervals are short until diagnosis is achieved and neoplastic lesions excluded. Thereafter small asymptomatic cysts can be followed up yearly with an USS to detect enlargement.

Post-operative follow-up

Review histology. Detect general complications of surgery like wound healing. Give regular USS to detect recurrence, or reserve until symptoms recur.

Parasitic cysts – Hydatid cysts

These are caused by ingestion of vegetables and water contaminated (usually by dogs) with the eggs of the parasite *Echinococcus granulosus* (unilocular cyst, good prognosis) or *E. multilocularis* (multiple cysts, poor prognosis).

History

General health is good. In all ages pain, jaundice, and ascites are uncommon. Patients usually present with a painless liver mass or complications. A history of contact with dogs or sheep is usual. Patients occasionally complain of right upper quadrant (RUQ) pain.

Examination

There is a smooth, rounded tense mass. If there is secondary infection there may be hepatomegaly, rigors and pyrexia and deep-rooted continuous pain. Jaundice is infrequent.

Complications

Intrabiliary rupture of the cyst produces biliary colic, jaundice and fever. Vomitus may contain hydatid cysts and membranes.

Intraperitoneal rupture leads to severe pain and shock with urticaria and pruritus.
Intrathoracic rupture produces bile-stained sputum.

Investigations

AXR shows calcified reticular shadow. Following intrabiliary rupture there may be gas in the cyst. Ultrasound shows an echogenic cyst.

FBC shows eosinophilia in 25%. Complement fixation test for hydatids is positive in 93%. Enzyme-linked immunosorbent assay (ELISA) gives positive results in 90% of cases (so 10% of patients can be false negative). Casoni's test has been largely abandoned. LFTs are usually abnormal and may demonstrate an obstructive picture.

Treatment

Cysts with extensive calcification are usually sterile and best left alone.

- ✧ Medical treatment consists of albendazole: 30% of cysts disappear, 30–50% show reduction and 20–40% remain unchanged.
- ✧ Radiological teatment consists of the PAIR routine: percutaneous fine-needle puncture, aspiration, injection of hypertonic saline and reaspiration. There is a small but definite risk of anaphylaxis and a theoretical risk of peritoneal seeding.
- ✧ Surgical treatment consists of removing the cyst entirely, cystectomy with removal of the germinal and laminated layers and preservation of the host-derived ectocyst. Alternatively it may be possible to enucleate the cyst. Cysts complicated by secondary infection require surgical drainage. Treatment by partial liver resection may be required, especially if the cysts are large and/or multiple. Remember to administer a course of albendazole before PAIR or surgery.

Follow-up

Follow up at short intervals until diagnosis is achieved. Then treatment is arranged.

Post-operative follow-up

Check pathology results. Detect general complications of surgery. Ascites may complicate this surgery and may indicate disseminated disease. Repeat USS until resolution of the cyst is confirmed, then discharge with advice.

Benign solid tumours
Haemangioma (vascular malformation)

These are blood-filled endothelial lesions with fibrous tissue. If big enough they produce size effects of pain, vomiting and elevation of diaphragm. There may be a palpable abdominal mass, which, if large, may produce heart failure in children and be associated with skin lesions in 85%. A bruit is audible in 15%. Rupture is rare. Lesions are hyperechoic on USS. CT scans with intravenous (IV) contrast are usually diagnostic. If doubt still exists, a labelled red cell scan is performed.

MRI can be useful in confirming the disease when it is equivocal on other imaging modalities. Where the diagnosis is certain and the risk of bleeding minimal, lesions can be observed. If large and peripherally placed, it may be suitable for surgical resection. If it is difficult to differentiate from neoplastic lesions, surgical resection is indicated.

Hamartoma

This is a congenital condition of normal tissues with disorderly arrangement. It presents as large liver masses in children, which produce pressure effects (pain, vomiting). Patients complain of an expanding abdomen with a mass. CT scan is diagnostic. Treatment is by surgical excision if the diagnosis is clear. Occasionally these are sarcomatous.

Adenomas and focal nodular hyperplasia

These are very similar in pathological terms.

✧ Adenomas are variable in size (4–30cm) and 90% occur in women between the ages of 30–60. There is an association with long-term use of oestrogen contraceptive pills. Thirty per cent rupture or haemorrhage and can be difficult to distinguish from low-grade hepatoma. There is an increased risk of rupture in pregnancy. Adenomas are pre-malignant.
✧ Focal nodular hyperplasia (FNH) occurs in the same patients, is not pre-malignant and may be observed without serious risk. If haemorrhage occurs, successful management can be ligation of the feeding vessel or wedge resection.

History

Take a general liver history. Most patients will be women aged from 30–60 with a history of oral contraceptive use. A third present with an abdominal mass, a third with rupture and a third are incidental findings. Symptoms are commonly vague – upper abdominal pain and discomfort.

Examination

Perform a general examination. Evidence of jaundice and anaemia may be present. The liver may be focally enlarged.

Investigations

LFTs are usually normal. FBC may reveal anaemia due to bleeding. Adenomas appear solid on ultrasound and have a characteristic arteriographic appearance. FNH also has a characteristic CT appearance with the presence of a central scar. Open/laparoscopic liver biopsy for histology can be performed where the diagnosis is unclear, but adenomas can be difficult to distinguish from well-differentiated hepatocellular carcinoma.

Treatment

Ruptured and bleeding lesions are excised as emergencies. Hepatic arterial embolisation can be useful in stopping bleeding. Intracapsular haemorrhage presents as an expanding tumour and requires partial liver resection. FNH does not need any treatment once confirmed on imaging, whereas adenomas should be excised as they are pre-malignant.

Follow-up

Patients with multiple adenomas need prolonged follow-up with repeated imaging. In females, stop the oral contraceptive pill. If diagnosis is certain then it is acceptable to monitor lesions every 6–12 months with ultrasound scans. If static or diminishing in size then operation may be deferred.

Post-operative follow-up
Enlargement of residual adenomas requires elective excision.

Adenomatous hyperplasia
This refers to sizeable nodules which develop in chronic liver disease. They may have pre-malignant potential and require long-term follow-up. Cholangioma and biliary cystadenoma are rare lesions.

Primary malignant tumours of the liver
The commonest tumour is primary hepatocellular carcinoma. Its incidence and geographical distribution parallels that of hepatitis B infection. It usually develops on a background of cirrhosis, but can also develop in a normal liver. Other rarer tumours include hepatocellular cholangiocarcinoma. This rare tumour shows features of both hepatocellular and cholangiocarcinoma and is thought to represent a coincidental occurrence of both. Cystadenocarcinoma tends to present as a large cystic tumour in adults. Sarcoma arises from the connective tissue elements of the liver and presents as a rapidly enlarging lesion associated with hypoglycaemia. Angiosarcoma is associated with the occupations linked to vinyl chloride production or ingestion of arsenic or anabolic steroids. It is an aggressive tumour.

In children the main tumours are hepatocellular carcinoma and hepatoblastoma. Hepatoblastoma tends to occur by the third year and produces increased levels of alpha-foetoprotein and gonadotropins, occasionally causing sexual precocity. Liver resection produces long-term survivors in 30%.

Hepatocellular carcinoma
Objectives
Diagnose hepatocellular carcinoma (HCC), differentiate from other causes of liver tumours, localise and stage the tumour, determine resectability, treat the tumour.

History
Take a general liver history. In areas of the world that screen for hepatocellular cancer the tumour may be detected when it is asymptomatic. In patients with the onset of liver cirrhosis, HCC is heralded by a worsening of liver function, producing ascites, jaundice, encephalopathy, and variceal bleeding. Patients may describe a feeling of a heavy mass within the abdomen dragging down, especially during exercise. General symptoms include anorexia, weight loss, abdominal or chest pain, vomiting, fever and weakness.

Examination
There is occasionally jaundice. There is abdominal distension and a liver mass. There is a bruit over the liver in 10% or friction rub is audible. Ascites is common and sometimes bloodstained. Additional infrequent clinical features include hypoglycaemia, hypercalcaemia, hyperlipidaemia and hyperthyroidism. Examine for features of liver failure and portal hypertension.

Investigations
LFTs are frequently abnormal. FBC may show either anaemia due to haemorrhage or polycythaemia from anomalous erythropoietin production. AFP is raised in one-third of cases. It is often high in undifferentiated disease and if it falls after resection it is useful as a marker for recurrence. Hepatitis B and C serology needs to be done in all patients. Clotting may be abnormal.
✧   Tumour markers are AFP and abnormal APT. Also measure CEA and carbohydrate

antigen 19–9 (CA 19–9) (markers for biliary-tract malignancies). Very high levels are associated with undifferentiated disease and a poor prognosis. This is a variable predictor for detection of hepatocellular carcinoma but any patient with chronic active hepatitis or cirrhosis who develops a rising level of AFP or a level exceeding 500 ng/ml should have investigations for the detection of hepatocellular carcinoma, e.g. USS.

✧ Tumour localisation: USS or CT scan are used to demonstrate size and position, multiple deposits and extrahepatic spread, e.g. porta hepatis. CXR may show direct diaphragmatic involvement or pulmonary metastases. Occasionally neither CT nor USS show a lesion in a cirrhotic patient who has a rising level of AFP. In these cases MRI may be useful or alternatively use a lipiodol-CT scan. Fine-needle aspiration cytology under USS or CT guidance has been advocated to differentiate HCC from other benign lesions in both cirrhotic and non-cirrhotic livers. However, there is a proven risk of seeding tumour along the needle track and it is only necessary if the diagnosis is in doubt.

Multi-slice helical CT scanners have reduced the need for arterioportography. For large posterior tumours consider imaging of the vena cava (cavography) to exclude caval involvement.

MRI scans carry a high diagnostic yield and can distinguish between benign and malignant lesions.

Pre-operative preparation

Correct fluid, electrolyte and clotting abnormalities. Determine the operative risk. Important considerations are that patients in Child's grades B and C have lost 50–60% of liver parenchyma already and patients with cirrhosis may not be able to regenerate liver tissue.

Treatment – surgical

Surgical resection is the optimal treatment and small tumours (smaller than 5cm) carry the best prognosis. Favourable results have also been obtained with local ablative techniques such as alcohol injection and radiofrequency ablation (RFA). Recently investigated modalities, e.g. radio-labelled ablation, laser photocoagulation and electrolysis, may become important.

Liver transplantation is a recognised treatment of HCC arising in a cirrhotic liver. Consideration is based on the Milan criteria: a single lesion less than 5cm or no more than three lesions less than 3cm. The University of California, San Francisco (UCSF) expanded criteria have included patients not meeting the Milan criteria.

Unresectable lesions

✧ Chemotherapy: both systemic and regional hepatic artery infusions give poor results, with response rates as low as 10–15%, but sorafenib has been recently associated with a small survival benefit. Immunotherapy, e.g. interferon or cytokines, has not proved helpful.

✧ Chemoembolisation: transarterial embolisation of tumours with gelatin sponge with or without added transarterial chemotherapeutic agents may give symptomatic benefit, with slight improvement in overall survival in some studies. Microspheres containing cytotoxic drugs can be given via the hepatic artery.

✧ Radiotherapy: external beam radiation causes radiation-induced hepatitis and is rarely used. Microspheres containing radioisotopes like yttrium-90 can be injected via the hepatic artery.

Follow-up

Intervals should be short (1–4 weeks) until the diagnosis and treatment plan have been decided. Many of these patients will have been followed up for cirrhosis.

Post-operative follow-up

Check the histology for the pathology and adequate resection margins. Common post-operative complications include the development of liver failure and intra-abdominal fluid collections. Investigate as indicated. The most common serious complication is tumour recurrence. Monitor serum AFP levels and perform serial USS of the liver every 4–6 months. Further resection, if recurrence is localised, can be performed and has been associated with extended survival. Median survival for these patients is in the region of one year.

Metastatic disease of the liver

Direct invasion can occur from adjacent organs such as the stomach, pancreas and hepatic flexure of colon. Most common tumours are metastatic from distant organs.

Objectives

Diagnose metastatic lesions, differentiate suitable lesions for resection, stage the tumours, treat the tumours.

History

Take a general liver history. Many are asymptomatic. There may be a history of previous malignancy. If large, expansion of the liver may cause pain in the abdomen and back. Flatulence and nausea may be features and lead to decreased appetite and weight loss. Eventually malnutrition and cachexia develops. Symptoms of cirrhosis may be present.

Examination

Perform a general examination. There may be evidence of weight loss. Hepatomegaly may be present. Examine for underlying features of cirrhosis.

Investigations

USS will detect metastases larger than 1cm diameter and, combined with CT scan, will reduce the false negative rate. LFTs may be normal. Serial CEA detects 30% of metastatic livers with normal USS (false positive rate is 15%). Laparoscopy should ideally be combined with intra-operative laparoscopic USS and liver biopsy.

Treatment – surgical

Fewer than 5% of liver metastases are suitable for resection. Surgical resection of the liver is usually confined to metastatic colorectal, neuroendocrine or congenital tumours. Rarely, other metastases may be considered for resection. Resection is contraindicated if less than 25% (fewer than two segments) of the liver can be left. Likely residual volumes can be calculated from CT images. Liver resection for colorectal metastases carries less than 5% peri-operative mortality and a five-year survival of 35–45%.

Other treatments

- ✧ Chemotherapy: regional hepatic artery infusion or systemic chemotherapy produces the same poor two-year survival. Intraperitoneal infusion has also been used.
- ✧ Chemoembolisation: transarterial chemoembolisation (TACE) using gelatin sponge with 5FU, doxorubicin and cisplatin is beneficial in ocular melanoma, advanced carcinoid syndrome and islet cell tumours. Complications include postembolisation

syndrome (nausea and vomiting, fever, abdominal pain and ileus), infarction of gall bladder, pancreatitis and bleeding.

✧ In-situ ablative techniques are receiving much interest in the literature. These techniques of cryotherapy (to produce an ice ball), radio-frequency, microwave and laser therapy (to produce thermal necrosis) and electrolytic destruction have yet to be tested in prospective randomised trials but are now commonly used as adjuncts to surgical treatments or in patients deemed unresectable.

Follow-up

Follow up at short intervals until suitability for resection is determined. Arrange operative or non-operative treatment as appropriate.

Post-operative follow-up

Check the histology for the pathology and adequate resection margins. Common post-operative complications include the development of liver failure and intra-abdominal fluid collections. Investigate as indicated. Monitor for recurrences with regular USS every 3–6 months, checking CEA levels. Occasionally re-resection is indicated.

The biliary tract

Liver, pancreatic and biliary disorders are closely related and should be considered together. For instance, a lesion in the head of the pancreas may cause obstruction of the biliary tract, which affects the function of the liver. One of the first objectives of the assessment is to determine which system contains the primary disorder and then determine what effect this has had on the function of the others.

Assessment of biliary tract disorders
Biliary history

Start with a general gastrointestinal history. When responses indicate a possible biliary problem, a more detailed biliary history is required. This may also mean a liver and pancreatic history. The two main indicators of biliary disease are pain and jaundice, and gallstones are the commonest cause.

✧ Biliary pain is colicky, severe and occurs in the right upper quadrant. It may radiate around to the back. Colicky pain is caused by the gall bladder contracting to try and overcome an obstruction. Eventually the contraction relaxes and the acute pain is relieved, leaving a dull ache until the next contraction starts. If the obstruction is caused by a gallstone, the stone may be expelled and the bout of biliary colic resolves until the next stone produces another episode. If the stone becomes impacted, inflammation and infection of the biliary tract can ensue. In the gall bladder the result is cholecystitis and the pain becomes constant. If the bile ducts are affected, jaundice and cholangitis may be produced.

✧ Jaundice: obstructive jaundice typically causes pale stools and dark urine and often causes pruritus. An enquiry into possible liver and pancreatic disease is indicated. Usually, jaundice caused by gallstone disease is associated with episodes of biliary colic. The onset of painless jaundice may indicate a neoplastic cause.

✧ Rigours: a history of fever with rigours indicates infection of the biliary tree, and when combined with pain and jaundice (Charcot's triad) indicates an infected, obstructed biliary tree that requires urgent treatment (decompression) to prevent septic shock.

✧ Risk factors: ask about previous biliary interventions or surgery. Recurrent biliary symptoms may be due to complications of these original treatments. There may be a family history of gallstones or there may be some inherited disorder that predisposes to the formation of gallstones, e.g. haemolytic anaemia, hyperlipidaemia, ileal disease or surgical resection, cirrhosis or cystic fibrosis.

Biliary examination

Perform a general and gastrointestinal examination, but in particular look for signs of jaundice and liver disease. Between episodes, abdominal examination may be normal. An enlarged palpable gall bladder in the presence of jaundice is indicative of a neoplastic cause rather than stone disease (Courvoisier's law). Severe inflammation of the gall bladder with adherent omentum may also produce a mass in the right upper quadrant; however, all masses should be considered to be malignant until proven otherwise. Rectal examination revealing the typical pale, toothpaste-consistency stools is typical of obstructive jaundice.

Investigation of biliary tract disorders
Laboratory investigations
Urinalysis

The presence of conjugated bilirubin indicates obstructive jaundice, although in some conditions associated with excess bilirubin production this will result in some bilirubin in the urine.

Biochemistry

❖ Release of integral membrane enzymes: cholestasis and obstructive jaundice are associated with an increased alkaline phosphatase. Gamma GT is particularly raised in alcoholic liver disease. Minor increases in ALT and AST occur in cholestasis and chronic liver disease. Significant increases are associated with acute hepatitis or with liver cell necrosis of any cause. Secondary tumour deposits cause a rise in alkaline phosphatase and gamma GT and a small rise in bilirubin.
❖ Tests for urea and electrolytes may indicate electrolyte abnormalities, particularly hyponatraemia and hypoglycaemia. Evidence of raised urea and creatinine levels may indicate impaired renal function associated with liver disease.

Haematology

FBC may reveal anaemia of chronic disease or indicate blood loss from the biliary system into the gastrointestinal tract. Other abnormalities of the blood cells may be detected, such as haemolytic anaemia, leukaemia and lymphoma. Clotting, particularly the INR, may be abnormal in liver and biliary disease.

Immunology

Hepatitis serology: screen for hepatitis B and C. Also screen for autoimmune disease and primary biliary cirrhosis.

Imaging techniques
Ultrasound

For technique, request form, results.
❖ The advantage of USS is that, as the first-line investigation, it is a very good non-invasive technique for visualising the presence of stones, gall bladder disease, dilatation of biliary tract and hepatic parenchymal disease. Also possible is ultrasound-guided biopsy of the liver and pancreas. A common hepatic duct with a diameter over 10mm is deemed dilated. A diameter above 15mm indicates significant organic disease. However, there is a 5–10% incidence of ductal stones in a common bile duct (CBD) of 5mm diameter. Other causes of duct dilatation include pancreaticobiliary cancer, chronic pancreatitis, congenital cystic disease and parasitic infestation.

❖ The disadvantages are that accuracy is dependent on the experience of the operator; and it may be unsatisfactory in obese patients, following previous surgery, or in the presence of ascites or gaseous distension of upper abdominal viscera. In these cases do a CT scan.

CT scan

For technique, request form, results.

❖ The advantages are that intravenous contrast can be given to outline the vessels and focal lesions within the liver and multiple scans can be performed to give non-contrast, arterial, venous and delayed phases of scanning; modern multi-slice spiral CT scans can be performed quickly (15–30 seconds) using 5mm cuts, giving more detail and allowing more sophisticated reconstruction; when used with contrast, CT is more sensitive than ultrasound at determining the nature of lesions within the liver, especially differentiating between small tumours cysts or abscesses; and CT is better for detection of solid lesions in the extrahepatic bile ducts (cholangiocarcinoma), pancreas and liver. MRI is useful in hilar carcinoma and primary carcinoma of the gall bladder, where it is superior to CT in assessing the presence and extent of extra-mural invasion.

❖ The disadvantages are that it is expensive and it uses ionising radiation.

MRI

For technique, request form, results.

❖ MRI is useful in hilar cholangiocarcinoma and primary carcinoma of the gall bladder, where it is superior to CT in assessing the presence and extent of extramural invasion. Newer techniques include MRCP, which may supersede diagnostic ERCP.

❖ The disadvantages are that it is expensive and time-consuming; and many patients find the experience unpleasantly claustrophobic.

PTC

Ultrasound is used to identify the dilated biliary system. Under local anaesthetic a needle is inserted through the liver parenchyma into the dilated bile duct and contrast agent is injected under X-ray screening to visualise the biliary system. Where an obstruction is detected a percutaneous drain can be inserted to continue drainage after the procedure. Prior to procedure cover with antibiotics and correct any clotting abnormalities.

❖ The request form is the radiology/ultrasonography request form.

❖ Results are as a written report and selection of X-ray images.

❖ The advantages are that it is used for visualisation of the biliary tract in the jaundiced patient, transhepatic drainage and insertion of endoprosthesis. In practice PTC is used when ERCP has failed, or for insertion of stents for palliation of large bile duct obstruction due to inoperable/incurable malignancy. It can be better at biliary drainage and visualisation of the biliary tree than ERCP for hilar cholangiocarcinoma.

❖ The disadvantages are complications including septicaemia, haemorrhage into peritoneal cavity and haemobilia, biliary peritonitis, intrahepatic arterioportal fistula, pneumothorax and contrast reactions.

ERCP

ERCP is performed using a large-bore side-viewing endoscope. The scope is passed through the stomach into the second part of the duodenum. The duodenal papilla is cannulated and contrast is injected under X-ray screening. The pancreatic and biliary duct system is visualised.

❖ The request form is the endoscopy/radiology form. It is a joint procedure between the radiology department and the endoscopy service.

✧ Results are as a written report and selection of ERCP images.
✧ The advantages are that it can be performed in all cholestatic jaundice patients irre-spective of whether the ducts are dilated or not; it also gives views of the stomach and duodenum; the pancreaticogram can be performed; certain lesions can be treated or palliated during the procedure – stone removal, endoscopic nasobiliary drainage, stent insertion for inoperable malignant large bile duct obstruction; and ERCP is good for diagnosis of ductal calculi, tumours of bile duct and pancreas and sclerosing cholan-gitis. In patients with complete biliary obstruction the proximal biliary tree may not be visualised and PTC is then indicated.
✧ The disadvantages are complications, which include pancreatitis (1–2%). If sphinc-terotomy is also performed complications rise to 6–10% and include haemorrhage, acute pancreatitis, cholangitis, retroperitoneal perforation, impacted Dormia basket, acute cholecystitis and gallstone ileus. Technical failure may result in patients with duodenal stenosis, previous Billroth II and duodenal diverticula and in an unco-operative patient.

Biliary manometry

This technique is performed at ERCP. The common bile duct is cannulated and the pressure in the bile duct is measured.

Request form and results are as for ERCP.
✧ The advantage is that it is good for investigation of patients with biliary dyskinesia (persistent pain after cholecystectomy) to characterise abnormalities of the sphincter (stenosis, dyskinesia). Measures are basal sphincter pressure, rate and progression of sphincter contractions and response to morphine and cholecystokinin. Dyskinesia is diagnosed by increased basal pressure, altered frequency and amplitude of phasic contractions and reversal of normal peristaltic direction.
✧ The disadvantages are as for ERCP. Results can be difficult to interpret.

Laparoscopy

Under general anaesthetic a laparoscope is inserted through a small sub-umbilical incision. It can be used as an investigative technique and can be combined with laparoscopic ultrasonography, cholangiography, biopsy or cytology.
✧ No request form. It is a surgical operation.
✧ The results is a written operation note, sometimes with photographic images.
✧ The advantages are that it allows visualisation of the liver, gall bladder, extrahepatic biliary system and pancreas and peritoneal lining; it can diagnose hepatic disease, primary neoplasms, secondary tumour deposits in the liver and peritoneum, and it enables biopsy of these lesions for histology; it also enables staging of hepatobiliary and pancreatic tumours; and it is useful for liver biopsy in chronic liver disease with a high risk of bleeding – haemostasis can be achieved and observed.
✧ The disadvantage is that it requires a general anaesthetic and is therefore associated with GA complications.

Biliary scintiscanning

The technique uses ^{99m}Tc-labelled compounds of iminodiacetic acid (HIDA, DISIDA, PIPIDA). HIDA is injected intravenously, taken up by hepatocytes, and then secreted into bile ducts and concentrated in a functioning gall bladder.
✧ Request form is for radioisotopes (medical physics department).
✧ Results are as a written report and selection of images.
✧ The advantages are that if the compounds are not taken up by the gall bladder, the most likely diagnosis is cholecystitis (false positives – chronic cholecystitis, gallstone pancreatitis, patients with alcoholic liver disease, patients receiving parenteral

nutrition); if the gall bladder is visualised, then it is 100% certain that it is not cholecystitis; it is routinely used in the jaundiced neonate for diagnosis of biliary atresia; and it is also useful for the functional evaluation of surgically constructed bilioenteric anastomoses.

✧ The disadvantage is the use of radioactivity. It is not used routinely – only for specific indications.

Intra-operative cholangiography and choledochoscopy

These techniques are used intra-operatively to assess the biliary system to identify abnormal anatomy or the presence of stones and to confirm their absence or complete removal.

Disorders of the biliary tract
Cystic disease of the biliary tract

Choledochal cysts include bile duct dilatation, choledochocele, bile duct diverticulae and/or liver cysts. There is increased incidence in the Japanese and 60% of cases occur in the first 10 years. Complications include cholangitis, pancreatitis, hepatic abscess formation and cholangiocarcinoma.

History

Symptoms of increasing jaundice, right upper quadrant pain and complications.

Examination

Cholestatic jaundice, abdominal mass and tenderness.

Investigations

USS and CT gives the diagnosis. MRCP or ERCP defines the anatomy.

Treatment

Treatment is surgical excision of extrahepatic biliary tree and reconstruction in the form of a hepatico-jejunostomy, with or without liver resection, and drainage of simple liver cysts. Surgery is recommended even in asymptomatic patients to reduce long-term risk of cholangiocarcinoma.

Gallstones

Gallstones are very common (18.5% in autopsy studies). There are three types:
✧ cholesterol: often radiolucent, multiple or large and single
✧ pigment: associated with infection or with haemolytic disease
✧ mixed.

Risk factors

Gallstones are more common in females and are associated with obesity, increasing age, genetic and ethnic factors, refined diet high in animal fat, diabetes mellitus, ileal disease and resection, haemolytic states, infection of biliary tract, parasitic infection, cirrhosis and cystic fibrosis.

Differential diagnosis

Most gallstones are clinically silent. Common co-existing causes of abdominal pain include colonic motility disorders and diverticular disease, gastritis and peptic ulceration, reflux oesophagitis and hiatus hernia, pancreatitis, colonic cancer, renal disease and ischaemic heart disease. In addition to gall bladder imaging, an OGD (or barium series) and barium enema may be necessary in patients undergoing elective cholecystectomy for chronic symptoms.

Silent gallstones

The vast majority will not cause symptoms or complications during life. Therefore there is no indication for cholecystectomy in the management of asymptomatic gallstones, except in acromegalic patients on long-term somatostatin analogue where gallstones can get very large; and in diabetic patients with gallstones.

Symptomatic gallstones – acute cholecystitis

This often presents with admission to hospital with acute abdominal pain, where the relevant investigations are performed and treatment is arranged.

Chronic cholecystitis

Cholecystectomy for gallstones is one of the commonest operations performed in the Western world. Partly this is because ultrasound is widely used for the investigation of abdominal pain and is very sensitive at detecting gallstones. Once detected, gallstones can be difficult to exclude as the cause of the pain until they are removed.

Objectives

Diagnose gallstones, differentiate from other causes of abdominal pain, treat gallstones.

History

Take a general biliary history. Typically, patients report recurrent attacks of epigastric or right hypochondrial pain, often radiating to the right side of the back or shoulder blade. Bouts of pain last several minutes to hours; they may subside or progress to acute cholecystitis. Nausea and vomiting may accompany each episode. Jaundice and dark urine may follow an acute attack and indicate a CBD stone. Intolerance to fatty foods, abdominal distension and belching can occur with the same frequency in the general population as they do in patients with gallstones.

Examination

Perform a general examination. Look for jaundice and signs of liver disease. Examination may be normal or there may be tenderness in the right upper quadrant. Occasionally adherent omentum to a previously inflamed gall bladder may produce a right upper quadrant mass.

Investigations

LFTs may be normal or demonstrate obstructive jaundice. USS detects gallstones and the presence of a dilated CBD. OGD and/or barium enema is used in selected patients to exclude co-existing disorders.

Treatment

Treatment is usually surgical. The current surgical standard is laparoscopic cholecystectomy. Advantages claimed for the laparoscopic approach include less pain, absence of ileus, day-case surgery, back to work in 10–14 days, less wound infection, less chest infection and less wound dehiscence. Warn the patient that the operation may be converted to an open procedure if there is dense fibrosis in Calot's triangle, severe adhesions from previous surgery, Mirizzi's syndrome or severe acute disease with inflammatory oedema. Conversion rate is widely reported as 5%.

Mini-cholecystectomy is an open cholecystectomy via a 5cm subcostal incision with use of a circular retractor. There is little evidence now to support its routine use.

Follow-up

Straightforward cases can be reviewed in 4–6 weeks with the results of investigations. If there are atypical features to the history or examination, review sooner.

Post-operative follow-up

Review uncomplicated cases in 4–6 weeks after surgery with histology. If histology confirms chronic cholecystitis and the patient is symptom-free, discharge. Complications include wound infection, incisional hernia and wound pain. Long-term complications include duct injury (which may present as progressive jaundice); damage to duodenum, jejunum and colon; and abscess formation around lost stones.

Persistence of original symptoms may be due to residual stones or alternative causes of abdominal pain and is known as post-cholecystectomy syndrome.

Other treatments for gallstones

Remember, cholecystectomy is the treatment of choice.

Cholecystolithotomy

This procedure is indicated in patients with a previous vagotomy for ulcer disease in the presence of a functioning gall bladder (demonstrated on biliary scintiscan). Vagotomised patients frequently develop symptomatic gallstones, but if a functioning gall bladder is removed a high percentage develop debilitating explosive diarrhoea. Therefore cholecystectomy is not performed and removal of the stones followed by oral bile salt therapy is the appropriate treatment. However, cholecystectomy is the right treatment if the gall bladder is non-functioning.

Dissolution by methyl tert-butyl ether (MTBE)

This dissolves cholesterol stones in hours via a pigtail catheter inserted radiologically in the gall bladder. It is left in the gall bladder a few hours then aspirated. It may cause damage if it escapes into the CBD or duodenum – it is best used in a non-functioning gall bladder. The main indication for use is in poor-risk patients or those who have had a previous vagotomy.

Extracorporeal shock wave lithotripsy

There is successful stone fragmentation in 80% of patients with solitary small gallstones. It fails if stones are larger than 3cm, multiple or calcified. Repeat treatments are frequently required. Maintenance therapy with bile salts is required. Recurrence rates are 50% at five years. Therefore the current role is restricted to fragmentation of occluding ductal calculi in jaundiced patients. It is not routine – 50% of patients require additional procedures to achieve stone removal.

Oral dissolution

This is only applicable to patients with a functioning gall bladder (on biliary scintiscan). Chenodeoxycholic and ursodeoxycholic oral bile salts result in dissolution after several weeks or months. Maintenance with ursodeoxycholate is then required. Recurrence is 12.5% after the first year, 61% by the eleventh year. The technique fails if the gallstone load is large (larger than 3cm or multiple) and/or stones are calcified. Bile salt therapy is restricted to patients in whom cholecystectomy is contraindicated, either as a primary treatment or after gallstone extraction, fragmentation or dissolution by MTBE.

Acalculous chronic gall bladder disease

There are two variations:
- adenomyomatosis of the gall bladder: diverticular formation of the epithelial lining
- cholesterolosis of the gall bladder: epithelial cells and macrophages in the gall bladder mucosa become laden with cholesterol, inducing chronic inflammation – the strawberry gall bladder.

Objectives

Diagnose the cause, differentiate from other causes of abdominal pain including gallstone disease, differentiate from cancer of the gall bladder, treat the cause.

History

Vague symptoms similar to chronic cholecystitis, but no gallstones.

Examination

This may be normal or there may be tenderness in right upper quadrant.

Investigations

USS normal or thickening of the gall bladder wall.

Treatment

Treat with cholecystectomy.

Follow-up

Straightforward cases can be reviewed in 4–6 weeks with results of investigations. If there are atypical features to the history or examination, review sooner.

Post-operative follow-up

Review uncomplicated cases in 4–6 weeks after surgery with histology. If histology confirms chronic cholecystitis, and the patient is symptom-free, discharge.

Mucocele of the gall bladder

There is a grossly distended gall bladder associated with cystic duct obstruction, usually by a stone, but it does not result in inflammation or infection. The gall bladder is filled with mucoid material.

Objectives

Diagnose mucocele, differentiate from other causes of abdominal pain and from cancer of the biliary tract, treat mucocele.

History

Take a biliary history. Patients are usually elderly and present with a painless mass in the right hypochondrium. There may be a history of acute pain in the right upper quadrant, like biliary colic or acute cholecystitis.

Examination

Patients are usually not jaundiced. Look for a painless mass in the right upper quadrant.

Investigations

LFTs are usually normal. USS shows distended gall bladder but normal CBD diameter.

Treatment

Treat with cholecystectomy.

Follow-up

Follow up at short intervals of 2–4 weeks until malignant obstruction of the biliary system is excluded.

Post-operative follow-up

Review in 4–6 weeks after surgery with histology. If histology confirms chronic cholecystitis and the patient is symptom-free, discharge.

Ductal calculi

These are mostly in the CBD; 5% are in intrahepatic ducts, more commonly in the left system of ducts. They arise as either secondary calculi from migration of gallstones or as primary calculi arising *de novo* within bile ducts. The predisposing factors to primary duct stones include stasis in the biliary tract caused by strictures, parasitic infestations, recurrent pyogenic cholangitis and indwelling stent. Stone impaction may result in progressive jaundice, cholangitis, gallstone pancreatitis, secondary biliary cirrhosis and portal hypertension.

Objectives

Diagnose the cause, differentiate from other causes of pain/jaundice, treat the cause.

History

Take a general biliary history; 15–20% of duct stones are asymptomatic. Symptoms include recurrent bouts of biliary colic (with or without jaundice), episodic upper abdominal pain and dyspepsia.

Examination

Perform a general examination. Examination may be normal. The patient may or may not be jaundiced. Examine for scars from previous biliary surgery, tenderness in the RUQ and evidence of liver disease.

Investigations

LFTs reveal obstructive jaundice. USS detects a dilated bile duct system. MRCP defines the anatomy and the obstruction, whereas ERCP does the same but can be combined with sphincterotomy or endoscopic stent placement.

Treatment

Ductal calculi found incidentally during intra-operative cholangiography

Stones less than 2mm diameter can be left alone, as more than 95% pass spontaneously. If they become symptomatic, remove them at ERCP. Stones larger than 2mm and smaller than 10mm can be removed by intra-operative duct exploration (laparoscopic or open) or by post-operative ERCP. Post-operative ERCP stone extraction is likely to fail for stones larger than 10mm diameter, and these are best removed surgically.

Ductal calculi without previous cholecystectomy

A cholecystectomy and common bile duct exploration can be performed either open or laparoscopically. In young patients with small CBD, explore and clear the duct and insert a T-tube. If there are multiple ductal calculi and/or a grossly dilated duct, some form of drainage may be required, e.g. hepatico-jejunostomy Roux-en-Y. If the patient is elderly or a poor operative risk, then perform ERCP and stone extraction, and reserve cholecystectomy for those who develop symptoms.

Patients with ductal calculi prior to laparoscopic cholecystectomy

Two procedures are possible.
- Pre-operative ERCP and sphincterotomy – but this carries the risk of combined morbidity of two procedures and the unknown risk of sphincterotomy in the under-50 age group.

✧ Combined open or laparoscopic cholecystectomy and exploration of common bile duct.

Ductal calculi discovered after cholecystectomy and exploration of CBD

Missed stones are rare where intra-operative choledochoscopy is used, but the incidence increases to 8% for completion T-tube cholangiography.

Treat by post-operative ERCP and sphincterotomy utilising flushing and drug-induced relaxation of the sphincter of Oddi. Other alternatives include dissolution with MTBE or percutaneous stone extraction via the T-tube tract, performed after 4–6 weeks of tract maturation. If stones are not detected during or soon after surgery (if cholangiogram was not performed or a T-tube was not inserted at operation), recurrent symptoms from missed stones usually occur within two years of cholecystectomy. Ductal stones presenting beyond this period are generally considered to be primary.

Recurrent ductal calculi

These are often multiple and associated with gross dilatation of the bile duct with or without duct stenosis. Duct stenosis may be primary (papillary stenosis) or secondary to previous bile duct exploration. Treat by either ERCP and sphincterotomy or surgically with hepatico-jejunostomy Roux-en-Y.

Multiple intrahepatic calculi

These are common in the east, associated with strictures of the hepatic ducts. Treatment is standard operative choledochotomy and stone extraction, transhepatic lithotomy and resection of the involved lobe.

Follow-up

Follow up at short intervals of 1–4 weeks until cancer is excluded and to prevent deterioration from jaundice. Consider admission and further investigation as an in-patient if the patient is frail or shows evidence of liver dysfunction.

Post-operative follow-up

Follow up until the patient is symptom-free and LFTs return to normal. When stable, discharge with advice regarding late development of bile duct strictures.

Cholangitis

Cholangitis is infection of an obstructed biliary tract. Systemic symptoms result from bacteraemia secondary to cholangiovenous reflux induced by biliary hypertension. Most commonly the obstruction is due to a stone; bile duct strictures; tumours of the bile duct and pancreatic head; and periampullary lesions. Less commonly it is due to bilioenteric anastomoses, spontaneous bilioenteric fistulas, cystic disease of the biliary tract and duodenal diverticula.

History

Take a general biliary history. The classical Charcot's triad of symptoms are pain in RUQ, intermittent fever/rigours and jaundice. Rigours are severe and nausea and vomiting are frequent.

Examination

Perform a general examination. Commonly there is tenderness in the right upper quadrant. Clinically apparent jaundice may not be present in the early stages.

Investigations

Treatment should not wait for the results of investigations. LFTs and USS confirm the diagnosis. Perform blood cultures, FBC, coagulation screen and U&E to detect renal impairment.

Treatment

Treatment is admission to hospital and resuscitation with oxygen, intravenous fluids and antibiotics; and urgent biliary decompression, e.g. ERCP and sphincterotomy/stent or percutaneous transhepatic biliary drainage. Specific treatment is then directed at the underlying cause. Watch out for concomitant renal failure.

Follow-up

Depends on the underlying condition and the treatment performed.

Post-operative follow-up

If a cholecystectomy and exploration of common bile duct was performed, this is followed up in the usual way: review histology, determine the presence of complications. Discharge once the patient is symptom-free and no other treatment is indicated. Advise regarding the late development of strictures.

Bilioenteric fistulas

Bilioenteric fistulas are an abnormal connection between the biliary system and other viscera. Bilioenteric fistulas can be classified as either internal or external.
- ✧ External fistulas communicate with the skin and are caused either by trauma or as a complication of surgery or therapeutic intervention, e.g. T-tube, stents, cholecystectomy.
- ✧ Internal fistulas occur between a variety of organs and are caused by a variety of pathologies (*see* Table 8.3)

TABLE 8.3 Causes of internal biliary fistulas.

INTERNAL BILIARY FISTULAS	PATHOLOGY
Bilioenteric	
Cholecystoduodenal	Gallstones
Cholecystocolic	Gallstones, carcinoma
Cholecystogastric	Gallstones, carcinoma, peptic ulceration
Choledochoduodenal	Ductal calculi, iatrogenic, duodenal ulcer, carcinoma
Bilio-bilial	
Cholecystocholedochal	Gallstones (Mirizzi's syndrome)
Others	
Broncho/pleuro-bilial	Trauma, operative injuries, liver abscesses/hydatid, subphrenic abscess
Cholecystorenal	Gallstones

Objectives

Diagnose fistula, determine underlying pathology, treat fistula, treat the underlying cause.

History

Take a general biliary history. Symptoms of non-malignant internal fistulas involving the gall bladder are similar to chronic cholecystitis, but jaundice and cholangitis are more common.

Examination

Perform a general examination. Examine for jaundice or evidence of underlying sepsis. Examine the chest. Examine for abdominal masses or tenderness.

Investigations

LFTs show general derangement, USS and AXR may show gas in the biliary tree. FBC may reveal anaemia and a raised WCC. U&Es may reveal renal impairment and blood cultures.

Treatment

Treat the underlying gallstone disease with cholecystectomy and closure of the fistula. For Mirizzi's syndrome, leave a cuff of gall bladder to close the fistulous opening. CBD is explored through a choledochotomy lower down. Management of bronchobiliary fistulas consists of adequate drainage of the hepatic/subphrenic abscess and decompression of the biliary tract.

Follow-up

Follow up at short intervals of 1–2 weeks to confirm the diagnosis, to prevent deterioration from the underlying condition and to exclude neoplastic causes. Consider admission for investigation and treatment.

Post-operative follow-up

This depends on the treatment and procedure performed. Review with regard to the histology and post-operative complications related to cholecystectomy and exploration of bile ducts. Monitor for the detection of bile duct stenoses with regular estimation of LFTs, USS and MRCP if necessary. Discharge once the patient is symptom-free and LFTs are normal, with advice regarding the late development of bile duct stenoses.

Gallstone ileus

This rare condition is caused by an intraluminal intestinal obstruction by a large gallstone subsequent to the establishment of a fistula, usually between gall bladder and duodenum.

History/examination

There is a history of gall bladder disease and it presents with small bowel obstruction. Elderly patients present with small bowel obstruction and air in the biliary tree.

Investigations

LFTs, USS, AXR shows air in the biliary tree. CT scan for anatomical information.

Treatment

Treat with surgery – enterolithotomy, check for other gallstones in the gut. The cholecysto-duodenal fistula should be left intact unless at a specialist centre.

Follow-up/post-operative follow-up

Follow up as for bilioenteric fistula.

Post-cholecystectomy syndrome

This syndrome is the persistence of symptoms referable to the biliary tract after cholecystectomy (excludes diseases outside the biliary tract). A careful history and investigation with laboratory tests, MRCP and/or ERCP is advised in all patients. Common causes are the following.

✧ Retained or recurrent calculi: diagnose and treat by ERCP.
✧ Gall bladder or cystic duct remnants: diagnosed if operative note indicates leaving gall bladder remnants behind or cholecystotomy was performed. USS and ERCP are useful to confirm diagnosis and exclude other causes. Treat by cholecystectomy.
✧ Bile duct strictures and other unrecognised iatrogenic injuries (choledochoduodenal fistula).
✧ Papillary stenosis, sphincter of Oddi dysfunction (SOD) syndrome and biliary dyskinesia.

Papillary stenosis
Fibrosis or fibromuscular hyperplasia of the sphincter of Oddi.

History
Pain similar to chronic cholecystitis.

Examination
Normal, or slight tenderness in right upper quadrant.

Investigations
LFTs show a slight derangement, including hyperbilirubinaemia and raised alkaline phosphatase. USS may demonstrate duct dilatation. ERCP shows the transduodenal segment of duct wider than the intrapancreatic segment. Biliary sludge and small calculi are often present. The resting sphincter pressure is raised and the normal phasic sphincter activity is lost.

Treatment
Treat with ERCP and sphincterotomy or with operative transduodenal sphincteroplasty.

Biliary dyskinesia
There is persistent pain after cholecystectomy but no abnormality on examination and routine investigations. The following abnormalities are demonstrated during ERCP manometry:
✧ elevated resting pressure
✧ tachyarrhythmia (increased phasic activity of the sphincter)
✧ retrograde contractions of the sphincter
✧ paradoxical response to cholecystokinin.

Treatment
Treat with ERCP and sphincterotomy.

Benign bile duct strictures
Most common causes are secondary to operative trauma. Untreated, the late consequences are liver fibrosis, secondary biliary cirrhosis and development of portal hypertension. Strictures may develop many years after cholecystectomy. Alternatively, damage to the CBD or CHD may present in the immediate post-operative period with development of an external biliary fistula associated with sepsis and development of subphrenic/subhepatic abscess. Peritonitis may occur and jaundice is often present but may not be severe or progressive. Other causes of bile duct strictures include: penetrating and non-penetrating abdominal injuries, chronic duodenal ulcer, chronic pancreatitis, recurrent pyogenic cholecystitis and parasitic infestations, sclerosing cholangitis.

Objectives

Diagnose stricture, detect the underlying cause, differentiate from neoplastic causes, detect liver dysfunction, treat stricture, treat the underlying cause, correct liver dysfunction.

History

Take a general biliary history. Commonly there is a history of previous biliary surgery. Determine the details of this: ask about length of stay and whether there were any complications at the time. The patient may complain of colicky RUQ pain similar to chronic cholecystitis or may present with mild painless jaundice. Ask about symptoms which would suggest any of the other causes.

Examination

Perform a general examination. May be normal or mildly jaundiced. Tenderness may be present in the RUQ.

Investigations

LFTs show raised bilirubin and alkaline phosphatase. USS may show a dilated intrahepatic duct system and evidence of portal hypertension. In stable patients MRCP is an excellent non-invasive method of visualising the biliary tree. ERCP or PTC or both can be further used to determine the relevant anatomy of the abnormality and provide information to assist reconstruction and treat the underlying condition. Liver biopsy may be indicated if cirrhosis is suspected.

Treatment

Treat with ERCP – balloon dilatation and indwelling stent for several months. But the majority of injuries require surgical repair in a specialist centre, as the correct treatment depends on accurate classification of the injury (e.g. Bismuth classification I –V). Numerous surgical procedures are possible depending on the exact injury, but most involve the use of a Roux-en-Y hepatico-jejunostomy. Best results are obtained with the first surgical repair and so should be performed in a specialist centre.

Follow-up

Follow up at short intervals of 1–4 weeks until diagnosis is confirmed and malignant causes excluded. Following repair of bile duct injuries there is a high incidence of further stricture formation and the development of biliary cirrhosis and portal hypertension. Therefore, these patients require long-term follow-up with USS and LFTs at regular intervals.

Sclerosing cholangitis

This is an obscure disorder of uncertain aetiology that results in progressive fibrous obliteration of the biliary tract. It is currently considered to be an autoimmune disorder. There were previously two categories: 'primary' where there was no previous biliary surgery or biliary tract disease; and 'secondary' where there was previous biliary surgery or biliary tract disease. However, both categories are often associated with inflammatory bowel disease (usually ulcerative colitis, occasionally Crohn's). Classification is based on the extent of involvement of the biliary tree: total diffuse, localised hilar, diffuse intrahepatic, diffuse extrahepatic and localised extrahepatic distal.

The disease progresses inevitably to cirrhosis and development of portal hypertension. Patients have a high risk of developing cholangiocarcinoma.

Objectives

Diagnose sclerosing cholangitis (especially in patients with UC or Crohn's), exclude cholangiocarcinoma, classify the disease, detect the degree of liver impairment, treat sclerosing cholangitis, treat the liver impairment.

History

Take a general biliary history. Look for vague ill health, asthenia, pain in the RUQ, jaundice, itching, pyrexia and attacks of rigours.

Examination

Perform a general examination. Examine for jaundice, anaemia and signs of liver disease. Examination may be normal but the liver is palpable and tender, the spleen is enlarged and jaundice is present in approximately 50%.

Investigations

LFTs show a cholestatic pattern but the alkaline phosphatase is often elevated out of proportion to the bilirubin. Most patients are hepatitis B surface antigen (HBsAg) negative. Antimitochondrial, anti-smooth muscle and antinuclear antibodies are absent – if present, suspect primary biliary cirrhosis. MRCP/ERCP/PTC show ducts are smaller in number and size with stricture formation. Saccular dilated areas between strictures are seen in diffuse disease. Differentiation from hilar and diffuse cholangiocarcinoma is difficult even with histology obtained from biopsies, or cytology from brushings at ERCP.

Treatment

Pruritus is controlled by cholestyramine and ursodeoxycholate. Cholangitis episodes are managed by intravenous antibiotics with or without stenting. Progressive jaundice and recurrent cholangitis are indications for surgical intervention. The aim of surgical treatment is to treat dominant strictures.

In the absence of cirrhosis, occasionally good results in localised disease have been obtained by ERCP or percutaneous balloon dilatation and stent insertion. Surgical options include Roux-en-Y hepatico-jejunostomy or intra-operative dilatation and external stent insertion. The stent is left in for 12 months and progress assessed by cholangiograms performed through the stent.

Diffuse disease or the presence of cirrhosis requires hepatic transplantation. Unexpected cholangiocarcinomas have been reported in 8% of livers removed during liver transplantation.

Follow-up

Follow up at short intervals until diagnosis is confirmed and cholangiocarcinoma excluded. Then follow up long term. Treat mild cases expectantly and monitor for the development of complications.

Post-operative follow-up

This depends on the operation and procedures performed. Review with histology and for the detection of complications of biliary surgery. Then provide long-term monitoring for the recurrence of symptoms or development of stenoses, using LFTs and USS, ERCP. Take a HIDA scan if stenoses of bilioenteric anastomoses are suspected.

Biliary disorders in AIDS

AIDS patients are prone to developing acute acalculous cholecystitis, papillary stenosis and abnormalities of the bile ducts similar to sclerosing cholangitis. Papillary stenosis and cholangiopathy produce symptoms of pain and raised bilirubin and alkaline phosphatase, and are diagnosed by ERCP and treated appropriately. The treatment for acalculous cholecystitis is cholecystectomy.

Recurrent pyogenic cholangitis

Recurrent pyogenic cholangitis is prevalent in Southeast Asia. It may occur in immuno-compromised people. There are recurrent bouts of bacterial cholangitis leading to formation of pigment stones and strictures. It affects intra- and extrahepatic ducts with a predilection for the left lobe of the liver.

History

Attacks of RUQ pain and rigours. May develop jaundice.

Examination

May be normal or tender RUQ. Mild jaundice.

Investigations

Investigate with obstructive LFTs and duct dilatation on USS. Diagnosed by ERCP.

Treatment

Treatment is surgery (of strictures and stones).

Duodenal diverticula

Duodenal diverticula are present in 12.5% of patients undergoing ERCP. They are usually asymptomatic but their significance in this situation is that they are associated with an increased incidence of post-procedural bacterial infection and can make ERCP technically difficult to perform.

Haemobilia

This is rare upper gastrointestinal bleeding originating from the biliary system. Causes include iatrogenic percutaneous radiological intervention; liver biopsy; blunt or penetrating trauma; extrahepatic bile duct tumours. Diagnosis and treatment is by selective mesenteric angiography and embolisation.

Tumours of the gall bladder
Benign tumours

Benign tumours are adenomas and papillomas. They are usually an incidental finding on USS during investigation of RUQ pain. Treatment is by cholecystectomy to exclude carcinoma. At post-operative follow-up determine that no malignant focus was detected and that excision was complete.

Carcinoma of gall bladder

This is often incidental on the histology report after cholecystectomy. Female to male ratio is 3:1 and it is more common in the over-65 age group. Gallstones are present in 75–90% of cases. The majority are adenocarcinomas. Rare types are neuroendocrine tumours and melanoma. If detected pre-operatively these tumours can be difficult to differentiate from Klatskin tumours or even Mirizzi's syndrome.

History

Often presents as chronic cholecystitis. Additional non-specific symptoms may be anorexia, nausea and vomiting and weight loss.

Examination

Normal or inflammatory mass in the RUQ or acute cholecystitis. In advanced cases there may be jaundice, enlarged liver and a palpable gall bladder. In very advanced cases there may be ascites. Anaemia is present in 50% due to haemobilia.

Investigations

LFTs may have raised alkaline phosphatase even if bilirubin is normal. FBC may show iron-deficiency anaemia. USS tends to identify only advanced cases. CT scan is more informative. AXR occasionally identifies the intramural calcification of a 'porcelain' gall bladder. Porcelain gall bladder is a pre-malignant condition. ERCP/PTC are usually needed to define these lesions. Also, the involvement of segment V duct by a gall bladder mass is indicative of cancer.

Staging

Staging is as follows.
- ✧ I: confined to mucosa/submucosa.
- ✧ II: involvement of the muscle layer.
- ✧ III: serosal involvement.
- ✧ IV: spread to cystic node.
- ✧ V: invasion of liver and adjacent organs.

Treatment

Stage I–II disease is treated by cholecystectomy. Porcelain gall bladders require resection. Stage III-IV needs extended right hepatectomy with excision of the biliary tree and lymphadenectomy. Response to radiotherapy and chemotherapy is poor.

Follow-up

Follow up at short intervals until diagnosis is confirmed and treatment is instituted.

Post-operative follow-up

Review within 2–4 weeks with histology and complete the staging process. Detect any post-operative complications. Thereafter follow-up is long term to detect recurrence and institute palliative therapy. Overall five-year survival is 5%. For surgically resectable cases it is 25%. Prolonged survival has been recorded for types I and II.

Tumours of the bile ducts

Benign tumours

These are adenomas and papillomas – rarer than carcinomas. They have a tendency to recur after excision. They present with jaundice and haemobilia (anaemia).

Malignant tumours (cholangiocarcinoma)

The tumours are classified according to position.
- ✧ Intrahepatic: minor hepatic ducts.
- ✧ Proximal: right and left hepatic ducts, hilar confluence and proximal common hepatic duct (Klatskin tumours).
- ✧ Middle: from distal common hepatic duct, cystic duct and confluence with common bile duct.
- ✧ Distal: from common bile duct to periampullary region.

There are three forms.
- ✧ Stricture: difficult to differentiate from sclerosing cholangitis.
- ✧ Nodular: form extraductal nodules.
- ✧ Papillary: friable tumour in the distal duct tends to produce haemobilia.

Cholangiocarcinomas grow slowly, infiltrate locally and metastasise late. They have a special predilection for perineural spread and rarely metastasise beyond the liver.

Objectives
Diagnose tumour, differentiate from other lesions, classify tumour, determine resectability, treat tumour, follow up to detect recurrence.

History
Take a general biliary history. The main presentation (90%) is with progressive, obstructive jaundice accompanied by itching and anorexia. They may also complain of a dull upper abdominal pain. Alternatively, presentation may be acute, with cholangitis or cholecystitis. Duration of symptoms is usually short and measured in months.

Examination
Perform a general examination. Anaemia may be due to haemobilia, especially with periampullary lesions. Stools may have a silvery appearance due to steatorrhoea and blood. Hepatomegaly may be present or there may be a palpable gall bladder in distal tumours. There may be a scar from previous cholecystectomy (an operative cholangiogram should never be passed as normal unless there is adequate and complete filling of the intrahepatic biliary tree).

Investigations
LFTs may show an obstructive pattern with a raised alkaline phosphatase and bilirubin and low albumin indicating impaired nutritional status. FBC may reveal an iron-deficiency anaemia. Clotting may be abnormal. CEA and CA19 are often elevated. USS identifies dilatation of biliary tree.

A triple-phase CT scan gives more detailed information about anatomy and the extent of arterial and venous involvement. CT can also be used for needle biopsy to confirm the diagnosis. MRCP can now give a detailed pre-operative road map of the biliary system.

ERCP/PTC are needed for decompression of the biliary tree and transbiliary biopsy can be performed. Coeliac axis angiography is sometimes performed to delineate vascular anatomy and tumour involvement at the hilum, although colour Duplex is a less invasive alternative.

Treatment
Surgical resection gives the best chance of cure and also offers the best means of palliation. Hilar lesions are treated by an extended right or left hepatectomy with resection of the caudate lobe and by resection of tumour and extrahepatic biliary tree with hepatico-jejunostomy.

Mid-duct tumours can be treated by extrahepatic biliary tree excision alone, provided the proximal resection margins are negative.

Periampullary tumours need a pancreatico-duodenectomy. Approximately 20% of lesions are resectable.

Irresectable lesions are treated by a surgical biliary bypass (Roux loop to segment III duct) or by percutaneous transhepatic or endoscopic stenting. Intracavity irradiation through stents is possible.

Photodynamic therapy can be used to treat unresectable tumours. This involves the administration of a photosensitising drug that accumulates in cancer cells, followed by exposure of the tumour to the appropriate wavelength of light. This results in tumour destruction by the activation of the photosensitiser. These tumours have a poor response to chemotherapy.

Follow-up
Follow up at short intervals (2–4 weeks) until diagnosis is established and treatment is instituted.

Post-operative follow-up
Follow-up is long term at regular 3–6 monthly intervals. Five-year survival is 30% for distal and periampullary tumours. If there is diffuse intrahepatic disease, most patietns die within one year. Five-year survival for proximal lesions is 5–15%. Recurrence of jaundice may indicate anastomotic stenosis or tumour recurrence, which can be treated by stenting.

Biliary parasites
Ascaris lumbricoides
Presentation is with biliary colic, pancreatitis, cholangitis, cholecystitis and eosinophilia. Plain radiography may show calcified worms and ultrasound can show linear filling defects that move. Treatment is ERCP, and removal of worms with laparotomy is only performed following endoscopic failure. Antihelminthic therapy kills the worms but they still need to be removed.

Clonorchis sinensis
This causes cholangitis and septicaemia. It is associated with development of bile duct carcinoma. It is diagnosed by finding typical ova in the faeces. It can be treated by chloroquine 300 mg for 2–6 months but relapse is common. The bile ducts must be cleared of worms and stones (surgically if endoscopic methods fail).

The pancreas
The pancreas serves endocrine and exocrine functions. The common bile duct runs through it. It is in close proximity to the stomach, duodenum, small bowel, large bowel, spleen, kidneys, portal vein and vena cava, while being tucked away in the retroperitoneum. Unfortunately the gland is prone to inflammation and tumour formation.

Tumours in the head of the pancreas and lesions of the body and tail of the pancreas present with very different symptoms and signs. Lesions in the head of the pancreas tend to obstruct the common bile duct and present with obstructive jaundice, while lesions affecting the body and tail of the gland have a more insidious presentation with weight loss and pain as their primary symptoms.

Lesions of the exocrine pancreas produce symptoms and signs of malabsorption, while lesions of the endocrine pancreas produce a variety of endocrine syndromes, e.g. diabetes mellitus and a wide range of syndromes associated with autonomous secretion of pancreatic and enteric hormones, e.g. insulinoma, gastrinoma, glucaconoma.

Inflammation of the gland is known as pancreatitis. Acute pancreatitis may be severe and life-threatening. Chronic pancreatitis can run a relapsing course with gradual destruction of the whole gland.

Assessment of pancreatic disorders
Pancreatic history
Start with a general gastrointestinal history. When responses indicate a possible pancreatic problem, a more detailed pancreatic history is required.
- Pain: site, severity, radiation, exacerbating and relieving factors.
- Jaundice: general questions regarding the aetiology of jaundice. Is the jaundice painless?
- Endocrine function: symptoms attributable to diabetes mellitus or, if indicated, symptoms associated with rare disorders, e.g. insulinoma, Zollinger-Ellison.
- Exocrine function: symptoms of weight loss and malabsorption, fat intolerance, frequent greasy stools that are difficult to flush away and foul smelling.

✧ Aetiological factors for pancreatitis: gallstones, previous biliary surgery or interventions, alcohol intake, hyperlipidaemia, hypercalcaemia, medications.
✧ Effect on other organs: symptoms attributable to liver failure, biliary obstruction, portal hypertension and hypersplenism, gastric outlet obstruction.

Pancreatic examination

Perform a general examination and in particular look for signs of weight loss, anaemia and jaundice; evidence of liver disease; upper abdominal mass; liver and spleen enlargement; portal hypertension; palpable gall bladder.

Investigation of pancreatic disorders

The methods of investigation include imaging, assessments of endocrine and exocrine function, analysis of serum markers of pancreatic disease and pancreatic biopsy for cytology/histology.

Laboratory investigations

Haematology

FBC may reveal anaemia due to a haemobilia or chronic disease. Leucopenia and thrombocytopenia may indicate hypersplenism secondary to splenic vein thrombosis. Clotting may be impaired in the presence of liver disease.

Biochemistry

✧ Liver function tests may reveal a cholestatic picture with a raised alkaline phosphatase. Raised bilirubin may indicate bile duct obstruction, while a raised gamma GT may indicate alcohol abuse.
✧ Blood sugar may reveal diabetes mellitus.
✧ Serum amylase is particularly useful in the acute setting for the diagnosis of acute pancreatitis but is not elevated in chronic pancreatitis. A raised serum amylase may be a marker of pancreatic trauma. Serum lipase is more sensitive and specific in the diagnosis of acute pancreatitis, but not routinely available.

Exocrine Function

Faecal fat excretion

A stool examination for fat is useful only for malabsorption. However, 80% of pancreatic secreting capacity may be lost without detection by the test.

Direct measurement

Direct measurement of pancreatic, digestive and secretory function is mainly used as a research tool, but these are the best tests for diagnosis of pancreatic exocrine insufficiency. The concentrations of bicarbonate and pancreatic enzymes are measured in duodenal juice after stimulation by a meal (Lundh test) or injection of secretin/cholecystokinin (secretin-pancreozymin test).

The faecal elastase test is easy to perform. Absence of elastase in faeces indicates exocrine insufficiency.

✧ No request forms are available. Specialised tests are not routinely available.
✧ Results are given as a written report.
✧ The advantage is that it provides a direct measurement of pancreatic exocrine function.
✧ The disadvantages are that the tests are invasive, expensive and only available in specialised centres.

Endocrine function

Fasting levels of glucose and/or hormones secreted by islets – insulin, proinsulin, C-peptide, glucagon, somatostatin and gastrin – are measured.

Provocative tests are used to measure serum level if fasting levels are not conclusive. For example, calcium perfusion of insulinomas and gastrinomas at angiography can cause a spurt of hormone release.

✧ There is no request form. Specialised tests are arranged by a clinician with a special interest or direct contact with a clinical biochemist to discuss the conditions for performing the tests.

✧ Results are given as a written report.

✧ The advantage is that direct information regarding the level of hormones often provides the diagnosis.

✧ The disadvantage is that specialised tests are not routinely available. They often require specialised biochemical analysis.

✧ Tumour markers include CEA and CA19-9.

Imaging techniques

Indirect imaging

Abdominal X-ray

An AXR may visualise the effect of the pancreas on adjacent organs, e.g. the colon cut-off sign may indicate displacement, stricture or fistula of the transverse colon. Calcification usually indicates chronic pancreatitis (though occasionally radiating sunburst calcification may be seen in cystadenoma or cystadenocarcinoma). A CXR may occasionally demonstrate a pancreatic pseudocyst in the posterior mediastinum.

Small bowel contrast series

This may show effacement or hypertrophy of folds in malabsorption secondary to chronic pancreatitis. Enlargement of the pancreatic head may cause widening of the C-loop of the duodenum and/or displacement of the angle of Treitz, e.g. advanced pancreatic carcinoma. Contrast studies may also reveal post-bulbar duodenal ulceration, which is characteristic of Zollinger-Ellison syndrome.

Direct imaging

Direct imaging of pancreatic parenchyma is provided by USS, CT and MRI. ERCP images the pancreatic duct system. Angiography images the pancreatic and peripancreatic vasculature. The newer techniques of MRCP and endoscopic ultrasound (EUS) are being increasingly used.

Ultrasound

Acoustic water-based gel is applied and an ultrasound probe manipulated over the abdomen by the sonographer.

✧ The request form is from radiology/ultrasound (check if your department uses the same or different forms).

✧ Results are in a written report compiled by the radiologist or sonographer and a selection of ultrasound photographs.

✧ The advantages are that it is a non-invasive technique. Indicators of pancreatic disease include diffuse or localised atrophy, alteration of texture and dilated bile duct. Abnormal dilatation of the pancreatic duct may be a result of cancer or chronic pancreatitis. EUS is excellent for chronic pancreatitis and endocrine tumours.

✧ The disadvantages are that it is operator dependent; the non-visualisation rate is 10–15%; only 50% of changes caused by chronic pancreatitis are detected by USS; and there is poor visualisation in the obese and when gaseous distension of the bowel is present.

CT scan

Multislice helical CT scanners can now examine the pancreas with 5mm slices and when combined with contrast, arterial and venous phase images can give detailed pancreatic anatomy.

✧ The request form is from radiology or is a specific CT request form.
✧ Results are as a written report by the radiologist and a selection of still CT images.
✧ The advantages are that it gives better visualisation of the gland than USS, especially in the presence of ascites or obesity and it is better at detection of calcification, gas, dilatation, small intrapancreatic pseudocysts and thicker walls of pancreatic abscess. The most valuable sign is localised or diffuse enlargement of the gland.
✧ The disadvantages are the use of radiation and that the procedure is expensive.

ERCP

A large-bore side-viewing endoscope is passed into the second part of the duodenum. The duodenal papilla is cannulated and contrast injected under X-ray screening. The pancreatic and biliary duct system is visualised. Brushings or biopsy can be performed to provide a tissue diagnosis. A stent can be placed.

✧ The request form is an endoscopy/radiology form. This is a joint procedure between the radiology department and the endoscopy service.
✧ Results are in a written report and selection of ERCP images.
✧ The advantages are that it allows diagnosis of a wide range of pancreatic conditions; the obtaining direct tissue samples; and the placing of a stent to relieve obstruction. It is good for diagnosis of ductal calculi, tumours of the bile duct and pancreas and sclerosing cholangitis.
✧ The disadvantages are complications, including pancreatitis(1%) – if sphincterotomy is also performed complications rise to 6–10% and include haemorrhage, acute pancreatitis, cholangitis, retroperitoneal perforation, impacted Dormia basket, acute cholecystitis and gallstone ileus; technical failure may result in patients with duodenal stenosis, previous Billroth II and duodenal diverticula – and in an unco-operative patient. In patients with complete biliary obstruction the proximal biliary tree may not be visualised and PTC is then indicated.

Angiography

Angiography generally requires admission to hospital, although some centres do this as a day-case. Under local anaesthetic, the femoral artery is cannulated and a catheter manipulated into the coeliac and superior mesenteric arteries. Contrast is injected and X-rays taken.

✧ The request form is from radiology.
✧ Results are in a written report from the radiologist and a selection of angiography images.
✧ Useful signs include arterial encasement – narrowing or irregularity of a vessel caused by invasion of tumour. Smooth encasement may be caused by chronic pancreatitis. Major venous involvement may indicate similar disease but is not as reliable. Angiography defines arterial variability for resection purposes.
✧ The disadvantages are that it is an invasive technique; and risks include haematoma at the puncture site. It is being replaced by reconstruction of vascular anatomy from CT or MR images, and by Duplex ultrasound. Angiography still has a role in localising pancreatic neuroendocrine tumours such as insulinomas, using selective calcium stimulation.

Diagnostic laparoscopy and intra-operative ultrasound

Under general anaesthetic a laparoscopy is performed, which enables direct visualisation of the intra-abdominal structures, in particular the liver and biliary system. Through a second port a special intra-operative ultrasound probe is inserted, which enables ultrasound images of the pancreas to be obtained. Biopsy of lesions can be performed under direct vision. The yield is higher the greater the extent of the exploration done by the surgeon.

✧ There is no request form.
✧ Results are an operation note and a selection of printed ultrasound images.
✧ The advantages are that direct visualisation of the liver can be obtained, which may reveal multiple small metastases; and better ultrasound images of the pancreas can be obtained. This can give valuable information regarding resectability before resorting to a full laparotomy.
✧ The disadvantage is that it is an invasive operative procedure.

Disorders of the pancreas
Congenital anomalies of the pancreas

✧ Ectopic pancreas presents with abdominal pain similar to peptic ulceration. It occasionally causes interference with gastric emptying.
✧ Annular pancreas may present with vomiting, with or without bile. Fifty percent of cases present in the newborn, where urgent operation is needed. The other 50% present between the ages of 20 to 70, when inflammation of the pancreas leads to constrictive symptoms.
✧ Accessory main pancreatic duct (pancreas divisum) is the result of the non-union of the dorsal and ventral portions of the pancreas. Patients most commonly present with recurrent pancreatitis or a single episode of pancreatitis, which is initially thought to be idiopathic. Diagnosis is by MRCP, where separation of the main and accessory pancreatic ducts is seen. ERCP can also be diagnostic, and therapeutic by endoscopic accessory duct sphincteroplasty. Open accessory duct sphincteroplasty can be performed.

Pancreatitis

Acute pancreatitis usually presents as an emergency admission with the typical abdominal pain and enzyme changes.

Although pain is a common feature of chronic pancreatitis, it can present in the outpatient department with signs of pancreatic endocrine and exocrine insufficiency and little in the way of serum enzyme changes. Chronic relapsing pancreatitis describes a condition of repeated attacks of acute pancreatitis, usually resulting in gradual destruction of the gland.

Risk factors are alcoholism, biliary tract disease, trauma (surgical, blunt, penetrating, ERCP), drugs (thiazides, steroids), metabolic disorders (hyperparathyroidism, hyperlipidaemia), infections (mumps, coxsackie B virus, mycoplasma pneumoniae, infectious mononucleosis, septicaemia), congenital mechanical obstruction of pancreatic duct (pancreas divisum), periampullary carcinoma, hereditary pancreatitis and vascular disease.

Acute pancreatitis

Patients with acute attacks are treated as an in-patients. Once the symptoms subside, patients are reviewed in the outpatient clinic.

Objectives

The outpatient consultation has three main objectives.

✧ Determine the underlying cause of the pancreatitis.
✧ Arrange treatment of the underlying cause to prevent further attacks.
✧ Detect any complications of pancreatitis, e.g. pseudocyst, pancreatic abscess.

Determine the underlying cause

Often this will have been identified during the in-patient episode, but the outpatient visit gives an opportunity to review the history now the patient is under less stress in order to identify any other significant factors: e.g. gallstones and alcohol consumption may co-exist.

Treatment of the cause

Each of the causes of pancreatitis can be dealt with as follows.
✧ Alcoholism: estimation of weekly alcohol consumption (truthful or untruthful); smell of alcohol on breath (or alternatively smell of strong mints); gamma GT levels, urine or serum ethanol levels. May respond to explanation, but usually need referral to a psychiatrist with an interest in alcohol abuse.
✧ Biliary tract disease: has the in-patient ultrasound scan given all the information necessary to arrange treatment, e.g. laparoscopic cholecystectomy? In cases of previous pancreatitis some assessment of the common bile duct is mandatory to exclude ductal stones, even in the face of normal common bile duct diameter and LFTs. For example, MRCP or pre-operative ERCP with or without sphincterotomy, intra-operative cholangiography or both.
✧ Trauma: it would be wise to repeat imaging, USS and/or CT, now the acute inflammation has settled, to determine whether trauma has resulted in distortion of the biliary system that will lead to long-term problems or require long-term follow-up. LFTs should also be monitored. MRCP with or without secretin will determine if there is duct disruption. ERCP may give similar information; however it is invasive (and may have been the cause of the trauma in the first place).
✧ Drugs: once again review the history, examination and investigation findings to confirm that pancreatitis can be ascribed to this cause. Repeat the investigations if in any doubt. Arrange for these drugs to be avoided or administered under close medical supervision in future.
✧ Metabolic disorders: perform serum calcium levels, serum parathormone levels and fasting serum lipids. Treat as appropriate.
✧ Infections: review the history, examination and investigation findings. Viral titres often need repeating 4–6 weeks after the acute episode to provide a diagnosis.
✧ Have the remaining causes been excluded, especially pancreas divisum and periampullary carcinoma, by ERCP? At ERCP, biliary manometry can also be performed to exclude sphincter of Oddi dysfunction and to sample bile to exclude bile crystals (microlithiasis) as a cause of pancreatitis.

Complications of acute pancreatitis

Any patient who has a persistence or reappearance of the inflammatory manifestations of acute pancreatitis must be suspected of developing a pancreatic pseudocyst or a pancreatic abscess. Other local complications of pancreatitis include haemorrhage, peptic ulceration and erosions, left-sided portal hypertension and variceal haemorrhage and vascular complications.

Pancreatic pseudocyst

Pseudocysts are thought to arise secondary to pancreatic duct disruption and leakage. These are not true cysts because they lack an endothelial lining.

Objectives
Diagnose pseudocyst, differentiate those suitable for conservative therapy, monitor for the development of complications, treat pseudocyst.

History
Recurrence of pain, nausea and vomiting, anorexia, weight loss.

Examination
Tender upper abdomen. Sometimes a tender mass.

Investigations
Leucocytosis, hyperamylasaemia may be present. USS or CT scan is diagnostic. Air within a pseudocyst suggests an abscess. USS may also detect a splenic artery aneurysm and portal hypertension. In chronic or recurrent pseudocysts an ERCP will exclude pancreatic duct stenosis as an aetiological factor.

Treatment
✧ Acute pseudocysts should be managed expectantly for 4–6 weeks, as spontaneous resolution sometimes occurs and surgical therapy is more effective if the cyst wall has been given time to mature.
✧ Chronic pseudocysts are usually asymptomatic and no recent attack of pancreatitis can be identified, but there may be a history of blunt abdominal trauma. Spontaneous resolution is rare and there is a high risk of complications (e.g. haemorrhage – erosion of major vessels, rupture, infection and local pressure effects) if treatment is delayed.
✧ Other factors for consideration in the treatment of pseudocysts are the following.
  ∝ Size: those smaller than 6cm may be observed and expected to resolve. Larger ones will probably need surgical drainage.
  ∝ Development of symptoms: compression of adjacent organs or indicative of an impending complication such as rupture, haemorrhage and infection.
  ∝ Maturity: acute 4–6 weeks.
  ∝ Vascular complications: CT angiography or intra-arterial angiography identifies a subgroup of patients with vascular complications associated with acute pancreatitis, including pseudoaneurysms and left-sided portal hypertension from splenic vein thrombosis. Presence of a pseudoaneurysm is rare. Treatment is angiography and embolisation or, if this fails, open exploration and exclusion of the aneurysm or pancreatic resection, as opposed to internal drainage of a pseudocyst. Presence of portal hypertension may be an indication for splenectomy with or without gastric devascularisation if there have been repeated gastric fundal variceal bleeds that have failed endoscopic treatment.
  ∝ Site of pseudocyst: retrograde enlarging anteriorly responds to a posterior cysto-gastrostomy. A cyst around the head of the pancreas close to the duodenum can easily be drained by cyst duodenostomy. Large cysts bulging into the transverse mesocolon can be drained using a Roux-en-Y loop for a cystjejunostomy. Cysts in the tail or body of the pancreas require a distal pancreatectomy or longitudinal pancreatico-jejunostomy. Infected or ruptured cysts or acute cysts with thin friable walls are best drained externally with wide-bore drains. In many instances the resulting pancreatic fistula will gradually close spontaneously. Occasionally a second procedure is needed to implant the fistulous tract into a Roux-en-Y loop of jejunum.

Percutaneous drainage of a pseudocyst

Indications for this procedure include the following.

✧ Patient is unfit for, or refuses, an operation.
✧ Acute fluid collection that is rapidly enlarging and needs external drainage.
✧ Infected pseudocyst that needs external drainage in a very sick patient.
✧ A pseudocyst that is in an unusual location (e.g. mediastinum, pelvis) and is not readily amenable to internal drainage.

Prior to drainage an MRCP or ERCP is required to delineate pancreatic duct anatomy. If the pseudocyst does not connect with the pancreatic duct, external drainage can be considered. If the pseudocyst connects with the pancreatic duct, drainage must be internal. Pseudocysts can also be drained by percutaneous cyst gastrostomy or via EUS-guided stenting of the pseudocyst into the stomach or duodenum.

Surgical drainage of a pseudocyst

This should also deal with the gall bladder if it has been identified as the original cause of pancreatitis.

Open: via an upper abdominal incision, lesser sac pseudocysts can be drained by a posterior cyst gastrostomy; pancreatic head or uncinate process pseudocysts can be drained into the duodenum; pseudocysts bulging through the transverse mesocolon can be drained by a cystjejunostomy.

Follow-up

Review with ultrasound scans to ensure those pseudocysts being managed conservatively are resolving. If there is no resolution after six weeks, consider surgical or radiological intervention if they are large or symptomatic.

Post-operative follow-up

Review within four weeks after surgery and at regular intervals (3–6 monthly) thereafter. Determine the success of the operation and detect any complications. Review histology of the pseudocyst wall to exclude a neoplastic cyst. Repeat abdominal USS to confirm that the pseudocyst is resolving if there are persistent symptoms (cysts can still recur despite surgery).

Complications include those of laparotomy and general anaesthesia. More specific complications depend on the procedure performed. Persistent leakage of fluid from a wound or drain site may indicate a pancreatic fistula. Send fluid for amylase concentration analysis. It is very high if from a pancreatic fistula. Pancreatic fistulas require admission for further assessment and treatment. Other complications include gastric outlet or small bowel obstruction related to the surgical procedure.

Pancreatic abscess

Pancreatic abscess is caused by extensive pancreatic and peripancreatic necrosis with formation of a peripancreatic fluid collection that gets secondarily infected (usually by *E. coli*, enterococci or fungi). It develops after the second week of acute pancreatitis and carries a high mortality/morbidity. Occasionally an infected pseudocyst may lead to an abscess.

Objectives

Diagnose pancreatic abscess, differentiate from pseudocyst, treat.

History

Take a general pancreatic history. Pancreatic abscess usually becomes apparent 2–5 weeks after an attack of pancreatitis as the attack appears to be resolving. The patient complains of increasing fever, pain and tenderness.

Examination
Perform a general examination. Patients with pancreatic abscess will look unwell, with evidence of sepsis. An abdominal mass may be palpable.

Investigations
Investigate with FBC, looking for leucocytosis or hyperamylasaemia; blood cultures are usually negative in the early stages. AXR shows soap-bubble appearance of a retroperitoneal abscess in less than 20% of cases. USS or CT scan is usually diagnostic. CT scan detection of air in the pancreas is diagnostic, or it may detect areas of low attenuation with contrast, which suggests necrosis.

Treatment
- ✧ Radiological: percutaneous drainage with wide-bore drains. Two drains can be placed side by side for irrigation and drainage. A sample should be sent for amylase and microbiology and appropriate antibiotics started. Will require follow-up scans and drain adjustment with or without further drainage.
- ✧ Surgical: retroperitoneal debridement and drainage.

Follow-up
Investigation of these patients is usually performed as an in-patient investigation.

Post-operative follow-up
Patients are usually in hospital for long periods until they recover from the acute episode. Possible long-term consequences of pancreatic debridement are endocrine and exocrine deficiency, for which insulin and pancreatic enzyme supplements may be necessary, and pancreatic fistulae.

Recurrent pancreatitis
More than one attack of acute pancreatitis needs further investigation for aetiology. If the cause is unclear, think of rarer causes of recurrent pancreatitis such as the following.
- ✧ Stenosis of the sphincter of Oddi, e.g. fibrosis after passage of a stone. This is diagnosed by ERCP and treated by ERCP sphincterotomy. If this fails or the problem recurs, open sphincteroplasty can be performed.
- ✧ Pancreas divisum: the duct of Wirsung is very small, therefore the duct of Santorini becomes the major ductal system, but it has a small papilla, therefore there is relative stenosis. This predisposes to pancreatitis. Divisum is found in 3–4% of the population, but in approximately 12% of patients with idiopathic pancreatitis. Thus the relationship between pancreas divisum and pancreatitis is unclear and surgical treatment carries a poor prognosis. Diagnosis is made at ERCP when pancreatic stenting may alleviate symptoms. Acessory duct sphincteroplasty can be performed at ERCP or at open surgery if relief has been obtained after a trial of a pancreatic stent.
- ✧ Biliary microlithiasis: biliary crystals can be seen at EUS or on microscopy of a bile sample taken at ERCP. Treatment involves cholecystectomy and/or endoscopic sphincterotomy.

Chronic pancreatitis and chronic relapsing pancreatitis
This condition may present with frequent attacks of pancreatitis requiring admission to hospital, or it may be insidious in onset with increasing pancreatic insufficiency. Unlike acute pancreatitis, gallstones are thought to be an uncommon aetiological factor.

Instead alcohol is the prime aetiological factor in 60–70% of cases, with no cause found in 30–40%. Rare causes such as pancreas divisum, neoplasia, trauma, cystic fibrosis and radiotherapy are responsible for the rest. Family history is very important: in younger patients with a strong family history, suspect familial pancreatitis.

Objectives
Diagnose chronic pancreatitis, exclude pancreatic cancer, identify underlying aetiological factor, detect pancreatic insufficiency, treat pancreatitis, treat aetiological factor, treat pancreatic insufficiency.

History
Take a general pancreatic history. Patients may complain of repeated bouts of upper abdominal pain which may or may not be related to alcohol ingestion. The pain may radiate to the back or shoulder tip and is constant and dull. Patients avoid lying on their backs, as this makes the pain worse. Initially pain is intermittent and episodic, progressing to constant pain. On questioning, the patient may admit to stools which are pale, bulky, oily or difficult to flush away. Symptoms due to the onset of diabetes mellitus are unusual in the early stages.

Patients may give a history of weight loss due to exocrine insufficiency and/or anorexia and nausea. Jaundice may be caused by biliary duct obstruction due to inflammation and fibrosis in the head of the pancreas. Similarly, signs and symptoms of gastric outlet obstruction may result from an inflammatory mass in the head of the pancreas. Haematemesis may be due to oesophageal varices. Take a detailed history of alcohol consumption. Take a detailed family history.

Examination
Perform a general examination. Look for evidence of weight loss, malnutrition, jaundice and/or stigmata of liver disease. Erythema ab igne from frequent application of a hot water bottle is often seen. Examination may be normal, but examine for a palpable epigastric mass representing an inflamed or fibrosed pancreas or a pseudocyst. Rupture of a pseudocyst may produce ascites. Splenomegaly usually indicates splenic vein thrombosis.

Investigations
Serum amylase may be normal and LFTs may indicate cholestasis. Blood sugar may be abnormal, as may clotting. FBC may reveal leucopenia and thrombocytopenia indicating hypersplenism. Faecal elastase will identify exocrine insufficiency. USS and CT scan can identify features suggestive of chronic pancreatitis and detect complications such as a dilated biliary tract and splenic vein thrombosis. MRCP can delineate biliary and pancreatic duct anatomy. EUS can be used to exclude a neoplasm as well as obtaining tissue for histology to exclude neoplasia or autoimmune disease.

Treatment – medical
Control pain and treat endocrine and exocrine insufficiencies. Treat any drug or alcohol addiction.
- Pain: usually requires opiates starting with dihydrocodeine (DF118) or codeine for mild to moderate pain, increasing to buprenorphine (sublingual), pethidine or morphine sulphate (MST). NSAIDs may increase the risk of gastrointestinal haemorrhage. Coeliac plexus blocks can be performed via EUS and can reduce opiate requirements, but recurrence of symptoms may occur in time.
- Exocrine insufficiency: Creon® and pancreatin contain enteric-coated microspheres that prevent deactivation in the stomach and allow a normal fat intake, which is

important for maintenance of weight and correction of malnutrition. Fat-soluble vitamin supplements are necessary.

✧ Endocrine insufficiency: diabetic control is usually obtained with oral hypoglycaemics but sometimes insulin is necessary. Blood-sugar control can be difficult in the presence of variable food intake due to the pain induced by eating. Therefore careful monitoring is required.

Treatment – surgical

Operations are considered mainly for the relief of pain, but no surgical procedure can restore endocrine or exocrine function. Rehabilitation must be planned in advance and there must be absolute avoidance of alcohol.

Indications for surgery

✧ Intractable pain (consider disruption to patient's life, narcotics needed to control the pain, control of alcoholism, age and general condition of patient).
✧ Development of complications, including the following.
 ∝ Lower bile duct obstruction: ERCP to exclude other causes and cancer. Relief of obstruction may relieve the pain.
 ∝ Duodenal obstruction: rare in chronic pancreatitis. Exclude cancer by biopsy. Treat non-cancerous cases by gastrojejunostomy.
 ∝ Vascular involvement: pseudoaneurysms and portal hypertension.
 ∝ Pancreatic cysts, pseudocysts, abscess, pancreatic ascites and pleural effusions.
 ∝ Presence of a dominant mass leading to suspicion or fear of cancer.
 ∝ Portal vein compression/mesenteric vein thrombosis.
 ∝ Pancreatic duct stricture with upstream dilatation with or without pancreatic duct stones.
 ∝ Colonic stricture.

Surgery/intervention

Isolated pancreatic stricture can be treated at ERCP, or if this fails and there is upstream duct dilatation, perform longitudinal pancreatico-jejunostomy.

For a mass in the head of the gland, perform pylorus-preserving pancreatoduodenectomy (PPPD) or standard Whipple's or Beger's operation (duodenum-sparing pancreatic head resection to be considered only if absolutely sure it is not malignant).

Inflammation restricted to the body and tail of the gland may be treated by distal pancreatectomy.

Whole gland disease may very, very rarely be treated by total pancreatectomy with or without islet cell autotransplantation (depending on pre-operative endocrine testing).

Open coeliac plexus block can be combined with open procedures.

Other procedures like cholecystectomy and parathyroidectomy should be performed for their own indications. These procedures will not affect the natural history of chronic pancreatitis.

Thoracoscopic splanchnicectomy for pain relief is effective, although the results may only last 12–18 months.

Follow-up

Follow up at short intervals of 2–4 weeks until pancreatic neoplasia is excluded. Then follow up long term at regular intervals to monitor pain control, endocrine and exocrine insufficiency and abstinence from alcohol. Monitor weight and nutritional status, including vitamin deficiencies.

Post-operative follow-up

Assess the patient for success of the operation in relieving pain (approximately 70% of patients) and for the development of complications, both expected (endocrine and exocrine insufficiency) and unexpected (pancreatic fistula, small bowel obstruction). Follow-up is long term for detecting and managing endocrine and exocrine insufficiency. Gradually increase the intervals as the patient stabilises (1–6 months).

Neoplasms of the exocrine pancreas

Benign neoplasms are rare and seldom of clinical significance unless they become very large and impinge on adjacent structures (CBD, duodenum, stomach or main pancreatic duct). They include adenoma, cystadenoma, lipoma, fibroma, leiomyofibroma, myoma, haemangioma, lymphangioma, haemangioendothelioma and neuroma. They usually need resection to confirm their benign nature.

Pancreatic cancer

Pancreatic ductal adenocarcinoma constitutes 80–90% of all primary malignant tumours arising from the gland and accounts for 10% of all cancers of the digestive tract. When cancer arises in the head (70%) it must also be differentiated from cancer arising in the ampulla, duodenum or lower common bile duct, which has a much better prognosis than true pancreatic adenocarcinoma. The rare mucinous cystic neoplasms (mucinous cystadenoma/adenocarcinoma) have a good prognosis if completely resected.

Pancreatic cancer is more common in older people. It has an increased incidence in smokers, diabetics (pancreatic cancer can cause diabetes mellitus), alcoholics and in those with hereditary pancreatitis.

Carcinoma of the head of the pancreas
History

The term 'periampullary' does not differentiate between carcinomas of the duodenum, pancreas, common bile duct or ampulla, but all these tumours present with similar symptoms. Jaundice is present in 90% and is classically described as painless, although pain can be present in up to 70% of patients. Severe pain radiating to the back is a sinister symptom suggestive of retroperitoneal tumour infiltration. Weight loss and anorexia are common even in the early stages. Nausea and vomiting, epigastric bloating and change of bowel habit can be reported. Haematemesis and melaena occur in late cases due to direct invasion of mucosa or portal hypertension secondary to portal vein compression by the tumour. Chills and fever due to cholangitis can occur.

Duodenal cancer can present with iron deficiency anaemia caused by occult GI bleeding or with symptoms of gastric outlet obstruction. Fluctuating jaundice is a characteristic of ampullary tumours, as are silver stools – steatorrhoea combined with GI blood loss.

Examination

Perform a general examination. Examination may be normal or jaundice and a palpable gall bladder (Courvoisier's sign) may be present in 25%. The liver is enlarged on palpation in up to 80% of patients at presentation.

Carcinoma of the body and tail of the pancreas
History

There is pain and weight loss. Jaundice is uncommon and may indicate involvement of the porta hepatis. Pain is usually dull, vague in the epigastrium or back. Can be episodic and related to meals, or constant and severe. Partial relief may be obtained by flexing the trunk forward. Severe pain may indicate extension of the tumour into perineural tissues, lymphatics and posterior retroperitoneum. Weight loss may be severe and rapid. Haemetemesis and melaena may occur.

Examination

Perform a general examination. There may be evidence of weight loss, but otherwise examination may be normal. Occasionally there may be migratory thrombophlebitis (Trousseau's sign), indicating advanced cancer. Early cases have few signs. Late signs are an abdominal mass or liver metastases. A rectal shelf may be evident on rectal examination in the rectovesical/vaginal pouch. Other late signs are ascites and an enlarged lymph node in the supraclavicular fossa.

Investigations

Ninety per cent of patients are diagnosed too late. Always suspect pancreatic cancer in patients with seemingly recent symptoms, absent physical signs and negative routine X-ray investigations.

FBC may reveal iron-deficiency anaemia. Blood sugar testing may detect diabetes mellitus or impaired glucose tolerance in 15% of patients. LFTs may indicate a cholestatic picture. Faecal elastase test may be abnormal.

USS is a good initial imaging technique and can usually identify a pancreatic mass, bile duct dilatation, liver metastases, ascites, extrapancreatic spread and portal hypertension.

Contrast enhanced CT scan is the gold standard for diagnosis and accurate staging of the disease. ERCP may be necessary to decompress the biliary tree, and it enables cytology. Alternatively, percutaneous needle biopsy under USS/CT control for diagnosis in potentially incurable cases avoids a diagnostic laparotomy. In cases where this is not possible a laparoscopic biopsy is less invasive than open operation.

Markers for pancreatic cancer, e.g. CA-19-9 and CEA, may be raised and may fall to normal after resection, providing a means of monitoring recurrence if levels rise again.

Pancreatitis can co-exist with all cancers and there may be gallstones – the presence of one does not exclude the other. Truly representative needle biopsies of the pancreas are often hard to obtain because of sampling error and confusion between tumour and associated pancreatitis.

Staging

The main objective is to detect irresectable disease – vascular invasion (portal vein, SMA, coeliac or hepatic artery) and metastases to the liver, peritoneal cavity, coeliac nodes or beyond. These can usually be detected by CT.

Tumour size greater than 3cm, invasion of contiguous organs like the duodenum or colon, and enlarged lymph nodes within the resection field are not contraindications to surgery. EUS can provide detailed assessment of vascular involvement and when combined with biopsy can give histological diagnosis. Staging laparoscopy can exclude liver and peritoneal metastases and when combined with intra-operative ultrasound can give further accurate staging.

Treatment – surgical
Pre-operative preparation

A good state of nutrition and hydration supplemented with intravenous fluids, elemental diet and multivitamins is required. Correct any clotting deficiency with vitamin K or FFP. If the serum bilirubin is high (greater than 200 umol/l), or in the presence of sepsis, hepatorenal failure, severe cardiopulmonary disease expected to respond to medical management and severe malnutrition, a temporary percutaneous or transhepatic biliary decompression should be considered.

Exclusions for surgery

Apart from irresectable disease, exclusions are very elderly or frail patients with multiple systemic disorders or a life expectancy of less than five years.

Surgery

Surgery is Whipple's pancreaticoduodenectomy or PPPD or total pancreatectomy. Whipple's operation is indicated for tumour confined to the duodenum, ampulla of Vater or lower CBD. However, if the rest of the gland is severely affected by pancreatitis, total pancreatectomy may be the better option. If frozen section confirms cancer at the resection margin a total pancreatectomy may occasionally be necessary. A suspected cancer of the body and tail is treated by a distal pancreatectomy. If unresectable or metastatic, a palliative biliary and gastric bypass is performed.

Follow-up

Follow up at short intervals (1–4 weeks) in cases where cancer is suspected.

Palliation

✧ Relief of jaundice, pruritus or impending cholangitis: ERCP/PTC and biliary stenting or hepatico-jejunostomy.
✧ Relief of duodenal obstruction: endoscopic or radiological stenting or open/laparo-scopic gastrojejunostomy.
✧ Relief of pain: coeliac plexus block (50 ml of 50% alcohol plus 20 ml of 6% phenol). External beam radiotherapy.
✧ Unfit for surgery: ERCP sphincterotomy and biliary stent.
✧ Stent blockage: indicated by recurrent jaundice and cholangitis. ERCP and change of stent.

Post-operative follow-up

Review to determine the success of the operation and to detect any complications. Review the histology to determine whether resection margins are clear of tumour. Examine for the general complications of a laparotomy and general anaesthesia. Small bowel obstruction may be due to recurrent tumour or adhesions – laparotomy is indicated to establish the diagnosis and relieve obstruction. Biliary obstruction may be due to tumour recurrence or anastomotic stricture. Exclude endocrine and exocrine pancreatic insufficiency.

Monitoring of recurrence

All patients should be referred for adjuvant chemotherapy following surgery. Single agent gemcitabine has a survival benefit versus no chemotherapy. Patients with locally advanced disease may have a response to combination chemoradiotherapy, whereas patients with metastatic disease should be offered palliative chemotherapy. A small number of patients have increased levels of tumour marker such as CA 19-9 or CEA levels pre-operatively and serial monitoring post-operatively is useful.
✧ Management of pancreatic endocrine insufficiency: insulin.
✧ Management of pancreatic exocrine insufficiency: Creon®/pancreatin tablets, vitamins and antibiotics.

Prognosis

Operative mortality is 1–5% in high-volume centres. Five-year survival is 10–25% for pancreatic ductal adenocarcinoma, 40–50% for ampullary carcinoma and distal cholangiocarcinoma, higher for mucinous cystic neoplasms and neuroendocrine tumours. Most mortality occurs from two months to two years.

Lesions of the endocrine pancreas

Endocrine cancers are relatively slow growing and many apparently metastasise only to regional lymph nodes. This allows surgical cure in a sizeable proportion of patients.

Insulinoma

Hyperinsulinaemia causes symptomatic hypoglycaemia. It is caused by B-cell neoplasia (insulinoma) or rarely, B-cell hyperplasia/microadenomatosis. In adults 80% of insulinomas are benign solitary tumours, 10% are multiple and are part of MEN I and 10% are malignant. There is an even distribution of tumours in the head, body and tail of the pancreas.

Differential diagnosis

Includes brain tumour, epilepsy, alcoholism and drug abuse, fibrosarcoma and non-pancreatic tumours, glucocorticoid deficiency, diffuse liver disease and factitious hyperinsulinaemia due to insulin abuse.

Objectives

Diagnose the cause, differentiate from other causes, localise tumour, treat hypoglycaemia, treat tumour.

History/examination

Take a general pancreatic history and perform a general examination. There are symptoms of weakness, sweating, hunger, palpitations and trembling. The median time of onset of symptoms to diagnosis is two years, because of the rare diagnosis and non-specific nature of the symptoms. Determine the relationship of symptoms to exercise and food. Hypoglycaemia may occur after fasting or soon after eating (reactive hypoglycaemia). Fasting hypoglycaemia is more typical of an insulinoma, reactive hypoglycaemia occurring after meals is seen more commonly in alimentary disorders, e.g. post-gastrectomy. Examination may be normal.

Investigations

For definitive diagnosis, measure simultaneous insulin and glucose levels at the time of hypoglycaemia. A diagnostic 72-hour fast in hospital will detect all cases. Other causes of hypoglycaemia such as fibrosarcoma and non-pancreatic tumours, glucocorticoid deficiency or diffuse liver disease will not be associated with a raised insulin level. Occasionally provocative tests to induce hypoglycaemia are needed, but these are second-line investigations.

Diagnosis

A positive diagnosis is based on three elements:
- recognition of probable nature of patient's symptoms
- presence of Whipple's triad:
  - hypoglycaemic symptoms produced by fasting
  - hypoglycaemia documented during symptomatic episodes
  - symptoms relieved by glucose intake
- demonstration that plasma insulin concentration is inappropriately high for the existing levels of plasma glucose. An insulin (IU/ml) to glucose (mg/dl) ratio of greater than 0.3 indicates insulinoma.

Pre-operative localisation

Seventy-five per cent of tumours are less than 1.5cm and are not visible or palpable. EUS is particularly useful for endocrine tumours of the pancreas.

Angiography is the most reliable localising investigation, especially when combined with a calcium stimulation test. CT can detect less than 60% of tumours. MRI may be more reliable. If imaging is negative, selective venous sampling for insulin is necessary. However, at laparotomy a complete examination of the whole gland is needed, including the use of intra-operative ultrasound to exclude multiple tumours.

Treatment
Benign disease

Treat with the simple enucleation, or with Whipple's operation or distal pancreatectomy, depending on the size and location of the lesion. Beware of enucleating lesions close to the main pancreatic duct – a pancreatic leak or fistula may develop.

Multifocal malignant disease

This may require a total pancreatectomy. Ninety-five percent of patients are cured, 5–10% experience recurrent hypoglycaemia requiring re-operation. Surgical mortality is less than 5%.
- ✧ Diazoxide for control of pre-operative hypoglycaemia – needs careful monitoring.
- ✧ Octreotide – infusion or long-acting depot preparation. Streptozotocin for metastatic insulinoma.

Follow-up

Follow up at short intervals(1–4 weeks) until diagnosis is achieved. Consider admission to hospital, and monitor and treat hypoglycaemia.

Post-operative follow-up

Determine the success of the operation by the relief of symptoms. Check histology to confirm complete excision. Long-term follow-up is required for management of pancreatic insufficiency.

Gastrinoma (Zollinger-Ellison syndrome (ZE))

This consists of intractable peptic ulceration caused by excess gastrin secretion. Twenty-five per cent have MEN I (also parathyroid hyperplasia and pituitary prolactinoma). Of gastrinomas, 60–90% are malignant and 50–80% will have lymph node metastases at presentation. They arise in the pancreas in 75% of cases. Other sites are the duodenum, omental lymph nodes, liver and gastric antrum. These tumours are more often multiple than solitary.

Objectives

Diagnose gastrinoma, differentiate from other causes of recurrent ulceration, localise gastrinoma, treat gastrinoma, screen for MEN I.

History/examination

Take a general pancreatic history and perform a general examination. Patients may present with symptoms of dyspepsia and/or severe diarrhoea in 5–7%, usually over several years. Examination is frequently normal.

Suspect in any patient with:
- ✧ peptic ulcer disease refractory to treatment
- ✧ multiple ulcers or ulcers in unusual places (distal duodenum or jejunum)
- ✧ peptic ulcer disease with diarrhoea

✧ recurrence after operation

✧ strong family history of MEN I or other feature of MEN, e.g. hypercalcaemia.

Investigations

Perform an OGD to document the ulceration. Determine gastric basal acid output – evidence of acid hypersecretion such as a basal level of more than 15 mmol/l suggests gastrinoma.

A normal basal acid level makes ZE unlikely. In patients with high basal acid levels, measure fasting serum gastrin levels. Gastrinoma is characterised by a basal gastrin level greater than 100 pg/l in the presence of acid hypersecretion (must be measured without proton-pump inhibitor (PPI) medication, which increases gastrin levels). Levels greater than 500 pg/ml are almost diagnostic of gastrinoma and levels from 100–500 pg/ml are highly suggestive.

Basal gastrin levels are also raised in pernicious anaemia, atrophic gastritis and gastric cancer, but these conditions do not have acid hypersecretion. Conditions which have raised gastrin levels and acid hypersecretion include gastrinoma, retained gastric antrum after Billroth II, antral G-cell hyperplasia and gastric outlet obstruction. Gastrinoma can be differentiated from these conditions by the secretin stimulation test. After injection of secretin gastrin, levels rise to over 200 pg/ml in gastrinoma patients only.

Once gastrinoma is diagnosed MEN syndrome needs to be excluded – serum calcium, phosphate and plasma prolactin levels need to be measured.

Tumour localisation

Most can be localised by CT scan. However, tumours less than 7mm are not detected. MRI may improve visualisation. Angiography is not used, as gastrinomas are hypovascular. EUS is useful where available. Somatostatin receptor scintigraphy (octreotide scan) can be positive in up to 80% of patients.

Laparotomy and operative search with intra-operative ultrasound and OGD to detect duodenal wall tumours by transillumination.

Treatment

Patients with pre-operatively identified liver metastases or MEN I are treated medically with control of ulceration by omeprazole. In the absence of liver metastases or MEN I, medical therapy is used for 6–12 months. Young and fit patients undergo surgical exploration, after initial stabilisation on medical therapy. At operation, if complete tumour resection is possible this is performed. However, if complete removal is impossible, as much tumour as possible is removed. Post-operatively, medical therapy is reintroduced and continued for as long as symptoms are controlled. If medical therapy fails again, rarely a total gastrectomy may be considered. Similarly for patients where total tumour removal was performed, basal and stimulated gastrin levels are measured at intervals post-operatively. If gastrin levels are still raised, medical therapy is reintroduced and gastrectomy is considered for poorly controlled patients.

Old or poor-risk patients are continued on medical therapy for as long as symptoms are controlled. If at any stage medical treatment ceases to be effective the patients are explored surgically for the tumour. The tumour is resected if possible, otherwise a total gastrectomy is performed.

Palliation

Liver metastases and advanced disease: streptozoticin and 5FU chemotherapy. Octreotide for symptoms. Liver resection in selected cases.

MEN I

Perform parathyroid surgery first, which may relieve symptoms completely. However, this is often only temporary, so continue to follow up in the clinic and proceed to gastrinoma treatment if symptoms recur.

Follow-up

See treatment section.

Post-operative follow-up

See treatment section. Long-term surveillance is needed, as recurrences may be late. Successful removal of all gastrin-secreting tumours needs to be confirmed by serially negative plasma gastrin responses to secretin stimulation.

VIPoma

Rare primary lesion is in the pancreas in 80%, 20% are ganglioneuromas and neuroblastomas.

History/examination

The condition is characterised by watery diarrhoea.

Investigations

Diagnosed by increased VIP levels, hypokalaemia, achlorhydria and acidosis.

Localisation

Usually solitary and large, and can be detected by USS, CT or angiogram.

Treatment

Initially medical, by intravenous fluids and octreotide. Therapeutic options include surgical excision, debulking and medical treatment. Metastatic disease is treated by streptozotocin.

Follow-up

Long term to detect recurrence and deterioration in condition.

Glucagonoma

This is a rare condition arising in the A cells of islets. Seventy to eighty per cent are malignant, with 50% having metastases at the time of presentation.

History/examination

There is a characteristic skin rash, necrolytic migrating erythema, weight loss, diabetes mellitus, DVT, anaemia, hypoaminoacidaemia, glossitis and cheilitis. Diagnosis is based on a recognition of skin rash in combination with diabetes mellitus in a setting of a chronic wasting disorder.

Investigations

Glucagon levels exceed 1000 pg/ml. Other conditions associated with increased glucagon levels are diabetes, chronic renal failure, shock states (myocardial infarction (MI), septicaemia, burns) acute pancreatitis, cirrhosis, familial hyperglucagonaemia and exercise.

Localisation

Usually large, therefore USS or CT is reliable.

Treatment

Treat with topical steroids and intravenous amino acids. Octreotide is good at controlling symptoms in the pre-operative period and as palliation. Perform surgical excision or debulking (effective in symptom relief). If surgery is not an option then perform selective arterial embolisation and chemotherapy with streptozocin and 5FU.

Follow-up

Long term to detect recurrence or deterioration in clinical condition.

Multiple endocrine neoplasia I

This is an autosomal dominant familial disorder characterised by the development of synchronous and metachronous endocrine and non-endocrine tumours, but with considerable phenotypic variability.

Parathyroids are involved in 85% and the majority of lesions consist of hyperplasia. Pancreatic islets (30–80%) are inevitably involved and the commonest pancreatic tumour is the gastrinoma. Pancreatic tumours are usually multiple. Pituitary tumours are most commonly prolactinomas with growth-hormone tumours next (10–60%). Other occasional tumours are adrenocortical lesions (25%), thyroid nodules, bronchial and intestinal carcinoids and lipomas.

Investigations

All patients with endocrine pancreatic tumours should be investigated by testing of serum calcium and phosphate levels, plasma assays of parathormone, insulin, gastrin, glucagon, somatostatin, pancreatic polypeptide, prolactin, growth hormone, ACTH and cortisol, chromogranin A and MRI scan of pancreas, pituitary and abdomen. All family members should be screened.

Multiple endocrine neoplasia II

An autosomal dominant familial cancer syndrome characterised by the development of medullary thyroid cancer (90%), phaeochromocytoma (50%) and hyperparathyroidism (20–30%) with variable expression. Type A consists of hyperparathyroidism, medullary carcinoma of the thyroid and phaeochromocytoma.

Type A can be associated with cutaneous lichen planus and Hirschsprung's disease.

Type B has a low incidence of parathyroid diseases but multiple mucosal neuromas, intestinal ganglioneuromas leading to megacolon and constipation, a Marfanoid habitus and characteristic facies with thickened lips and alae nasi along with medullary carcinoma of the thyroid and phaeochromocytoma.

Investigations and screening

Calcitonin, CEA, metanephrine and normetanephrine both urinary and serum, ionised calcium, parathyroid hormone.

NINE

Colon, rectum and anus

Henry Tilney and Paris Tekkis

Introduction

Conditions affecting the colon, rectum and anus range from the trivial to the life-threatening. The knowledge of these conditions among the public is complicated by embarrassment and folklore. Many patients attending the surgical outpatients are concerned about the intimate nature of the examinations that they are likely to undergo and require careful reassurance. Certain groups of patients become very preoccupied with the maintenance of a 'regular bowel habit' and consult if there is any variation in what is perceived as normal, while reluctance to attend can result in others consulting only when symptoms are severe and tumours may be advanced. In addition to these difficulties colorectal cancer is one of the commonest malignancies and can mimic the presentation of nearly all other colorectal and anal disorders. The priority of investigation for many patients is to exclude colorectal malignancy, but the necessary tests are often unpleasant and invasive and their application to all patients with colorectal symptoms would be impractical. However, the diagnosis must always be kept in mind, especially if minor conditions do not respond to treatment. It is this combination of factors that makes the assessment of colorectal disorders particularly difficult. After introductions and putting the patient at ease it is important to ascertain what they are hoping for from their consultation, as investigations to exclude malignancy are sufficient to satisfy many patients, who are then content to manage their own symptoms with simple advice.

Assessment of colorectal disorders

Colorectal history

The history should include a basic history of the whole gastrointestinal (GI) tract, including questions about non-specific features such as malaise, weight loss and vomiting. When the responses indicate a possible colorectal problem a more detailed colorectal history is required. Abdominal symptoms include pain (ask about site, periodicity, aggravating factors and nature: constant or colicky), distension or borborygmi (noisy bowels). Ask about any medications, in particular the long-term use of laxatives or antidiarrhoeal drugs. Ask about urgency, tenesmus, wet-wind, incomplete evacuation and weight loss. A history of recent exotic travel may be relevant, and a careful family history with particular attention to colitis, polyposis syndromes and colorectal cancer is essential.

Abdominal pain

Typically, abdominal pain in colonic disorders is colicky. Visceral midgut pain is generally felt in the periumbilical region, while hindgut pain tends to lead to suprapubic discomfort. The left iliac fossa is a common site for pain and this may be associated with diverticular disease, although other diagnoses are not excluded. Colicky colonic pain may equally be a feature of benign irritable bowel syndrome or a stenosing carcinoma of the colon. Constant pain may indicate a complication of diverticular disease (e.g. localised or free perforation, abscess) or advanced bowel cancer with nerve involvement.

Alteration in bowel habit

There are a wide variety of bowel habits that may be considered normal, but a change may be an important symptom of colorectal disease, which can suggest bowel cancer. Time should be taken to identify the previous bowel habit, the new bowel habit, the timing of the change and the presence of constipation or diarrhoea. Enquire about the consistency and frequency of stool and whether this is associated with the passage of blood or slime (mucus).

Rectal bleeding

If rectal bleeding is part of the history ask about the timing of this and whether there have been any previous episodes of rectal bleeding. Is the bleeding bright red, dripping into the toilet as in haemorrhoids or mixed in the motion as with inflammatory bowel disease or malignancy? Is the bleeding painful, as with an anal fissure, or painless? Does bleeding only occur at defaecation or at times in between? Ask about the amount of blood, although patients commonly overestimate this. Does it drip into the toilet, are there dark clots (suggests bleeding higher in the colon) or is there just a smear on the toilet paper? Note that the history is not totally reliable in excluding a cancer of the bowel, which can present with any type of rectal bleeding.

Anal and perineal symptoms

These include pruritus (itching), pain and its relation to defaecation, discharge and bleeding.

Prolapse

Something 'comes down' at defaecation or on straining or coughing. These lumps may reduce spontaneously or require manual reduction.

Incontinence

Ask about timing and severity; incontinence to flatus, liquid stool, solid stool. Enquire regarding urgency, tenesmus, wet-wind and incomplete evacuation. A history of previous anal surgery or trauma is important, and in female patients a careful obstetric history is essential, noting the number and nature of previous deliveries, obstructed and prolonged labour, instrumental delivery and obstetric tears or the need for episiotomy.

Colorectal examination

General examination may reveal anaemia associated with neoplasia or inflammatory bowel disease. Dermoid cysts are associated with Gardner's syndrome; acanthosis nigricans and dermatomyositis with neoplasia; and pyoderma gangrenosum, arthropathy, uveitis and finger clubbing with inflammatory bowel disease. Examination of the gastrointestinal tract begins with the mouth, which may reveal oral Crohn's or the perioral pigmentation associated with Peutz-Jeghers syndrome.

Abdominal examination

Inspect the supine abdomen for stomas; the scars associated with previous colorectal surgery; evidence of distension; visible peristalsis; and a mass or other organomegaly. Palpation may reveal tenderness or a palpable sigmoid colon, which is common and a normal finding, especially in constipation. Neoplasm or diverticular disease may be associated with a bowel mass. The liver may be enlarged due to secondary spread from a bowel neoplasm.

Rectal examination

Explain the procedure to the patient, explain the justification for it and obtain verbal consent. Place the patient in the left lateral position with the knees flexed as far as possible into the abdomen. Cover the patient's legs with a blanket to minimise exposure. On inspection look for evidence of pruritus ani, perianal warts, perianal abscess, perianal haematoma, prolapsing haemorrhoids, thrombosed haemorrhoids, skin tags, anal fistulas, anal fissures (and the frequently associated 'sentinel tag'), anal cancer, rectal prolapse and faecal soiling of the perineum.

Ask the patient to bear down as if defaecating. Look for abnormal perineal descent, eversion of the anus, prolapsing haemorrhoids and other protruding lesions such as rectal prolapse or neoplasm. The pulp of a gloved lubricated index finger is used to palpate for the thickened cord of a fistula track or other abnormalities around the anus. The pulp of the finger is then pressed onto the anus until the sphincter relaxes and the finger is them slid into the rectum. Significant pain at this point may indicate an anal fissure and the examination may have to be deferred until it is less painful following treatment of the fissure, or if diagnostic concern is present then examination should be performed under anaesthetic. Note the state of the resting anal tone, which largely reflects the condition of the internal anal sphincter. Ask the patient to contract the anus (examining the 'squeeze pressure' provided by the external sphincter) and hook the finger over the puborectalis muscle. This indicates the uppermost limit of the external sphincters and can be used as a landmark to determine the position of lesions, e.g. lesions above this indicate supralevator disease.

The rectum should be assessed in relation to three parts: the lumen and its contents, the rectal wall and structures outside the rectum. Note the contents of the rectum and the consistency of the faeces. Consider the rectum in quadrants (front, back, left, right) and palpate each one in turn. Note the position of any abnormality in relation to a notional clock-face where the anterior wall is considered 12 o'clock and posterior 6 o'clock (as if the patient is viewed in the lithotomy position). Withdraw the finger and inspect it for blood, mucus, pus and the nature of the faeces.

Extra-intestinal signs of inflammatory bowel disease (IBD)
There are various eye and skin signs, which should be identified on examination in relation to Crohn's disease and ulcerative colitis.

Ophthalmic signs
There are generally seen in active disease and are more common in Crohn's than in ulcerative colitis.
- Episderitis: redness and soreness of the eye similar to conjunctivitis. This is the most common ophthalmic manifestation of IBD.
- Iritis and uveitis: this is less common. It is associated with reduced visual acuity and a painful red eye.

Cutaneous signs
- Erythema nodosum: painful, raised red lesions, often on the shins, most frequently associated with Crohn's disease, affecting 15% of sufferers. Mirrors disease activity and biopsy shows subcutaneous septal panniculitis with neutrophil infiltrate.
- Pyoderma gangrenosum: affects around 2% of those with IBD, especially Crohn's colitis. Lesions are deep ulcers with a necrotic base and an undermined purple edge. They characteristically occur on the lower limbs and can be single or multiple, but are also seen around stomas and surgical scars. Histology reveals a neutrophilic dermatitis.

Investigation of colorectal disorders
Laboratory investigations
Blood tests
Haematology
Full blood count (FBC) for iron-deficiency anaemia and white cell count and differential. Plasma viscosity, erythrocyte sedimentation rate.

Biochemistry

Liver function tests (LFT) for indicating metastases. Thyroid function tests may be useful in the assessment of constipation and diarrhoea. C-reactive protein (CRP) for inflammatory conditions including colitis.

Immunology

Alpha-foetoprotein (AFP) and carcinoembryonic antigen (CEA) may be raised in colonic neoplasms.

Faecal tests
Faecal occult blood

This guaiac-based test for peroxidase activity can be performed at home by the patient. The patient smears a faecal sample onto a pre-prepared card which is then returned to the laboratory, where the presence of blood can be detected. The presence of blood can occur in normal individuals but may be an indicator of gastrointestinal pathology, and a consistent finding requires further investigation. This test forms the first-line investigation in the UK National Bowel Cancer Screening Programme. It is a simple and quick screening test, sensitivity is 50–70% and about two-thirds of tumours are thought to bleed in the course of a week. There are false positives caused by ingestion of animal haemoglobin, nosebleeds and so on, and dietary restrictions are required for two days prior to testing. False negatives occur due to intermittent bleeding of the tumour. The test is of no use in patients with obvious rectal bleeding.

Microbiology

In patients with diarrhoea, potential infective causes should be excluded by a stool culture. Fresh faecal samples are required and if parasites are suspected these samples should be transported immediately to the laboratory for examination. Toxins produced by *Clostridium difficile* may be identified in patients with pseudomembranous colitis.

Imaging techniques
Proctoscopy

A rectal examination is performed prior to insertion of the proctoscope. The technique consists of insertion of either a metal or disposable plastic rigid tube fitted with a fibre-optic light source for inspection of the distal rectum and anus. The proctoscope is lubricated with water-soluble gel and inserted with the central obturator in place until the rectum has been entered, and then it is removed. The rectal mucosa is inspected as the instrument is slowly withdrawn. The patient can be asked to bear down to demonstrate prolapsing mucosa and haemorrhoids. This short instrument gives a good view of the distal rectum and anal canal and is particularly useful for the diagnosis of haemorrhoids. Injection or banding of the haemorrhoids can be performed through the proctoscope.

The procedure may be unpleasant for the patient. Only the distal rectum can be observed.

Rigid sigmoidoscopy

A rectal examination is performed prior to insertion. The sigmoidoscope is a rigid tube, made of metal or disposable plastic, with a removable central obturator. The longer length of the sigmoidoscope enables more of the rectum and lower sigmoid colon to be inspected, although in practice only the distal two-thirds of the rectum can frequently be assessed.

In addition to the fibre-optic light source there is a connection for air insufflation using a rubber bulb. The sigmoidoscope is inserted for a few centimetres through the anus, with anterior angulation of the scope being required to negotiate the 90-degree anorectal junction. The obturator is removed and the scope window secured to provide an air-tight seal. The rectal ampulla is inspected and the lumen of the bowel identified. Air is introduced via the instrument to open up the lumen ahead. Patients should be warned that air is being introduced and they may feel the need to pass flatus but ask them to try and retain the air if they can.

The instrument is advanced only when the lumen ahead is visible. More of the rectum and lower sigmoid can be inspected. The procedure can usually be performed in the outpatient department without bowel preparation (although a phosphate enema can be administered if necessary).

Biopsies can be taken from abnormal lesions. However, care should be taken when sampling mucosal lesions above 10cm because of the risk of perforation, especially if the bowel is inflamed. There is a risk of bowel perforation if not performed gently. It is uncomfortable for the patient, especially if too much air is introduced.

Flexible sigmoidoscopy

This involves insertion of a 60cm flexible fibre-optic sigmoidoscope via the anus, and it is frequently capable of evaluating the colonic mucosa as far as the splenic flexure. It is usually performed as a day-case procedure involving bowel preparation with phosphate enema just prior to the procedure. In some units flexible sigmoidoscopes are available for use in the clinic rooms or in a designated 'rapid access' endoscopy list running concurrently with the colorectal outpatient clinic. Patients who can be selectively asked to self-administer enemas at home on the basis of their referral letters can be investigated immediately. The steerable nature of the scopes enables the turns of the sigmoid colon to be negotiated. Once again air insufflation is used to open up the lumen ahead. The scope is advanced when the lumen ahead is visible.

Approximately 70% of colorectal carcinomas are within reach of the flexible scope. Biopsies can be performed and polyps excised. Bowel preparation (with an enema) is necessary; equipment is expensive and needs careful cleaning and maintenance. Not all of the colon is inspected.

Colonoscopy

Colonoscopy involves using a flexible fibre-optic scope that is longer than the flexible sigmoidoscope and allows the whole of the colon to be inspected successfully by experienced operators in 90% of cases. Formal bowel preparation is required in the days prior to the procedure through the use of purgatives, and intravenous sedation (usually with benzodiazepines and opiates) is used for the procedure itself. Patients who are sedated should be warned not to drive or operate machinery for 24 hours after the procedure. The scope is steerable and air insufflation is used.

The whole colon can be visualised and biopsies can be taken for tissue diagnosis. However, the technique is very much operator dependent and one must trust the opinion of the operator who makes the report. Therapeutic procedures such as polypectomy can be performed.

Being operator dependent, it requires training and an experienced practitioner. It is uncomfortable for the patient. Major risks, of which patients should be warned, include colonic perforation in 0.1% (rising to 0.3–4% following biopsy/polypectomy), and haemorrhage rates are quoted at 0.03% following diagnostic colonoscopy and 1.9% after polypectomy.

Double contrast barium enema

The procedure involves infusing barium contrast through a catheter into the rectum. The balloon on the catheter is inflated to prevent leakage. The patient is placed on a tilt table which is manoeuvred through different positions to coat the whole bowel in barium. Air is insufflated after evacuation of most of the barium to finely coat the bowel wall with barium and provide mucosal detail.

It provides fine mucosal detail as well as gross anatomy and shows fistulas not easily visible on colonoscopy. It involves a significant dose of X-rays; bowel preparation is required; and rates of colonic perforation between 0.01 and 0.04% are reported.

Abdominal ultrasound technique

This is a useful non-invasive technique for the investigation of abdominal pain in order to detect pathology in other organs, e.g. the gall bladder, although its ability to detect colonic pathology is somewhat limited.

Pre-operatively it can be used to detect liver metastases in patients with colorectal cancer, although its accuracy in this respect is considered inferior to that afforded by CT scans. Ultrasound can also be used intra-operatively for the same purpose. It is operator dependent and, therefore, may be poor at defining bowel pathology.

Endoanal/transrectal ultrasound

A specially designed lubricated rotating probe, confined within a fluid-filled sheath to maintain tissue contact, is inserted into the rectum. Alternating bright and dark rings represent the anal sphincters and layers of the bowel wall, and sphincter defects and the relation of tumours or fistula tracks to the muscles can be assessed.

Transrectal ultrasound is a specialised technique, but in the centres where it is used it has proved useful in determining the local spread of rectal cancers and in the assessment of perianal fistulas and anal sphincters. It is an uncomfortable technique for the patient, which occasionally needs to be performed under anaesthetic. It is operator dependent.

Computed tomography (CT) scan

The scan gives an accurate definition of anatomy. It is useful for defining the extent of local spread of tumours and for investigating potential metastatic deposits. It is commonly used to assess for complications of diverticular disease.

It is expensive and associated with high doses of radiation. Equivalent information can often be obtained by other means with lower radiation exposure.

Magnetic resonance imaging (MRI)

MRI detects minute quantities of energy released by hydrogen ions when they are forced to change direction by a strong magnetic field. The patient passes through the scanner, which is quite claustrophobic and noisy. The scan does not require exposure to ionising radiation. It provides detailed information, which is useful in assessing the nature and extent of complicated perianal and other fistulas. Reconstructions in multiple planes are possible, allowing excellent anatomical detail. It can be particularly useful in the assessment of rectal tumour encroachment on the mesorectal fascia (the circumferential resection margin), which can help to select those who would benefit from pre-operative radiotherapy, and in the investigation of complicated anorectal sepsis. It is expensive and time-consuming. Some patients find the experience intolerable.

Examination under anaesthetic

This may be useful for patients with very painful anal conditions preventing adequate examination and diagnosis in the outpatient clinic, or in cancer to assess rectal resectability.

Diagnostic laparoscopy

This can potentially be used for assessment of a number of pathologies including the assessment of liver metastases when combined with intra-operative ultrasound, although the technique is not as widespread as the practice of the 'staging laparoscopy' in the assessment of upper GI malignancies.

Physiological techniques
Anal manometry
This involves the insertion of air/water-filled balloon pressure measuring systems into the rectum. The pressure inside the rectum is recorded during different conditions. The maximum resting pressure reflects function of the internal sphincter while the maximum squeeze pressure indicates function of the external sphincter. Pressures decrease with age and are commonly reduced in incontinence.

Rectal compliance
A balloon is inflated in the rectum and the volume and pressure is recorded at first sensation and the maximum amounts tolerated. Compliance is decreased in inflammatory bowel disease but increased in patients with chronic constipation, who are used to harbouring large volumes of stool in the rectum.

Electromyography
This involves the insertion of fine electrodes into the anal sphincter muscles and is useful in identifying damage to the sphincters, although this is generally now regarded as a research tool.

Pudendal nerve latency
This is measured by the use of a disposable electrode attached to a gloved finger. The nerve is stimulated as it crosses the ischial spine, and the time taken for the impulse to travel to the sphincter is recorded. Prolonged latency is associated with faecal incontinence, rectal prolapse, solitary rectal ulcer syndrome, severe constipation and sphincter defects.

The rectoanal reflex
Normal reflex consists of an inhibition of sphincter contraction in response to inflation of a balloon in the rectum. The loss of this reflex is almost diagnostic of Hirschsprung's disease, but may also be absent in patients with rectal prolapse and incontinence if resting pressures are already low.

Anal sensation can be assessed in relation to a thermal or electrical stimulus applied to the anal mucosa. Reduced sensation may be an important factor in patients with incontinence, especially if they have had previous anal surgery.

Defaecating proctogram
Barium suspension is infused into the rectum, and the patients are recorded as they void this suspension. This simulates defaecation and is useful for demonstrating abnormal anorectal angles in patients with pelvic floor weakness or prolapse, rectoceles, or the function of ileoanal pouches. In patients with anismus or obstructed defaecation, the acute anorectal angle may be maintained during attempted defaecation due to paradoxical contraction of the external sphincter complex, and this can be demonstrated by the defaecating proctogram.

Colonic transit time
The patient ingests special radio-opaque markers that can be followed by plain abdominal X-rays. This technique may be used to diagnose slow transit constipation.

Disorders of the colon and rectum
Rectal bleeding

Most cases of rectal bleeding presenting to the surgical clinic are due to minor anorectal conditions that are easily diagnosed and treated. However, sometimes these minor conditions co-exist with other more serious pathology, such as colorectal cancer. Therefore, the more serious causes of rectal bleeding should be excluded in the middle-aged or older patient initially and in any age group where the symptoms fail to settle despite apparently adequate treatment, rather than attributing the symptoms to minor anal conditions. Causes of rectal bleeding, in decreasing order of incidence, include the following.

✧ Diverticular disease.
✧ Inflammatory bowel disease:
  ∝ Crohn's disease
  ∝ ulcerative colitis
  ∝ infective colitis
  ∝ ischaemic colitis.
✧ Neoplasia:
  ∝ benign polyps
  ∝ adenocarcinoma.
✧ Coagulopathy.
✧ Benign anorectal disease:
  ∝ haemorrhoids
  ∝ anal fissure
  ∝ fistula-in-ano
  ∝ rectal prolapse
  ∝ rectal varices
  ∝ solitary rectal ulcer.
✧ Arteriovenous malformation.
✧ Radiation proctitis/enteritis.
✧ Profuse upper gastrointestinal bleeding/small bowel bleeding including gastroduodenal ulceration, jejunoileal diverticula and Meckel's diverticulum.

History

Take a general colorectal history and anorectal history. Determine the type of bleeding, the timing and the amount. Determine whether the blood is separate from the stool or mixed in. Is the blood bright red or dark? Is there pain associated with the passage of blood?

✧ Haemorrhoids are associated with bright red rectal bleeding separate from the stool or coating it, on the paper or dripping into the toilet. Bleeding is usually painless and may be associated with prolapsing haemorrhoids.
✧ Anal fissure is associated with a smear of bright red blood on the paper and pain on defaecation.
✧ Rectal prolapse is associated with a serosanguinous discharge and the prolapse.
✧ Inflammatory bowel disease is usually associated with blood mixed in with stool, which may be loose or diarrhoea. It is associated with frequent, loose, bloody stools and the presence of mucopus in more severe cases. Systemic disturbance, abdominal pain, malaise and weight loss may also be features.
✧ Tumours vary in their presentation, depending on the site of the tumour and the rate of bleeding. Tumours near the anus tend to present with bright red bleeding similar to haemorrhoids. More proximal tumours may present with dark red bleeding, while caecal tumours may be insidious and only present with iron-deficiency anaemia.
✧ Diverticular disease or angiodysplasia may present with a history or episodes of brisk

rectal bleeding of large amounts or with the passage of a large dark red stool. This bleeding usually stops and stools return to normal before the next episode.

✧ Ischaemic colitis is associated with left-sided abdominal pain and blood-stained diarrhoea in elderly patients with evidence of atherosclerosis or previous aortic aneurysm repair.

✧ Radiation proctitis patients have a history of radiotherapy, possibly following resection of a rectal carcinoma.

Examination

Perform a general colorectal and anorectal examination. Examine for the presence of anaemia and all causes outlined above.

Investigations

Investigations are FBC to detect anaemia; inflammatory markers including erythrocyte sedimentation rate (ESR) and CRP; and stool cultures in the case of bloody diarrhoea.

Perform proctoscopy and rigid sigmoidoscopy in all patients. If indicated to exclude carcinoma or other underlying pathology, proceed to colonoscopy or flexible sigmoidoscopy and barium enema to look for more proximal colonic lesions.

Selective mesenteric angiography may be useful in identifying abnormal blood vessels associated with angiodysplasia, but is more useful in identifying actively bleeding lesions in the acute situation where rates of bleeding of 0.5–1.0 ml per minute can be detected. Bleeding as slow as 0.1 ml per minute can be detected by using radio-labelled red-cell scans.

Treatment

In young patients with haemorrhoids and no other suspicious features in the history it may be justified to treat the minor anorectal condition and review at 4–6 weeks to assess whether the bleeding stops. If the symptoms are persistent, or there are any features in the history that might suggest a malignancy is possible, direct visualisation of the colon should be performed early. Treat underlying causes as appropriate.

Follow-up

Following exclusion of serious underlying pathology, patients can be followed at six-weekly intervals until the cause of the bleeding has been successfully treated.

Diarrhoea

Diarrhoea can be defined as the passage of more than three loose stools a day or of a stool mass greater than 200 g/day. Diarrhoea can be classified as acute or chronic and the causes fall into several groups.

Acute diarrhoea is classified into the following groups.

✧ Infective or toxin diarrhoea:
  ∝ viral: adenovirus, Norwalk, rotavirus
  ∝ bacterial: *Campylobacter, Escherischia coli, Shigella*
  ∝ toxins: *Clostridium difficile, Staphylococcus* spp.
  ∝ parasites: *Entamoeba, Giardia.*

✧ Drugs: angiotensin-converting enzyme (ACE) inhibitors, antibiotics, digoxin, fluoxetine, lithium, metformin, non-steroidal anti-inflammatory drugs (NSAIDs), proton-pump inhibitors (PPI), ranitidine, statins, 5-aminosalicylates (5-ASA), alcohol, cocaine.

✧ Ischaemic colitis.

✧ Inflammatory bowel disease.

Chronic diarrhoea is classified as follows.
- Infection: *Giardia, Campylobacter, Salmonella.*
- Drugs (*see* above).
- Malabsorption: lactose intolerance, chronic pancreatitis, bacterial overgrowth, short gut, coeliac disease.
- Inflammatory bowel disease: Crohn's disease, ulcerative colitis.
- Metabolic disease: diabetes mellitus, hyperthyroidism.
- Neoplasia: bowel cancer, pancreatic cancer, carcinoid, VIPoma, medullary thyroid cancer, Zollinger-Ellison syndrome.
- Functional.
- Irritable bowel syndrome.
- Faecal impaction.
- Anal sphincter damage.
- Purgative abuse.

History

Take a general colorectal history. Ask about stool frequency and consistency. Ask about the duration of symptoms and associated blood or mucus. Differentiate from incontinence and the passage of frequent small hard stool with irritable bowel syndrome. How has the bowel habit changed, and over what period?

A short history may suggest an infective cause, but may also be the first presentation of inflammatory bowel conditions such as Crohn's. Evidence should be sought regarding travel abroad, food poisoning and diarrhoea among other family members or close acquaintances.

Food poisoning

Food poisoning is usually obvious from the history. Onset within 12 hours suggests a toxin cause, e.g. *Staphylococcus aureus* toxin or *Bacillus cereus. Vibrio parahaemolyticus* is responsible for most seafood poisoning and may be associated with vomiting and severe abdominal pain. After this time, and up to three days, *Salmonella enteritis* is the commonest cause.

Viral gastroenteritis

This is one of the commonest infections of the small bowel and causes vomiting, abdominal pain and diarrhoea. Characteristically the diarrhoea is profuse and watery.

Bloody diarrhoea

Bloody diarrhoea usually indicates large bowel infection, e.g. *Shigella* or *Entamoeba histolytica.*

Crohn's or ulcerative colitis (UC)

These conditions may be suggested by a positive family history, or symptoms of longer than 1–2 weeks' duration or frequent bouts of diarrhoea over time. Ask about other symptoms associated with these conditions: skin rashes, arthritis, iritis.

Previous surgery

Surgery on the stomach or small bowel such as partial gastrectomy or small bowel resection predisposes to conditions associated with diarrhoea such as dumping or short gut syndrome.

Malabsorption

This is suggested by chronic diarrhoea not associated with fever or blood in the stools, but with weight loss and signs of nutritional deficiencies. Stools are often described as pale and offensive, and oily droplets within the stool may have been noticed. Could the patient have exocrine pancreatic failure?

Ask about change of bowel habit and alternating constipation and diarrhoea, which suggests a possible colonic cancer. A long-standing history of alternating constipation and diarrhoea associated with left iliac fossa pain in older patients is suggestive of diverticular disease.

Ask about symptoms of hyperthyroidism. Ask about diabetes mellitus – autonomic neuropathy can be associated with diarrhoea.

Tuberculosis is a rarer cause of diarrhoea and may be associated with ethnicity or travel to or from areas where TB is common. Lymphoma may be suggested by a chronic history of weight loss and night sweats.

A drug history is important. In particular ask about antibiotic therapy and other drugs associated with diarrhoea.

Rare causes such as carcinoid tumours may be associated with other symptoms such as severe flushing and recent-onset asthma. Zollinger-Ellison usually presents with severe peptic ulceration resistant to treatment.

Examination

Perform a general colorectal examination. Assess hydration and examine for pyrexia. Perform a rectal examination and proctoscopy/sigmoidoscopy to identify inflammatory mucosa or other lesions, and obtain a stool sample for microbiology. Perform a rectal biopsy for a diagnosis of inflammatory mucosa.

Investigations

Exclude infection and inflammatory bowel disease.

Food poisoning can be confirmed by sending stool and food samples for microbiology.

If parasites are suspected, the stool sample should be transported to the laboratory immediately for inspection – ask for ova, cysts and parasites.

Perform a rectal biopsy for histology to differentiate inflammatory bowel disease from infective causes of bloody diarrhoea (*Shigella*, *Entamoeba histolytica*) and to differentiate between Crohn's and ulcerative colitis.

Use abdominal X-ray (AXR) to exclude dilated colon, e.g. toxic megacolon in severe ulcerative colitis.

Colonoscopy/barium enema is used to exclude carcinoma if indicated. Care should be taken in the colonoscopy of acute colitics due to the risk of perforation, but in those over the age of 45 with chronic diarrhoea, imaging of the entire colon is mandatory to exclude malignancy.

If malabsorption is suspected, perform a faecal fat estimation and if confirmed investigate further to identify the underlying cause.

Routine blood tests include *Salmonella* titres and amoebic serology if suspected; blood cultures if pyrexial; FBC; ESR/CRP; thyroid function tests; blood sugar; antiendomysial or anti-tissue transglutaminase antibodies (for coeliac disease); serum albumin; iron studies; folate and B12 levels.

Treatment

Food poisoning and infective diarrhoea can be managed with isolation, fluid resuscitation and other supportive measures until the episode subsides. Antibiotics are prescribed where indicated for severe infection with *Shigella* or *Campylobacter*. Travellers' diarrhoea is most commonly caused by *E. coli* and can be treated with trimethoprim or ciprofloxacin.

The management of Crohn's and ulcerative colitis, irritable bowel syndrome, colorectal carcinoma, diverticular disease, malabsorption, hyperthyroidism, carcinoid syndrome and Zollinger Ellison syndrome will be described under the relevant sections.

Follow-up

Follow up at short intervals until the cause is identified and serious causes are excluded. There may be an indication for in-patient management in severe cases to avoid dehydration and facilitate prompt investigation.

Constipation

There is a wide range of normal bowel frequency, from two to three times a day to once a week. However, defaecation less than twice a week or straining at stool for more than 25% of bowel movements merits consideration, as do a sensation of incomplete defaecation and excessive time spent attempting to open the bowels. Symptoms are said to have a prevalence of 2–28%. Most cases (50–60%) are simple/functional constipation with normal transit times and need no investigation as they respond to dietary manipulation and laxatives. In 10–15% there is slow transit constipation, which often requires long-term laxative use.

Causes of chronic constipation include the following.

+ Idiopathic slow transit constipation: the colon may be normal or have a variety of physiological derangements.
+ Colorectal disease: underlying bowel disorder, the most important of which is cancer. Other conditions that can cause constipation are irritable bowel disease, diverticular disease, Crohn's ulcerative colitis, ischaemic colitis, hernias and volvulus.
+ Anal pathology: anal fissure, anal stenosis, anterior mucosal prolapse, haemorrhoids, descending perineum syndrome, perianal abscess, rectocoele, anal cancer.
+ Neurological disease or injury:
   ∝ peripheral: Hirschsprung's, autonomic neuropathy, Chagas disease
   ∝ central: cerebrovascular accident, cerebral tumours, Parkinson's disease, meningocele, multiple sclerosis, paraplegia
   ∝ muscular: dermatomyositis, systemic sclerosis.
+ Metabolic disease, e.g. diabetes mellitus, hypothyroidism, hypercalcaemia.
+ Psychiatric illness, depression or debility.
+ Gynaecological pathology: large fibroids, ovarian cysts.
+ Drugs, e.g. codeine preparations, morphine, antidepressants, iron, anticholinergics.

History

Take a general colorectal history. Determine what the patient means by constipation. Determine the time-course of the symptoms – sudden onset, especially in patients over 50, is more indicative of a serious underlying cause, as are other alarm symptoms including rectal bleeding and weight loss. Ask about the frequency of stool, the amount and the consistency. The passage of small amounts of hard faeces suggests constipation. Pain on passing faeces suggests anal pathology.

Ask about change in bowel habit – is this a recent problem or has it been going on for years? Ask about abdominal pain and bloating or alternating bouts of diarrhoea. Ask about medications. Ask about lifestyle – some work conditions or poor toilet facilities may lead to prolonged avoidance of defaecation, which predisposes to constipation. Ask about obstetric and gynaecological history to identify possible birth injury from instrumentation or gynaecological pathology associated with constipation, e.g. ovarian cysts. Ask about the other causes of constipation.

Examination

Perform a general examination. Examine for anaemia, jaundice, hypothyroidism and weight loss. Perform an abdominal examination: palpable masses may be faecal, diverticular, neoplastic or gynaecological in origin. Perform a rectal examination and remember to examine for conditions such as faecal impaction, perianal scars, fissures, haemorrhoids, prolapse or neoplasm. Assess perianal descent (the extent to which the anus descends on bearing down – normally 1–3.5cm). Excessive descent (greater than 3.5cm or below the plane of the ischial tuberosities) suggests perineal laxity and can lead to a sensation of incomplete evacuation and/or mucosal prolapse.

Investigations

Proctoscopy, sigmoidoscopy and AXR (dilated colon and faecal masses) should be performed on everybody. Patients with loss of haustral pattern or megacolon/rectum on X-ray are unlikely to respond to simple laxatives and further investigation is indicated.

Gross structural abnormalities and colonic strictures can be excluded using a double contrast barium enema. Colonoscopy should be reserved for those in whom colorectal cancer or inflammatory bowel disease need exclusion (alarm symptoms are sudden onset after 50 years of age or a significant family history of colorectal neoplasia or inflammatory bowel disease).

Urea and electrolytes including calcium, blood sugar and if indicated thyroid function tests, parathormone and serum porphyrins for metabolic and endocrine causes are performed.

Colonic transit time studies are useful for those with normal diameter colons and persistent symptoms.

Anorectal physiology and electromyography of puborectalis and external anal sphincter are useful for suspected abnormalities of the defaecation mechanism.

Full thickness rectal biopsy under general anaesthetic is used to exclude adult Hirschsprung's disease (absent anorectal reflex on anal physiology). Samples are sent fresh for immediate acetylcholine analysis.

Treatment

Older patients or patients who present with sudden-onset constipation need urgent investigations including barium enema/colonoscopy to exclude underlying cancer or other serious pathology. In younger patients with no other suspicious clinical features or older patients in whom serious underlying pathology has been excluded, more time is available for assessment and trial of therapies. Education regarding diet and exercise and what constitutes a normal bowel habit should be given.

If the problem is simply straining at hard stool without abdominal or anal pain, simple advice regarding fibre in the diet removes the need for further assessment unless the condition fails to respond. Increase the amount of fibre in the diet – give a dietitian referral or high-fibre diet sheet. Prescribe ispaghula husk. Lactulose softens a hard stool. Senna increases bowel contractility to expel the stool (care is needed in long-term use). Glycerin suppositories and arachis oil enemas are useful to soften hard stool impacted in the rectum. Phosphate enemas can be useful to clear more stubborn stool extending into the sigmoid colon.

In those with established defaecatory disorders, biofeedback may be useful, but when there is established intractable constipation, an initial purge with potent osmotic laxatives may be required, followed by regular high doses of more gentle osmotic laxatives with or without stimulant laxatives. However, care should be exercised, especially in the elderly, who may require in-patient treatment and an intravenous drip.

Laxatives are unlikely to be effective if the haustral pattern of the colon has been lost or there is megacolon or megarectum. In these patients anorectal manometry is useful to identify underlying disorders such as Hirschsprung's. Patients who have an absent rectosphincteric reflex and evidence of megacolon/rectum should undergo a full thickness rectal biopsy to exclude Hirschsprung's.

Patients with severe idiopathic constipation should undergo colonic transit studies and anorectal physiology studies, as there are a number of abnormalities of defaecation that can be diagnosed, such as an increased anorectal angle caused by abnormal contraction of the puborectalis muscle at defaecation; failure of the pelvic floor to relax on attempted defaecation – the outlet syndrome; abnormal perineal descent; and pudendal nerve neuropathy.

Surgery

Hirschsprung's short segment disease can be treated with an anorectal myectomy, rectal myectomy or anal sphincterotomy. Distal disease can be treated by a 'pull-through' operation.

Anorectal myectomy may be effective in the 'outlet syndrome' (contraindicated if marker studies indicate severe colonic inertia).

Surgery is rarely used in severe idiopathic constipation except in the most serious and persistent cases, e.g. ileostomy, irrigating caecostomy, percutaneous endoscopic colostomy (PEC) with anterograde irrigation.

In those with refractory slow transit constipation and no defaecatory disorder, colectomy and ileorectal anastomosis is occasionally indicated, but only after more than one expert opinion has been obtained.

Follow-up

After the exclusion of serious underlying pathology, most patients can be discharged to the care of the GP, following simple advice on diet and laxatives. In those with refractory constipation, further follow-up should be guided according to the results of special investigations.

Post-operative follow-up

Review with histology to confirm the diagnosis and determine the success of the operation. Detect any complications of general anaesthesia and of the specific procedure. For 'pull-through' operations, check the histology to confirm that normally innervated bowel had been reached. Residual Hirschsprung's can be a cause of residual constipation.

Chronic megacolon

Chronic megacolon is an abnormally dilated colon or rectum with loss of haustral pattern. It may affect the total colon or segments. Causes are congenital (Hirschsprung's) or acquired.

Acquired causes include the following.

- ✧ Obstruction: chronic anal stenosis, strictures (ischaemic), annular neoplasms.
- ✧ Chagas disease.
- ✧ Hypothyroidism.
- ✧ Neurological disorders: spina bifida, cauda equina, paraplegia, Parkinson's.
- ✧ Psychological disturbances.
- ✧ Idiopathic: no underlying cause. Adynamic bowel syndrome may affect the colon only, with normal rectum, or it may present as megarectum with variable colon in continuity. Rectal capacity and sensation are diminished but sphincteric responses and rectal biopsy are normal.

History

Take a general colorectal history. Patients may present with similar symptoms to chronic constipation or faecal incontinence due to overflow secondary to faecal impaction. Those with idiopathic megacolon may describe abdominal pain and distension in the context of chronic constipation.

Examination
Perform a general colorectal examination, looking for the same abdominal and perianal conditions as are associated with chronic constipation.

Investigations
Investigate with proctoscopy, sigmoidoscopy and AXR. X-ray reveals abnormally dilated large bowel and loss of haustral pattern. Give colonoscopy/barium enema to exclude underlying organic disease in older patients and other age groups where indicated. Perform anal physiology studies. Exclude Hirschsprung's with full thickness rectal biopsy in selected patients.

Treatment
Treat underlying conditions. Otherwise treat medically with colonic washouts, disimpaction of faeces and, in severely symptomatic patients, surgical treatment bowel resection. Generally the longer the history, the worse the outcome, but procedures including colectomy with ileorectal anastomosis and restorative proctocolectomy have good reported outcomes, with permanent stomas affording a generally good quality of life in those in whom initial surgery has failed.

Follow-up
Following the initial consultation, serious underlying causes, suggested by the history and clinical examination, should be excluded. Chronic and idiopathic causes can be reviewed at 3–4 monthly intervals to assess the efficacy of conservative treatments. Discharge with advice to the GP on future management and discharge once organic causes have been excluded and the condition stabilised, or offer surgery in an appropriately counselled patient when all other avenues of treatment have failed.

Rectal inertia
Mainly seen in children where the rectum is over-stretched by repeatedly inadequate evacuation.

History
There is chronic constipation in apparently healthy individuals, with mild abdominal distension and occasional perianal soiling. Older children and adults may have psychological problems. Differentiation from Hirschsprung's may be difficult, but Hirschsprung's normally presents with problems from birth, while rectal inertia presents only after toilet training.

Examination
Abdomen is flat but faecal masses are palpable in left colon. Make rectal examination to exclude underlying physical problems like anal fissure or anal stenosis. There may be evidence of soiling, poor anal tone and hard faecal masses.

Investigations
In cases that do not respond to medical treatment examine under anaesthetic and take full thickness rectal biopsy.

Treatment

Empty the bowel by saline rectal washouts (in-patient if necessary for 2–3 weeks). If indicated perform manual evacuation, then recommence toilet training at regular intervals. For adults, continue the use of phosphate enemas or suppositories. Do not stimulate the proximal colon with laxatives as it may aggravate the condition.

Follow-up

There is usually a chronic history so there is no urgency for investigation unless the history and examination suggest suspicious features. Investigations and trials of treatment can be performed at 1–3 monthly intervals until symptoms are controlled. Discharge once stable on medication.

Diverticular disease

Colonic diverticula are false, pulsion diverticula consisting of mucosa and serosa, which form at areas of structural weakness of the colonic wall where the vasa rectae penetrate the muscularis propria to supply the mucosa. The condition is thought to be a consequence of the Western diet, with a relative lack of vegetable fibre, although structural changes in the colonic wall associated with aging and disordered motility (hyperelastosis and altered collagen structure) are thought to contribute.

Diverticulosis describes the presence of diverticula, and is very common, affecting more than 60% of those over 70 years. Around 90% of people are said to be asymptomatic, perhaps explaining how relatively infrequently people are admitted with symptomatic diverticula (diverticular disease), given the high prevalence.

The term 'diverticulitis' implies infection and inflammation in association with diverticula. Right-sided diverticula are common in the Orient, while in the West left-sided diverticulosis is more typical. The condition typically starts after age 30 and peaks in 60s–70s, but younger patients do present acutely with complicated diverticular disease. Severity ranges from episodes of mild discomfort to the onset of complications which include perforation, abscess formation, intestinal obstruction, fistulation into neighbouring organs and haemorrhage. Carcinoma of the colon can co-exist with diverticular disease.

History

Take a general colorectal history. Symptoms may be episodic and recurrent and include mild to severe left iliac fossa (LIF) or lower abdominal pain, dull and constant, lasting hours to days and precipitated by diet or stress. There are sheep-dropping faeces, with occasional mucus and diarrhoea.

The following symptoms may suggest the onset of complications.

✧ Perforation: severe constant pain in the lower abdomen and feeling systemically unwell.

✧ Intestinal obstruction: history of increasing constipation and abdominal distension associated with colicky abdominal pain. Diverticular strictures are related to scarring following previous episodes of diverticulitis, and distinction from malignant strictures can often only be finally made after histological examination of the resected specimen.

✧ Fistulation can occur into the colon, small intestine, uterus, vagina, abdominal wall and bladder. Fistulae form when an inflamed diverticulum adheres to an adjacent organ and a pericolic abscess ruptures into it. May present with symptoms of chronic ill-health, low abdominal tenderness, intermittent diarrhoea, pneumaturia and faecal vaginal discharge.

 ∝ Colovesical: urgency and dysuria (recurrent urinary tract infections (UTI)), pneumaturia and faecaluria.

    ∝ Colovaginal: air and faeces per vagina, much more common following a previous hysterectomy.
- Haemorrhage: there may be a history of episodes or brisk bright-red bleeding per-rectum.
- Caecal or right-sided diverticula is found in one-third of diverticular patients: shows appendicitis-type symptoms.

Examination

Perform a general examination. In acute attacks there may be low-grade fever, tenderness and rigidity and occasionally a mass in the lower abdomen. Localised perforation and abscess formation may be suspected if examination reveals a localised mass, while free perforation into the abdominal cavity generally presents as an emergency with generalised peritonitis. Vaginal examination may reveal a foul, brown discharge. Abdominal distension and active bowel sounds may suggest intestinal obstruction. Rectal examination may reveal blood or pus.

Investigations

Flexible sigmoidoscopy shows the multiple openings of the diverticula, and in acute attacks may reveal an inflamed mucosa and oedema. Barium enema is not advisable in the acute phase, due to the risk of perforation, but is useful for investigation of chronic symptoms. Barium shows the typical out-pouchings and long constricted segments of bowel. Perform flexible sigmoidoscopy to exclude carcinoma within segments of diverticulosis. Take a mid-stream urine specimen for microscopy and culture to detect subclinical fistulation.

    CT is useful for assessment of adjoining organs for fistula and involvement of tissue planes, and the presence of an inflammatory phlegmon or abscess.
- Perforation: the presence of a localised mass or abscess can be confirmed on USS, but CT is increasingly used in the acute setting as it provides more information.
- Intestinal obstruction is usually diagnosed by plain AXR. Gastrograffin enema can confirm the diagnosis and identify the level of obstruction.
- Fistula: barium enema can define the tract, but such connections are commonly not seen even when they exist. Cystography and cystoscopy can be used to confirm and define colovesical fistulas and exclude primary bladder neoplasms.
- Haemorrhage: differentiate from vascular ectatic lesions. Use sigmoidoscopy to exclude bleeding from piles and use arteriography to exclude vascular ectatic lesions and potentially arrest bleeding in the case of massive diverticular bleeds.

Treatment

Diverticular pain

Colonic spasm rather than inflammation is relieved by faecal bulk-forming agents – Isogel, Fybogel, antispasmodics. Colonic resection only for severe cases requiring repeated admissions, or those with complicated disease (local or free perforation, stricture, fistulation). Elective resections are increasingly being performed laparoscopically.

Uncomplicated disease

Acute attack settles over 4–5 days and only 30% have recurrent symptoms. However, 5–10% become severe and need sigmoid colectomy.

Diverticular abscess

CT-guided percutaneous drainage and intravenous antibiotics should be the first-line treatment in those with localised signs and a confirmed abscess, with emergency surgery reserved for those with generalised peritonitis.

Complicated disease and peritonitis

Treat with Hartmann's procedure (resection and end colostomy) or colonic lavage, primary anastomosis and defunctioning ileostomy, depending on the extent of peritoneal contamination. If soiling is minimal then consideration can be given to omission of the defunctioning stoma.

Fistulation

Treat with elective sigmoid resection with primary anastomosis and repair of fistulous opening in the affected organ. In the case of colovesical fistula, no attempt is made to close the bladder but the urethral catheter is left for 10 days and many surgeons request a cystogram to ensure closure of the defect prior to catheter removal. However, in the elderly patient, or one unfit for surgery, a trial of conservative therapy with prolonged antibiotics may be justified.

Follow-up

Initial investigation should be tailored to exclude serious underlying pathology, and colonoscopy should be performed if concerning symptoms are present in patients over the age of 50 or who have a strong family history of colorectal cancer or inflammatory bowel disease.

In most patients the diagnosis can be confirmed by barium enema, and patients are seen once following this investigation to give simple dietary advice.

For those with complications, or two episodes of significant diverticulitis, surgical resection should be considered on an elective basis to prevent future emergency admissions and to reduce the likelihood of a Hartmann's procedure being required.

Post-operative follow-up

Review with the histology to exclude co-existent carcinoma. Examine for complications of laparotomy and general anaesthetic. If a Hartmann's was performed, determine the timetable for reversal or whether reversal is to be performed. Symptoms continue in 25% of patients after surgery and are thought to be caused by the underlying disordered bowel motility.

Polyps in the colon and rectum

A polyp is an abnormal overgrowth of the colonic mucosa and can be sessile (flat) or pedunculated (on a stalk). Polyps fall into the following categories.

- Inflammatory: occur in UC, Crohn's, diverticulitis, chronic dysentery and, rarely, benign lymphoid hyperplasia.
- Hamartomatous polyps: juvenile and Peutz-Jeghers (P-J) have significant malignant potential.
- Metaplastic polyps: size 1–2mm, rarely larger than 5mm; biopsy confirms the diagnosis and they need no ongoing observation.
- Adenomatous polyps: benign tumours composed of abnormal colonic glands. Classified according to the growth pattern of the glands: 75% are tubular adenomas, 10% villous and 15% tubulovillous adenomas. All have malignant potential.

Relationship of polyps to cancer

There is a strong relationship. Approximately 40% of patients treated for a polyp develop further polyps. Only 3% of adenomatous polyps are malignant, but a third of villous papillomas are malignant. The risk of malignancy increases with size, from 1% for polyps less than 5mm to 40% for polyps larger than 2cm and 60% for those greater than 3cm.

Familial polyposis – hereditary
Familial adenomatous polyposis (FAP)

FAP is characterised by hundreds of adenomatous colorectal polyps by the second or third decade of life. It is an autosomal dominant mutation of the APC gene at position 21 on chromosome 5q.

Screening should begin in the early teens for patients from affected families, whose information is collected in polyposis registries. To prevent the almost inevitable development of colorectal cancer, resection (restorative proctocolectomy or colectomy and ileorectal anastomosis, which necessitates ongoing rectal surveillance) should be performed as soon as practically possible following diagnosis.

Hereditary non-polyposis colorectal cancer (HNPCC)

HNPCC is responsible for 2% of colorectal cancer. It is characterised by early diagnosis of colorectal cancer (approximate age 45, compared with 65 for the general population). HNPCC is diagnosed according to the Amsterdam Criteria II, as follows.

- At least three relatives should have an HNPCC-associated cancer (colorectal, endometrial, small bowel, ureter, renal pelvis), of whom one should be a first-degree relative of the other two.
- At least two successive generations should be affected.
- At least one colorectal cancer should be diagnosed before the age of 50.
- FAP should be excluded.
- Tumours should be verified pathologically.

History

Take a general colorectal history and a careful family history. Polyps are usually asymptomatic and may present as anaemia due to occult bleeding. Retrograde propulsion of large pedunculated polyps may produce abdominal pain, spasm and colic and cause colocolic intussusception. Rectal lesions can cause tenesmus or change in bowel habit to diarrhoea. Mucous discharge may occur, especially with villous papilloma, which may lead to dehydration and electrolyte imbalance. Large papillomas may produce hypokalaemia, metabolic acidosis leading to symptoms of lethargy, muscle weakness, mental confusion and renal failure.

Examination

Perform a general examination. Examination may range from normal to signs of dehydration, anaemia, mental confusion and muscle weakness.

Investigations

FBC may reveal anaemia. Urea and electrolytes (U&E) may indicate dehydration or hypokalaemia. Rigid sigmoidoscopy may reveal the presence of rectal adenomas, which should prompt colonoscopy examination and polypectomy.

Treatment

Treatment of colorectal polyps and villous papillomas is by regular colonoscopy with intervals as specified by British Society of Gastroenterology guidelines. CT colonography or barium enema are alternatives for patients in whom colonoscopy is technically challenging.

Malignant polyps

Following colonoscopic excision of a malignant polyp, a decision must be made as to whether radical resection of the excision site is required. Considerations include the likelihood of the cancer being completely excised and the chance of lymph node metastases being present.

Favourable characteristics include:

- complete endoscopic resection with a margin of normal tissue
- cancers confined to the head of a polyp
- well or moderately differentiated tumours
- absence of lymphovascular invasion.

If doubt exists in patients fit for major surgery then radical resection of the site is indicated. This is technically easier if the site of the polyp is 'tattooed' with ink at the time of polypectomy, to ensure that it is removed and examined histologically.

Follow-up

All patients are followed up by regular colonoscopy, according to British Society of Gastroenterology guidelines.

Carcinoma of colon and rectum

The UK lifetime risk of colorectal cancer is around 5%, with nearly 35 000 new cases diagnosed in 2002, and it is responsible for 19 000 deaths annually. Seventy per cent of cases occur within reach of the 60cm flexible sigmoidoscope (i.e. distal to the splenic flexure). Rectal cancers, by definition, occur within 15cm of the anal verge. Overall five-year survival has improved from 22% to 50% over the last 10 years.

Predisposing conditions are genetic; dietary factors (increased animal fat and proteins); colorectal polyps; familial polyposis coli; radiation proctocolitis; previous ureterosigmoidostomy, ulcerative colitis (especially total colon involvement longer than 10 years – consider for prophylactic bowel excision); and schistosomiasis.

Staging of colorectal carcinoma

Dukes' staging (modified by Astler and Coller) is shown in Table 9.1.

TABLE 9.1 Staging of colorectal carcinoma.

UICC/TNM		DUKES' STAGE
Stage 0	Carcinoma in situ	
Stage I	No nodal involvement, no distant metastasis	A
	Tumour invades submucosa (T1, N0, M0)	
	Tumour invades muscularis propria (T2, N0, M0)	
Stage II	No nodal involvement, no distant metastasis	B
	Tumour invades into subserosa (T3, N0, M0)	
	Tumour invades into other organs (T4, N0, M0)	
Stage III	Nodal involvement, no distant metastasis	C
	1 to 3 regional lymph nodes involved (any T, N1, M0)	
	4 or more regional lymph nodes involved (Any T, N2, M0)	
Stage IV	Distant metastasis (any T, any N, M1)	D

Note: in the commonly used Astler-Coller modification of the Dukes' stage, C1 implies any lymph-node involvement, while if the apical lymph node removed (closest to the tie on the arterial pedicle) is involved it is classified as C2.

Modes of spread

Intramural spread may be transverse, lateral and radial. Most consider a longitudinal clearance of 2cm to be adequate. In rectal cancer, where 'total mesorectal excision' is the recommended method of excision, a circumferential resection margin (distance from the tumour to the nearest radial cut edge) of greater than 1mm is considered to be uninvolved.

Extension to adjacent structures

This applies more to the rectum than the colon.
- Anterior spread is to seminal vesicles and prostate in the male and to the posterior vaginal wall in the female.
- Lymphatic spread: rectal cancer occurs in 50% of pararectal nodes, to lower colic nodes, to inferior mesenteric nodes. Lateral lymph node spread is more common to the hypogastric lymph nodes (internal iliac nodes).
- Haematogenous spread is to the liver in 18–20% at presentation, the lung in 5%.
- Perineal spread, transperitoneal spread.

History

Take a general colorectal history. The onset is often insidious, but after that the development of symptoms depends on the site of the tumour. Enquire regarding predisposing conditions, e.g. ulcerative colitis, Crohn's, previous gastric surgery (which doubles the risk of colorectal cancer).

In addition to the polyposis syndromes, a positive family history is an important risk factor for the development of colorectal cancer. In one study with a baseline population risk of 1/50, the risk rose to 1/17 for any positive family history, 1/10 if one relative was affected below the age of 45 and 1/6 if two or more relatives were affected.

Caecal, ascending colon and hepatic flexure

Symptoms are insidious for a long time, with vague upper abdominal pain and flatulent distension, pallor, lassitude and general ill-health. Alteration in bowel habit is less frequent. Occasionally there is diarrhoea.

Transverse and descending colon

There is increasing constipation alternating with diarrhoea. Occasionally there is blood and mucus. May also present with fistulation, e.g. gastrocolic – vomiting faeces.

Sigmoid and rectal

Rectal bleeding is the most frequent presentation. It is usually slight, with alteration in bowel habit and spurious morning diarrhoea. The patient wakes and passes mucus in the presence of constipation and tenesmus. Severe pain may indicate extension into surrounding tissues and a poor prognosis. May also present with fistulation, e.g. colovesical.

Guidelines

Specific guidelines which identify those patients considered to be at high risk of colorectal cancer (and therefore warranting urgent referral and investigation) were published by the National Institute for Health and Clinical Excellence (NICE) in 2005. High-risk groups were identified as the following.
- Patients aged 40 and above with rectal bleeding and a change in bowel habit to looser stools and/or increased stool frequency persisting for six weeks or more.

✧ Patients aged 60 and above with rectal bleeding persisting for six weeks or more without a change in bowel habit but in the absence of anal symptoms.
✧ Patients aged 60 and above with a change in bowel habit to looser and/or more frequent stools persisting for six weeks or more in the absence of rectal bleeding.
✧ Patients with a right iliac fossa mass consistent with colonic involvement, irrespective of age.
✧ Patients with a palpable intraluminal (not pelvic) rectal mass.
✧ Men of any age with unexplained iron deficiency anaemia (haemoglobin <11 g/100 ml) irrespective of age.
✧ Non-menstruating women with unexplained iron deficiency anaemia (haemoglobin <10 g/100 ml)

Examination

Perform a general colorectal examination. Examine for the presence of jaundice, anaemia and weight loss. Perform an abdominal examination: examine for a palpable mass, e.g. in RIF due to caecal lesion; or enlarged liver indicating metastases. Perform rectal examination: 75% of all rectal tumours and approximately a third of bowel tumours can be palpated. Determine the location, mobility and extent of spread around bowel and into surrounding tissues.

Investigations

Do FBC, U&E, LFTs, CXR and ECG. Determine pre-operative CEA level. Perform Proctososcopy: determine size, site, extent and distance from anal verge. Flexible sigmoidoscopy needs bowel preparation with a phosphate enema. All patients suspected of possible carcinoma of the colon should undergo rigid sigmoidoscopy and barium enema or colonoscopy. Suspicious lesions detected on barium should undergo colonoscopy and biopsy. CT scans of the chest and abdomen are used to stage the disease (looking for liver and lung metastases) and to look for local complications such as duodenal or ureteric involvement. Alternatives include the use of liver ultrasound and CXR, but these are considered less sensitive.

Barium enema

Double contrast is more reliable but still has a false negative rate of more than 2%. Features of malignancy are mucosal destruction, abrupt cut-off of barium and localised lesion with sharp demarcation from the involved areas ('apple-core lesions').

Colonoscopy

This is generally considered the first-line investigation if there is a high suspicion of cancer, or if barium enema is equivocal. Full examination of colon should be made to demonstrate additional pathology, e.g. synchronous carcinoma (present in 2–5% of cases), diverticula disease. If it cannot be performed pre-operatively due to a stenosing primary lesion, arrange for full examination of the colon within three months after the operation to remove the primary lesion.

Endoluminal ultrasound

This is useful in rectal tumours for defining the involvement of the rectal wall and extent of extra-rectal involvement and adjacent lymph nodes.

MRI

This is increasingly used to locally stage rectal cancers, to determine their relationship to the mesorectal fascia and to select patients likely to benefit from pre-operative radiotherapy.

Treatment

All patients should be discussed at the multidisciplinary team (MDT) meeting (involving surgeons, oncologists, radiologists and pathologists, amongst others) where potential alternative management strategies can be discussed. Pre-operative radiotherapy may be recommended in patients with large rectal tumours where the potential circumferential resection margin is threatened. It is also considered when local excision of a small rectal cancer is contemplated in poor-risk patients. Ongoing trials may suggest a survival benefit for all rectal cancer patients undergoing curative surgery.

Bowel preparation

This varies widely according to local policy, but there is a current trend away from the use of mechanical bowel preparation, with its attendant side effects and negative impact on post-operative recovery, unless on-table colonoscopy is likely to be needed or there is a high likelihood of forming a defunctioning stoma, in which case many consider a column of faeces between the stoma and anastomosis to be undesirable. Right-sided colonic lesions do not require preparation. Bowel preparation agents include Picolax, Fleet, Klean-Prep and polyethylene glycol. All can cause electrolyte disturbances and dehydration, and patients should be given concurrent intravenous fluids to prevent profound drops in blood pressure on the induction of anaesthesia. Do not use in obstructing lesions – use on-table lavage instead.

Ward prophylaxis

Peri-operative antibiotics (commonly used but with little evidence except for a potential reduction in wound infection rates), deep vein thrombosis (DVT) prophylaxis with TED stockings and subcutaneous heparin.

Even in the presence of liver metastases the patient's best interests may be served by removal of the primary tumour.

Abdominoperineal resection

Used when the tumour is very close to the anal verge or invading the anal sphincters. End colostomy in the left iliac fossa.

Anterior resection

Used when the tumour is situated more proximally in the rectum such that adequate distal clearance can be attained with acceptable post-operative functional results. Sometimes a covering colostomy/ileostomy is fashioned to mitigate against the consequences of anastomotic leakage (stomas do not prevent leaks). Patients undergoing radical rectal surgery should be warned of the possibility of sexual and urinary dysfunction following surgery due to inadvertent damage to the pelvic nerves.

Locally advanced tumours

En bloc resection. Radical approach can give survival rate of 50% at five years depending on the stage.

Small cancers of the rectum

These are mobile in the rectal mucosa. They especially occur in the elderly. Perform local excision with a 0.5–1.0cm margin of healthy tissue. Transanal endoscopic microsurgery (TEM) allows accurate local full thickness excision but even in T1 lesions, lymph node metastases have been reported in up to 17% of patients with tumours invading the lower one-third of the submucosa.

Palliative transanal resection (often with a urological resectoscope – TART) can be used to palliate those with rectal cancers who are unfit for radical surgery.

Local radiotherapy is not widely accepted.

Multiple colonic tumours
Synchronous tumours: incidence is 2–5%, and they often require total colectomy.

Hepatic metastases – suitability for liver resection
The aim of liver resection (resectability) is to remove all macroscopic disease with clear margins, leaving sufficient functioning liver. Considerations include the following.
✧ Patients with solitary, multiple and bilobar disease who have had radical treatment of the primary colorectal cancer are candidates for liver resection.
✧ The ability to achieve clear margins (R0 resection) should be determined by the radiologist and surgeon in the regional hepatobiliary unit.
✧ The surgeon should define the acceptable residual functioning volume, approximately one-third of the standard liver volume, or the equivalent of a minimum of two segments.
✧ The liver surgeon and anaesthetist should make the clinical decision regarding fitness for surgery.
✧ If deemed medically unfit for surgery, patients should be considered for ablative therapy.
✧ Extrahepatic disease that should be considered for liver resection includes:
  ∝ resectable/ablatable pulmonary metastases
  ∝ resectable/ablatable isolated extrahepatic sites, e.g. spleen, adrenal or resectable local recurrence
  ∝ local direct extension of liver metastases to, for example, diaphragm/adrenal, that can be resected.

Follow-up
In suspected colorectal cancer, urgent endoscopic investigation should be performed and patients should be seen at regular appropriate intervals to give the results of biopsies and staging investigations and to agree a treatment plan. If surgery is indicated explain all possible procedures to the patient, including the possibility of a colostomy/covering ileostomy. Referral to the stoma service pre-operatively is helpful. There is a good case for colonoscopy screening for those patients with familial colonic polyposis, family history of colonic malignancy, previous colorectal cancer and adenomas and inflammatory bowel disease.

Inoperable and recurrent tumour
Provide regular review and discuss palliative chemotherapy with an oncologist. Consider involving the palliative care team early, as they can offer advice on the amelioration of symptoms as well as terminal care.

Monitor CEA and CA 19-9. If the levels of these markers rise it may indicate recurrence (assuming a high pre-treatment level fell to normal following initial surgery). However, a large number of recurrences are associated with no rise in their levels.

Post-operative follow-up
Review with the histology to determine adequate tumour resection; for grading and staging of the tumour; and to discuss subsequent oncological follow-up, although this is increasingly arranged during the MDT meeting. Examine for complications of laparotomy and general anaesthetic.

Complications of anterior resection include anastomotic leak, usually detected in an in-patient, but it may present later as a pelvic abscess/collection. Investigate by water-soluble enema to detect leak and CT scan to define collection. If anastomosis has been protected by a covering colostomy and the leak is small and the patient well, conservative management can be pursued and resolution expected. Defunctioned patients should have a water-soluble contrast enema arranged six weeks following surgery to exclude 'radiological' leaks prior to arranging reversal of the covering stoma.

Patients in whom direct evaluation of the entire colon was not possible prior to surgery (stenosing lesions, emergency surgery) should have a completion colonoscopy within three months to exclude a synchronous tumour not detected at operation.

Opinion is divided as to the most appropriate follow-up strategy following colorectal cancer resection. The benefits of intensive follow-up depend to a point on the fitness of the patient to undergo subsequent hepatic or pulmonary resections should metastases be diagnosed. In some studies the major benefit from following patients for five years following surgery has been psychological support, with very few asymptomatic recurrences being detected. To resolve this question the FACS Trial (Follow up After Colorectal Surgery) is ongoing to assess the cost-effectiveness of intensive versus minimal follow-up following resection of potentially curable colorectal cancer.

Most patients currently followed up in hospital undergo abdominal palpation to look for hepatomegaly, rigid sigmoidoscopy to assess for anastomotic recurrence in the case of low anastomoses, and regular ultrasound or CT scans according to local protocols.

Adjuvant therapy for colorectal carcinoma

Chemotherapy is generally considered for those with node positive disease (Dukes' C). five-year survival is 82% for Dukes' A, 69% for Dukes' B and 54% for Dukes' C.

Irritable bowel syndrome (IBS)

Generally, IBS describes a syndrome of recurrent symptoms of abdominal pain, bloating and/or altered bowel habit with no underlying organic disease. However, the lack of organic disease does not diminish the distress the symptoms can cause. Psychological factors and stress play an important role in the symptoms, although most patients have no obvious psychological or personality disorder. In middle-aged and older patients, a diagnosis of IBS should be made only after carcinoma or other organic disease has been excluded by the appropriate investigations. In younger patients, cancer is less likely but not unknown, and a difficult balance has to be obtained between unnecessary investigation and missing the occasional tumour. The less-experienced surgeon should probably err on the side of caution.

History

Take a general colorectal history. Classically, the IBS patient presents before the age of 35 and gives a history of recurrent abdominal pain that can occur at various sites around the abdomen. They may complain of abdominal bloating and describe some relief on passing flatus or faeces. Faeces are more frequent and smaller and may be loose or like string or sheep droppings. There may be associated passage of mucus and a feeling of incomplete evacuation. Typically the symptoms seem out of proportion to the patient's apparent well-being. Take a careful dietary history and note the intake of fibre. Take a history of smoking, alcohol consumption, ongoing stress and psychological disturbances past and present.

Ask about other psychological symptoms – anxiety, stress, depression drugs – and about referral to hospital to investigate similar anxiety-related symptoms affecting other body systems, e.g. difficulty swallowing. Coeliac disease is an important differential diagnosis and should especially be considered in the presence of mild anaemia.

Examination

Perform a general colorectal examination. Look to exclude underlying pathology. Determine the site of pain. Palpate for masses or palpable colon in the left iliac fossa, which may indicate thickening or spasm. Make a rectal examination to exclude rectal or anal pathology.

Investigations

Investigate with proctoscopy, sigmoidoscopy and AXR. If insufflation of air at sigmoido-scopy reproduces pain this is highly suggestive of irritable bowel syndrome. Further investigation e.g. colonoscopy/barium enema, ultrasound scan, is only indicated if underlying pathology is suspected, or in the presence of alarm features including onset after age 50, bleeding and weight loss. In patients without such features investigation should be kept to a minimum as they may simply increase the patients' anxiety.

Treatment

Give an explanation of symptoms, empathy and reassurance. A high-fibre diet may improve symptoms or make them worse, but is often tried initially. Sorbitol and caffeine may exacerbate symptoms. Peppermint oil may be tried to reduce gut spasm, as may anticholinergic drugs such as dicycloverine and hyoscine butylbromide, but there is no convincing trial evidence to suggest that they are better than placebo. Tricyclic antidepressants in low doses have been shown to be beneficial, possibly working via gut serotonin receptors. Some patients have a good result from cognitive behavioural therapy but often these are difficult patients to manage and they are victims of long-term management.

Follow-up

Once organic disease is excluded, further investigation should be kept to a minimum. After this, time should be given for dietary manipulations or other treatments to work, but if these fail patients may benefit from referral to physicians with a special interest in IBS.

Pneumatosis coli

These are gas-filled cysts found in the subserosal and submucosal planes. They are thought to result from lymphatic stasis, and the dilated channels then fill with gas.

History

The patient is asymptomatic or presents with colicky abdominal pain. A fulminant form exists, which may present with abdominal pain and bloody diarrhoea associated with pneumoperitoneum.

Examination

Examination may be normal or there may be evidence of abdominal distension.

Investigations

They are often detected as an incidental finding on AXR and barium enema.

Treatment

No active treatment is necessary. Cysts can be induced to disappear by oxygen therapy over 3–4 days. In fulminant disease the patient should be treated symptomatically, but if they deteriorate to the point of laparotomy the outlook is bleak and surgery generally involves excision of the affected segments and exteriorisation of both bowel ends.

Volvulus of the large bowel
Sigmoid volvulus

Predisposed by a long, redundant loop of sigmoid colon with a narrow base of attachment of the sigmoid mesocolon. It is classically seen in those with a long history of constipation and possibly laxative abuse, perhaps in long-term care due to neuropsychiatric disorders. Patients may present with an anticlockwise torsion of 180 degrees, which reverts spontaneously, leading to intermittent symptoms of abdominal pain, distension and constipation. If rotation of 360 degrees or more occurs, reduction is required to prevent perforation secondary to closed-loop obstruction. The chronic form may cause symptoms over many years.

History
Take a general colorectal history. In the chronic form patients may present to the outpatient clinic with a history of recurrent episodes of colicky central abdominal pain associated with distension and complete constipation. Motility disorders such as Hirschsprung's and Chagas diseases may predispose.

Examination
Perform a general examination. Examination may be normal between episodes, or during episodes there may be abdominal distension, tinkling bowel sounds and an empty rectum with blood on the glove.

Investigation
AXR shows a markedly distended loop of colon originating from the left iliac fossa and extending into the right upper quadrant ('coffee bean'). U&Es may reveal dehydration and other electrolyte abnormalities. FBC may reveal anaemia. Between episodes, barium enema may reveal a large redundant sigmoid loop, which suggests the diagnosis.

Treatment
Resuscitate if acute. Colonoscopic reduction is successful in 80%, but recurrence occurs in 90% and therefore it should be considered a temporary measure prior to definitive surgery.

Follow-up
Review for need for surgery. Because of the high rate of recurrence and the risks of emergency surgery, all but the very unfit should be considered for elective repair. Options include resection with or without stoma; fixation of the redundant loop (sigmoidopexy); or novel minimally invasive treatments such as percutaneous endoscopic colostomy (PEC), which involves fixation of the colonic loop to the anterior abdominal wall using PEG tubes.

Caecal volvulus
This occurs with a congenitally mobile caecum that twists up into the left upper quadrant of the abdomen. It often occurs in younger patients than does the sigmoid volvulus and it can be precipitated by pregnancy, recent surgery, left colonic obstructions and congenital malrotation/bands. The majority are really ileocolic; 10% are purely caecal; 11% of people have failure of fusion.

History
Patients may present acutely or with indolent obstructive symptoms with recurring vague indigestion and cramp-like abdominal pain.

Examination
Examination may be normal between episodes or the patient may present with abdominal distension arising from the right iliac fossa.

Investigations
During acute episodes, AXR reveals a large bowel loop arising from the RIF to the left upper quadrant. Between episodes a barium enema may reveal a chronically enlarged caecum, which suggests the diagnosis.

Treatment

Acutely colonoscopic decompression is not effective and surgery is required – options include right hemicolectomy, caecopexy and caecostomy.

Follow-up

Review with results, which may or may not suggest the diagnosis but should exclude other causes, e.g. cancer. Decide on need for surgery.

Post-operative follow-up

Review with histology to exclude the presence of co-existing carcinoma or other pathology. Detect any complications of laparotomy and large bowel resection.

Vascular lesions of the colon

The major vascular conditions affecting the colon can be classified as:
✧ ischaemic lesions of the large bowel
✧ angiodysplastic lesions of the colon.

Ischaemic conditions of the colon

There are three main causes of ischaemia and three main forms which present.
   The main causes of ischaemic colitis include the following.
✧ Thrombosis: arterial or venous, caused by arteriosclerosis, polycythaemia rubra vera, portal hypertension, malignant disease of the colon, hyperviscosity syndrome due to platelet abnormalities or high molecular weight dextran infusion.
✧ Emboli: left atrium (AF), left ventricle (MI), atheromatous plaque in the aorta.
✧ Vasculitis: polyarteritis nodosa (PAN), systemic lupus erythematosus (SLE), giant cell arteritis (Takayasu's arteritis), Buerger's disease, Henoch-Schönlein purpura.
✧ Surgical trauma to vessels: aortic reconstruction (with an inadequate marginal artery), resection of adjacent intestine.
✧ Non-occlusive ischaemia: shock-hypovolaemia or septic, congestive cardiac failure (an uncommon but frequently fatal complication of cardiopulmonary bypass).
✧ Spontaneous ischaemic colitis.

The three forms of ischaemic colitis are gangrenous, transient and stricturing.

Gangrenous

This presents with several days of abdominal pain and rectal bleeding. There is mild to moderate abdominal tenderness. Proctoscopy shows bleeding above the level of the proctoscope ('red-currant jelly'). The disease occurs most commonly at the splenic flexure (so-called 'Griffiths' point': the watershed between the superior and inferior mesenteric artery territories). On AXR, ischaemic colitis shows thumb printing, picket-fence thickening of folds and sacculation. Thumb printing is due to submucosal oedema and haemorrhage. Arteriography may show complete occlusion of the vessel. Colonoscopy may reveal haemorrhagic nodules and ulceration, but should be performed with care due to the risk of perforation.
   Treatment is initially supportive with total parenteral nutrition (TPN). If it deteriorates it needs surgery with resection of the bowel.

Transient

This occurs in patients who are middle-aged, with known peripheral vascular disease; collaterals form.

Stricturing

This may present with symptoms of chronic obstruction with a history of vascular disease (cardiac or peripheral). Strictures form due to scarring following the chronic ischaemia.

Vascular ectasia of the colon

This condition tends to affect the over-60 age group. They are acquired disorders, also known as angiodysplasia or arteriovenous malformations. They produce anaemia from chronic blood loss, generally of venous origin, or sudden haemorrhage. They are usually small and not detectable at operation and are only diagnosed by angiography. They mostly occur in the caecum and right colon. The cause is unknown but there is a 20% correlation between aortic stenosis and angiodysplasia. It is also associated with microaneurysm and collagen diseases.

History

Obscure colonic bleeding. There may be a history of intermittent episodes of fresh rectal bleeding.

Examination

Chronic cases may present with anaemia with otherwise normal examination findings. Acute cases may present with shock and fresh rectal bleeding.

Investigation

Give OGD and colonoscopy to rule out other causes of bleeding. Radio-labelled red-cell scans or selective mesenteric angiography can help to identify the site of bleeding and therapeutic angiography can be used to embolise the affected vessel.

Treatment

Treat with angiographic embolisation or segmental colectomy as guided by imaging studies.

Follow-up

Follow up at short intervals (1–4 weeks) until the cause is identified.

Inflammatory bowel disease (IBD): ulcerative colitis and Crohn's

IBD describes conditions associated with inflammation of the large bowel. The main differential diagnosis is between ulcerative colitis (UC) and Crohn's.

Other conditions that enter the differential diagnosis include tuberculous infections, amoebic dysentery, bilharzial infestations of the colon, *Salmonella* enteritis and colitis, *Campylobacter* infections, antibiotic-associated pseudomembranous colitis, necrotising enterocolitis, radiation-induced colitis and enteritis, ischaemic colitis (rare under age 60), complicated diverticular disease (especially with internal fistula), pneumatoides cystoides intestinalis (early stages) and primary cytomegalovirus colitis (can simulate or complicate UC).

Diseases that mimic Crohn's and exhibit similar X-ray signs include small bowel adenocarcinoma, lymphomas and small bowel phytobezoar.

Differentiation between ulcerative colitis and Crohn's

Crohn's disease can affect the entire gastrointestinal tract, from mouth to anus, and is characterised by discontinuous 'skip' lesions, while UC affects only the colon, except for backwash ileitis in patients with diffuse and severe disease who have an incompetent ileocaecal valve. It tends to do so in a confluent manner from the rectum, extending variable distances proximally (note that in some patients with UC there is relative 'rectal sparing'). UC and Crohn's describe a spectrum of disease, and those patients with colitis that cannot be differentiated into either category are labelled 'indeterminate colitis'.

IBD is covered in full in the section describing disorders of the small bowel.

Pseudomembranous colitis

This is a specific form of infective colitis generally seen in hospitalised patients receiving antibiotics. It is caused by *Clostridium difficile*. It is more common in elderly patients, after surgical intervention, in patients with intestinal neoplasm and in patients with atherosclerotic ischaemia.

History/examination

The mild form consists of watery mucoid diarrhoea which is offensive; the severe form results in toxic dilatation and a risk of perforation.

Investigations

It is diagnostic by colonoscopy and biopsies, where an off-white slough of necrotic mucosa and exudates (the 'pseudomembrane') is characteristic. Stool culture is used to identify *C. difficile* or its toxin.

Treatment

Give oral vancomycin for 1–2 weeks, or give intravenous metronidazole.

Neutropenic colitis

This may develop in patients undergoing chemotherapy. It is caused by super-infection, e.g. *Clostridium septicum.*

Rectal and anorectal disorders
Proctitis

Proctitis is an inflammation of the bowel similar to ulcerative colitis but inflammation is confined (initially) to the rectum and anal canal. The causes of proctitis can be divided into sexually transmitted infections, other infective causes, inflammatory bowel disease and trauma (mechanical, radiation).

✧ Sexually transmitted infections include gonorrhoea, herpes, *Chlamydia* and lymphogranuloma venereum. They are common in those engaging in unprotected receptive anal intercourse.
✧ Non-sexually transmitted infections include group 'A' *Streptococcus.*
✧ Inflammatory bowel disease: a non-specific variation of UC accounts for many cases of non-infective proctitis. While in most cases the course is benign, the condition may result in late rectal strictures. Crohn's and UC may also present initially with isolated proctitis.
✧ Trauma: often related to the insertion of foreign bodies into the rectum for sexual gratification or to radiation injury following radical radiotherapy for prostate cancer (*see* below).

History

Take a general colorectal history. Mainly in young adults, who present with rectal bleeding, diarrhoea, tenesmus and passage of mucus or mucino-sanguinous discharge. Take a sexual history to identify possible infective or factitious causes.

Examination

Perform a general examination. Examination may be normal but examine for general features of ulcerative colitis. In the rectal examination look for other perianal conditions.

Investigations

Sigmoidoscopy shows mucosa oedematous and hyperaemic. Perform biopsies for histology; colonic involvement is excluded by colonoscopy.

Treatment

Give bowel sedatives and stool softeners, prednisolone suppositories and enemas, sulphasalazine tablets or enemas. Any co-existent perianal disease (fissure, abscess, fistula, haemorrhoids) is treated by the appropriate surgical procedure.

Neutropenic anorectal infections

There is a high incidence of anorectal bacterial infections in neutropenic patients, caused by *E. coli*, *S. aureus*, *Klebsiella*. Diagnosis can be late in patients who are unable to mount a white cell response, and the development of large abscesses or necrotising fasciitis is possible. They are treated by intravenous antibiotics; by drainage of pus and limited debridement of slough and necrotic areas; and by formation of colostomy in cases where the condition progresses and conservative management fails.

Radiation proctitis

Rectal bleeding following pelvic irradiation has been reported in up to 95% of patients in retrospective studies, with symptoms peaking at one year from treatment and tending to resolve after 18 months. Some authors have suggested that up to 5–10% of patients require surgery for complications of radiation proctitis. There is increased incidence in diabetics and those with significant cardiovascular disease. Symptoms may appear within two weeks of treatment.

History

Symptoms are frequency, diarrhoea, rectal blood and mucus and tenesmus. Occasionally symptoms are delayed and the patient is found to have a large rectal ulcer which requires biopsy to exclude cancer.

Other symptoms may result from rectal fistulation into the vagina or urinary tract. There may also be damage to the small bowel and transverse colon.

Examination

Examine for lower abdominal tenderness. Rectal examination may be normal or an indurated area may be palpable. Look for blood on the glove on withdrawal.

Investigation

Investigate with sigmoidoscopy with biopsy for diagnosis and to determine the extent of the disease.

Treatment

Treatment is medical initially, using 5-ASA/steroid enemas if symptoms are persistent or troublesome. With severe symptoms consider topical formalin solution (requires anaesthetic) or laser coagulation. Formalin is effective in 80% of patients after 1–2 applications but 30% develop recurrent symptoms. Surgery is reserved for those with severe complications (perforation, fistula, stricture). Defunctioning sigmoid loop colostomy is provided for 6–12 months to rest the bowel. However, haemorrhage and tenesmus may continue.

Alternatively a Hartmann's procedure can be performed (although acceptable leak rates are reported in those with isolated segments of radiation injury undergoing primary anastomosis).

Follow-up
Flexible sigmoidoscopy and biopsy are needed to make the diagnosis, define the extent of affected bowel and exclude other causes such as cancer. Trial of medical treatment can be attempted in those with debilitating symptoms, but close review is required to monitor response. In severe cases consider admission for in-patient care.

Post-operative follow-up
Review with histology to confirm the diagnosis and detect complications of the procedure. Determine if the surgical procedure has been successful in relieving the symptoms and review accordingly. Decide whether to reverse any colostomies at 6–12 months. Symptoms should have settled completely before this is performed.

Involvement of the colon by gynaecological pathology
This is involvement of the sigmoid colon by ovarian carcinoma, which can present with symptoms suggestive of bowel cancer. Also, endometriosis can implant onto the serosa of the sigmoid colon and rectum and cause characteristic symptoms.

Endometriosis of the bowel
Although endometriosis (defined as the presence of functioning endometrial tissue outside of the uterus) occurs in 4–17% of women of reproductive age, only 5–10% of these will have colorectal involvement.

History
Take a general colorectal and gynaecological history. Dysmenorrhoea, dyspareunia, cyclical rectal bleeding (occurs in up to one-third of patients but very few have involvement of the bowel mucosa) and painful defaecation just before menstruation are characteristic. Pain is relieved once menstruation starts. Occasionally bowel obstruction is caused. Differential diagnosis includes malignancy (primary or metastatic), diverticulitis, IBD, pelvic inflammatory disease (PID) and radiation colitis.

Examination
Perform a general examination, including full abdominal and pelvic examination. Usually examination is normal and the diagnosis is suspected on the history.

Investigations
Sigmoidoscopy; laparoscopy and biopsy for histological diagnosis; joint care with gynaecologists.

Treatment
Treat with hormone manipulation initially (combined oral contraceptive pill, gonadotropin-releasing hormone (GnRH) analogues). Treat with Hysterectomy, oophorectomy and rectosigmoidectomy.

In younger patients, excise endometrial implants.

Follow-up
Follow up at short intervals until diagnosis is obtained.

Post-operative follow-up

Review with histology to confirm diagnosis. Recurrence requires further laparoscopy.

Rectovaginal fistulas

Causes include:
- ✧ obstetric injury
- ✧ IBD (Crohn's)
- ✧ radiation injury
- ✧ infection (cryptoglandular, Bartholin's gland, lymphogranuloma venereum)
- ✧ neoplasm (anal, rectal, vaginal)
- ✧ trauma (foreign body, iatrogenic: vaginal or anorectal surgery)
- ✧ congenital.

History

Take a general colorectal and gynaecological history. History will include the occurrence of a foul vaginal discharge resistant to normal therapy progressing to the passage of flatus or faeces per vagina. Symptoms may be intermittent or constant. Recent prolonged labour preceding the onset of symptoms may be a feature, as may recent perineal irradiation.

Examination

Perform a general examination including abdominal, rectal and vaginal examination.

Investigations

Rigid sigmoidoscopy may reveal the fistula. Some authors recommend the rigid sigmoidoscope to examine the vagina as well in this circumstance and it is better than the speculum at identifying the vaginal component of the fistula. Fistula may also be demonstrated by barium enema or vaginal contrast study. Examination under anaesthetic (EUA) may be required in difficult cases. Inserting a tampon into the vagina and instilling methylene blue into the rectum can help to prove the existence of a fistula that is hard to demonstrate.

Treatment

Treatment depends on the cause and height of the fistula. All sepsis should be adequately drained before attempts at repair are made. Very superficial tracks can sometimes be treated by simple fistulotomy; medical treatments such as infliximab may be useful in Crohn's fistulae. Defunctioning stoma should be considered for recurrent fistulae and complex cases.

Transanal repair: rectal advancement flap, sleeve (circumferential) advancement flap (used if defect is large).

Transperineal repair: laying open of fistula and immediate overlapping sphincter repair, transverse transperineal repair (fistula track divided along with perineal body and vaginal and rectal defects closed separately).

Transvaginal repair: inversion of fistula (into rectum), vaginal advancement flap.

Transabdominal repair: dissection of rectovaginal septum, interposition of omental or gracilis muscle flap, with or without limited rectal excision.

Follow-up

Follow up at short intervals until cancer is excluded. Prompt treatment is required to avoid complications from sepsis.

Post-operative follow-up

Review with histology to exclude cancer. Determine the success of the procedure and decide a date for possible closure of any covering colostomy.

Recto-urinary fistulas

Causes include diverticulitis, Crohn's, carcinoma, irradiation of the bladder and tuberculosis of the prostate. Most recto-urinary fistulas result from injury, mainly as a result of prostatic or urethral instrumentation. Retroprostatic fistulas are rare and result from complications of transrectal needle biopsy of the prostate.

History

Take a general colorectal and urological history. Usually there is a history of recurrent urinary tract infections or the passage of flatus (pneumaturia) or faeces (faecaluria) in the urine. Other features of the history may be suggestive of one of the causes above.

Examination

Perform a general examination. Examine for evidence of sepsis, anaemia and renal impairment. Examine for features of one of the underlying causes.

Investigations

Take FBC, U&Es and urine and blood cultures. Sigmoidoscopy may identify the fistula and help identify any underlying disorder. Contrast studies of the bowel may identify the fistula. CT scan may give more detailed information for planning definitive surgery.

Treatment

Treatment is by insertion of a urinary catheter and definitive diagnosis and treatment of the underlying pathology. Post-traumatic fistulas are amenable to direct repair either by perineal, trans-anal or trans-sphincteric approach.

Follow-up

Follow up at short intervals until cause is identified. Treatment should be arranged promptly to avoid the development of sepsis and deterioration in renal function.

Post-operative follow-up

Review with histology to confirm the diagnosis. Determine the success of the operation and detect any complications of the procedure.

Disorders of the anorectal musculature
Rectal prolapse

A partial prolapse involves the mucosa only; a complete prolapse involves the entire thickness of the rectal wall. In children under two, prolapse is not uncommon (it is often associated with a diarrhoeal illness or prolonged coughing) but usually resolves spontaneously (it is, though, associated with cystic fibrosis and so a sweat test should be performed). The differential diagnosis in adults includes haemorrhoids and large polypoidal tumours.

History

Take a general colorectal history. In children the prolapse is usually incomplete and has been noticed by the parent. Adults tend to complain either of the prolapse itself and resulting soiling of underclothes from mucus, blood and faeces, or a varying degree of faecal incontinence. The prolapse will tend to be noticed at defaecation or on coughing or straining.

Examination

Perform a general examination. In children the prolapse can be viewed when sitting the child on a potty. In adults the anus may be patulous with decreased tone. Active contraction of the anal sphincter onto the examining finger is weak. The patient experiences no discomfort on rectal examination, and anal and rectal sensation are decreased. Bearing down produces the prolapse. If complete, two complete layers of bowel wall are palpable between the fingers. Generally a prolapse of greater than 5cm in length is complete and less than 5cm needs careful examination to differentiate complete from incomplete. Procidentia of the uterus may often co-exist, and a combined approach to treatment between gynaecologist and surgeon is required.

Investigations
Proctoscopy and sigmoidoscopy are performed to exclude underlying rectal disorders. Anorectal physiology is useful to detect any underlying pathology, investigate the incontinence aspect of the disorder and plan appropriate treatment.

Treatment
For babies do nothing. It will spontaneously resolve. In children, if it is incomplete it is self-limiting; give laxatives and ensure regular defaecation with or without enemas. For older children inject sclerosants into the lower rectal mucosa.

In adults, if anal sphincter function is satisfactory and the prolapse partial (i.e. anterior mucosal prolapse) then a careful mucosal excision (similar to a haemorrhoidectomy) can be perfomed.

If poor sphincter tone is a contributory factor, sphincteric exercises may help.

Surgery
✧ Perineal procedures: Delorme's (mucosal stripping and muscle placation), Altemeier's (perineal rectosigmoidectomy).
✧ Abdominal procedures: include laparoscopic/open suture rectopexy, Ivalon® sponge/mesh rectopexy, resection rectopexy.
✧ Transabdominal rectopexy has a 90% success rate, but is a major abdominal procedure. There is a risk of sexual dysfunction, which needs to be included in the consent process. For frail or elderly patients, a Delorme's procedure may relieve symptoms and does not preclude a second procedure but has a high recurrence rate.

Follow-up
Intervals are short until serious underlying pathology has been excluded. Thereafter, a decision on surgical treatment or expectant management should be made.

Post-operative follow-up
Patients are reviewed to determine the success of the procedure and to detect any complications. After transabdominal rectopexy the commonest complication is constipation, which occurs in a third of patients. If prosthetic mesh has been used there is the risk of deep-seated infection, which, if it fails to settle, requires removal of the mesh. Some patients may complain of sexual and urinary disturbances due to disruption of the pelvic nerves.

Descending perineum syndrome
Excessive straining leads to a prolonged reflex inhibition of musculature with an abnormal descent of the perineum and bulging of the anterior rectal wall towards the anal canal.

History
Take a general colorectal history. There are generally non-specific symptoms of difficulty passing faeces, tenesmus and incontinence. Associations include a long history of

constipation, vaginal deliveries, previous rectal/perineal surgery, rectocoeles and enterocoeles.

Examination
Perform a general examination. On straining, the anus descends to 1cm below the inter-ischial line.

Investigation
Investigate with sigmoidoscopy to exclude rectal disease and detect any complications, e.g. solitary rectal ulcer. Anal physiology studies may be helpful in difficult cases, as may defaecating proctography.

Treatment
Advise the patient to avoid straining, give Bisacodyl suppositories and bulk-forming laxatives. Inject sclerosants or surgically excise any mucosal prolapse. Biofeedback may be beneficial.

Follow-up
Non-urgent review to determine the success of the treatment in helping defaecation. Once stabilised, discharge with advice.

Post-operative follow-up
Review to determine success of operation and detect any complications. Otherwise follow-up is the same as non-operative.

Solitary rectal ulcer
These may be multiple and not all cases have ulceration. Symptoms result from an internal rectal prolapse or intussusception, which causes trauma to the rectal wall. Persistent rectal symptoms are due to rectal ulceration, which is commonly situated 7–10cm from the anal verge on the anterior or anterolateral wall. There are well-defined indurated edges, with a grey base with surrounding mucosa which may look normal or oedematous or nodular. The mechanism of ulceration may be rectal prolapse, failure of relaxation of puborectalis muscle or insertion of foreign bodies.

History
Take a general colorectal history. This condition is characterised by a long history of prolonged and multiple visits to the toilet associated with prolonged, unproductive straining, although rectal bleeding and passage of mucus during and between defaecation may occur. There may be a deep-seated perineal pain and the sensation to defaecate may be so strong that the patient becomes desperate and inserts fingers or other objects into the rectum in an attempt to empty the already empty rectum.

Examination
General examination may be normal with some lower abdominal discomfort. Rectal examination reveals rectal soreness and an indurated area internally.

Investigations
Investigate with sigmoidoscopy and biopsies. Sigmoidoscopy reveals haemorrhage or oedema, or in 50% an ulcer adjacent to a valve of Houston on the anterior surface, approximately 5–8cm from the anal verge. This may look like a rectal carcinoma but repeated biopsy reveals only non-specific inflammatory changes or fibromuscular hyper-plasia of the lamina propria.

A defaecating proctogram may reveal an internal intussusception.

Treatment

Explain the condition to the patient. There is no medical therapy, although rectal steroids have been used. Biofeedback has been proposed to modify the harmful toilet habit. With severe symptoms use abdominal rectopexy to treat prolapse, or rectal excision and end-colostomy, although fewer than two-thirds of patients derived a benefit from rectopexy in some series.

Follow-up

Follow up at short intervals of 1–2 weeks until cancer is excluded. Thereafter see the patient after 1–3 months to try different therapies, assess severity of symptoms and decide on the need for surgery.

Post-operative follow-up

Review to determine the success of the procedure in relieving symptoms and to detect complications. Complications of rectopexy are described under rectal prolapse.

Faecal incontinence

This is the involuntary passing of flatus or stool. Its incidence is underestimated but may be up to 1–2%. Causes include old age, childbirth, chronic constipation, anal dilatation or fistula surgery, dementia and faecal impaction, low rectal tumours and autonomic neuropathy associated with diabetes mellitus. It can be classified as:

✧ traumatic: obstetric, surgical, accidental/war
✧ colorectal disease: haemorrhoids, rectal prolapse, IBD, tumours
✧ congenital: spina bifida, surgery for imperforate anus, Hirschprung's
✧ neurological: cerebral, spinal, peripheral
✧ miscellaneous: behavioural, faecal impaction.

Anal continence depends on a variety of mechanisms, including stool consistency, rectal capacity/compliance, sphincter function, anal sensation and an intact rectoanal inhibitory reflex. The underlying mechanisms in incontinence may include either damage to the anal sphincter or perineal descent due to excessive straining over many years leading to a traction neuropathy of the pudendal nerve.

Severity of incontinence

Browning and Parks' grades are shown in Table 9.2.

TABLE 9.2 Incontinence grades.

Grade A	normal continence to solid, liquid and flatus
Grade B	incontinence of flatus but no faecal leakage
Grade C	acceptable control over solid stool, but no control over liquid or flatus
Grade D	continuous faecal leakage

History

Take a general colorectal history. Enquire about the above causes and the severity of incontinence.

Examination

Perform a general examination. Examine for perineal scars from obstetric injury or fistula surgery. Note the degree of perineal descent at rest and on straining and any associated prolapse. Exclude abnormality of lumbosacral plexus.

In a rectal examination, look for faecal impaction or rectal tumours. Examine sphincter integrity at rest and on contraction.

Investigations

Investigate with proctoscopy and sigmoidoscopy.

If recognised causes of faecal incontinence are not found, the patient is said to have idiopathic faecal incontinence. Less severe cases require no further investigation and can be treated symptomatically with loperamide.

Severe cases

✧ Anal manometry measures the presence of and relaxation after rectal distension by balloon. Anal canal pressures at rest reflect activity of the internal sphincter (50–80cm H_2O) and voluntary contraction of the external sphincter (squeeze pressure) will increase the pressure of the anal canal to 150cm H_2O. It is used to diagnose a short and weak sphincter.
✧ Sphincter EMG can detect silent areas of a sphincter defect and localise the ends of the muscle pre-operatively. Also traction neuropathy of the pudendal nerve – some muscle fibres lose their innervation.
✧ Anorectal sensation: rectal compliance balloon or thermal stimulation.
✧ Trans-anal ultrasound to image defects in the sphincter.
✧ Defaecating proctogram to detect prolapse.

Treatment

Mild cases

Give counselling, and give constipating agents if loose stool is present. Advise physio-therapy with anal sphincter and pelvic floor exercises, or biofeedback methods. Leakage after passing motion may indicate incomplete evacuation, which can be treated by a glycerine suppository after each motion or by a daily phosphate enema.

Severe cases

Severe cases may require operative treatment with sphincter repair when defects are identified. Reconstructive options include graciloplasty or the insertion of artificial neo-sphincters. Sacral nerve stimulation has recently emerged as a potential new treatment.

Follow-up

Follow up at short intervals initially to assess severity and review with investigations. Mild cases can be discharged to the GP when serious underlying pathology has been excluded. Severe cases need a decision made regarding surgery when appropriate investigations have been completed.

Post-operative follow-up

Review to assess the success of the procedure and to detect any complications of the procedure. Recurrence not amenable to further surgery may require a stoma.

Anorectal suppuration and anorectal abscesses

These can be caused by both aerobic (*Staphylococcus*, *Streptococcus*, *E. coli* and *Bacillus pyocyaneus*) and anaerobic (*Clostridium welchii* and *Bacteroides*) bacteria.

Particularly susceptible are leucopenic, ulcerative colitis (15%), Crohn's (25%) and diabetic patients.

Perianal skin infections are caused by *Staphylococcus aureus* and nearly all heal with simple incision and drainage.

Perianal abscess of bowel origin starts internally in glands in the intersphincteric space (cryptoglandular). Spread to the skin immediately adjacent to the anus is termed a perianal abscess. Spread laterally into the buttock is termed an ischiorectal abscess. These may originate from high intersphincteric infection or from pelvirectal disease. These abscesses can be considered as perianal fistula in which the internal openings are small, cannot be found at operation and will heal spontaneously in the majority. In a minority the fistulous track will persist and require formal fistula surgery.

History
Severe throbbing pain, worse on sitting and coughing. Ask about a history of predisposing factors, e.g. malignancy, chemotherapy, UC, Crohn's or diabetes. Often will present as emergencies rather than to the outpatient clinic.

Examination
Red (may not be very red), tender, rounded swelling in the perianal area; there may be some degree of induration and later some fluctuation. Ischiorectal abscesses occupy a larger area to one side of the anus and sometimes may be bilateral.

* Submucous abscess presents as dull aching pain in the rectum with usually no external evidence of infection. Rectal examination may reveal a rounded smooth area of induration on one side of the upper anal canal and lower rectum. Pus may be seen draining from an internal opening.
* Pelvirectal abscess is normally a complication of pelvic sepsis. There are signs of infection with pyrexia, rigors, diarrhoea, weakness and lower abdominal tenderness or even a mass. Rectal examination shows it is tender high in rectum and may have a boggy swelling.

Investigation
Investigate with FBC to detect underlying leucopenic condition. Test blood sugar to detect diabetes mellitus. Perform examination under anaesthetic. Pus should be sent for microbiology. A sample of the abscess cavity wall should be sent for microbiology and histology.

Treatment
Examination under anaesthetic; perform incision and drainage. Perform rigid sigmoidoscopy and proctoscopy. Biopsies of inflamed mucosal lesions are taken if appropriate. Examine for the internal opening of a perianal fistula. If the internal opening of a fistula is seen it should be noted and left. Attempts to probe cavities for fistula tracks in the acute setting are likely to be rewarded only by the creation of new tracks through the friable indurated tissue, rather than by the identification of an existing track. Otherwise, incise and drain the abscess cavity. Underlying disorders are treated appropriately.

Post-operative follow-up
Review with the results of microbiology of the pus. Infections of *Staph. aureus* will all heal, and provided the wound is clean the patient can be discharged. Those with organisms of bowel origin should be followed up until complete healing is confirmed. Most will heal but some will not heal or will recur within a short time. These patients should be investigated for possible perianal fistula by EUA.

Anorectal fistulas
There is usually only one internal opening, but there may be more than one external opening. These usually start as a perianal abscess but the internal opening persists, or perianal gland infection persists as a source of sepsis. This is particularly likely to occur in the presence of some underlying disorder such as UC or Crohn's or with chronic infections such as TB, actinomycoses and lymphogranuloma venereum. Occasionally carcinoma of the rectum can present as a fistula.

Differential diagnosis

Exclude colloid rectal carcinoma, proctocolitis, Crohn's of small intestine, TB, actinomycosis and lymphogranuloma venereum.

Local conditions include pilonidal sinus, suppurative hidradenitis, chronically infected Bartholin's gland and vaginal and urethral fistulas.

Classification

Goodsall's rule relates the external opening of an anal fistula to its internal opening. Fistulas with external openings anterior to the inter-ischial line have their internal opening on the same radius. External openings posterior to the inter-ischial line form a horseshoe to open in the midline. Exceptions include anterior openings more than 3cm from the anus (which may be anterior extensions of posterior horseshoe fistulas) and anterior fistulas associated with other diseases, e.g. Crohn's, malignancy.

Fistulas are also classified according to height and relation to the anal sphincters:
- subcutaneous
- low intersphincteric: goes underneath the subcutaneous part of the external sphincter
- trans-sphincteric: track extends through the external sphincter
- anorectal opening between the rectum and exterior.

An alternative classification is the Park's classification. See specialised texts.

History

Take a general colorectal history. There may be a history to suggest an underlying disorder or previous acute perianal abscess followed by intermittent or persistent discharge or recurrent abscess.

Examination

Perform a general examination. Rectal examination may reveal the presence of single or multiple external openings. Granulation tissue may mark the opening or there may be the presence of pus. The external opening may have temporarily healed and be indicated by an area of reddish/brown induration. Induration may also be palpated inside the rectum, indicating the site of the internal opening. Try to determine the course of the track between the internal and external openings.

Ask the patient to squeeze the inserted finger to determine the relation of the primary track to the puborectalis sling, which correlates to the upper extent of the external sphincters. Then advance the finger to identify any induration above the levator muscles.

Investigations

The main investigation is the EUA. However, in complicated disease or in cases complicated by other diseases, fistulography may provide useful information as to the course of the track, especially if an internal opening has not been identified. MRI scanning has an increasing role in identifying the course of fistulas and excluding other disease, and, in experienced hands, endoanal ultrasound (often with hydrogen peroxide contrast) can give valuable anatomical information.

Treatment

Treat with surgery – EUA and treatment of fistula.
- Laying open.
- Seton insertion.
- Fibrin glue/fistula plug.

✧ Chronic: long-term metronidazole treatment.
✧ TB: treat active disease prior to treatment of fistula.

For UC/Crohn's it is necessary to get control of the primary disease first. However, resection of the ileocaecal region in Crohn's, with no other apparent disease of the bowel, often fails to heal perianal fistulas. Long-term treatment with metronidazole, salazopyrin or azathioprine is needed, however, it may lead to amyloid deposition and death from amyloid renal and cardiac failure. Therefore rectal excision and colostomy are acceptable alternatives. Infliximab may be used in an attempt to heal a fistula once any associated abscess has been drained.

Follow-up

If a fistula is suspected, the patient should go forward for EUA where it can be formally assessed. If symptoms are atypical it may be prudent to perform a flexible sigmoidoscopy first, or at the time of the EUA to exclude co-existing colorectal conditions.

Post-operative follow-up

If a seton has been inserted it will require attention (some patients are left long term with a seton to control their symptoms by establishing adequate drainage). Examine for evidence of ongoing sepsis or recurrent discharge, which may suggest unrecognised extensions of the original disease and require either repeat surgery or an MRI to diagnose.

Hidradenitis of the perianal skin

This is not a condition of bowel origin, but it tends to be referred to colorectal clinics because of the site. The condition consists of chronic inflammation of sweat glands leading to recurrent infection and abscess formation. The affected area begins as induration and may progress to sinus formation. The majority of cases occur in the axillae, but 30% are perianal. Differential diagnosis includes pruritus ani and perianal fistula.

History

Take a general colorectal history, which will usually be normal. There is a history of recurrent infections of the area, sometimes progressing to boils/abscess formation.

Examination

Perform a general examination. Examine the axillae to detect any disease there. The groins and perianal area may be indurated and show evidence of scarring and chronic inflammation. There may be multiple small boils with white heads and small amounts of pus in the sweat area of the groins and perianal area. Rectal examination is normal.

Investigations

Few investigations are needed for a diagnosis. Bowel investigations are indicated if the history/examination suggests a co-existing bowel condition. Microbiology of any pus should confirm skin bacteria only. Test urine to exclude glycosuria and also test blood sugar.

Treatment

In mild cases long-term antibiotics, e.g. erythromycin, may be effective in reducing the rate of infection, combined with conservative measures such as wearing loose airy clothing and daily washing. More severe cases require excision of affected skin and subcutaneous tissue to deep fascia with or without a split skin graft (plastic surgery referral).

Follow-up

Mild cases can be reviewed after 1–6 months to determine the effect of conservative measures. Failure of medical treatment or severe disease are indications to consider surgery.

Post-operative follow-up

Review with histology to confirm diagnosis. Detect recurrence or any complications of surgery, e.g. skin necrosis. Unless it is severe, skin necrosis can be treated conservatively with antibiotics and dressings. Extensive skin necrosis may require a plastic surgical opinion.

Pruritis ani

This is an itchy and irritated anus. Secondary causes include anorectal and dermatological disorders, but in many the underlying problem cannot be found. Minor degrees of faecal soiling can lead to irritation and scratching, or to overzealous cleaning and the application of inappropriate topical preparations. This in turn results in damage to the delicate perianal skin and further irritation, and a vicious circle results.

Dysfunction of the internal anal sphincter allows anal leakage, and skin tags prevent adequate cleaning of the anus, as do perianal warts. There may be mucus discharge from haemorrhoids, benign or malignant rectal tumours, anal fissures and fistulas. All may be made worse by the ingestion of spicy foods and caffeine.

Secondary causes can be classified as the following.
+ Fungal infection: secondary infection due to *Candida, Trichomonas* or *Tinea crura.*
+ Parasitic infestation: threadworms, scabies etc.
+ Other infections: gonococcal proctitis and *Condyloma acuminatum, Herpes simplex.*
+ Dermatological disorders: contact dermatitis, psoriasis, lichen planus, eczema.
+ Neoplasia: rectal adenoma, rectal adenocarcinoma, squamous cell anal carcinoma, malignant melanoma, Bowen's disease, Paget's disease.
+ Benign anorectal: haemorrhoids, fistula, fissure, prolapse, sphincter dysfunction, incontinence, radiation proctitis, ulcerative colitis.

History

Take a general and colorectal history to detect any of the causes outlined above. Perianal and anal itching may be severe and worse when warm. Enquire about the length of symptoms, change of bowel habit, diet, recent travel etc. In children, suspect *Enterobius* infestation. Enquire about an itchy or irritating rash elsewhere on the body.

Examination

Perform a general examination to detect any general skin conditions. Long-standing irritation causes excoriation and icthyosis, and the perianal skin is corrugated, making removal of faecal particles difficult. In advanced cases skin becomes atrophic and excoriated with oedema and thickening of the underlying dermis.

Examine the anus resting and straining. On rectal examination assess the anal tone and squeeze pressure. Palpate for polyps, fissures, fistulas and neoplasms.

Investigations

Perform urinalysis, blood sugar and FBC. Examine the affected area under a Wood's light. *Corynebacterium minutissimum* is diagnosed by the presence of bight pink-orange fluorescence (beware – Anusol fluoresces purple). Perform proctoscopy and sigmoidoscopy to detect any underlying colorectal condition, e.g. neoplasm, haemorrhoids, prolapse. Perform biopsies and arrange colonoscopy as indicated.

Biopsy affected skin if suspicious. Skin scrapings are taken for fungal elements.

For detection of threadworms in children, a piece of 'Sellotape' is applied to the anus and then stuck onto a clean glass slide. This is repeated for two days, in the mornings. Microscopy reveals the ova deposited on the perianal skin overnight.

Treatment

The aims are to decrease leakage, improve hygiene and prevent injury to perianal skin.

- Treat underlying conditions such as haemorrhoids, fissures and warts.
- Treat fungal infections with nystatin or clotrimazole. Treat threadworms with piperazine.
- Give advice on hygiene: gentle washing with water only, no soap, wet wiping after defaecation is more efficient at cleaning the anus than dry wiping, avoid vigorous rubbing, wear cotton underwear, no tights.
- Decrease leakage: modify diet to avoid spicy foods and fibre, reduce or abstain from alcohol and caffeine. Prescribe loperamide or codeine.
- Pruritus: avoid scratching. Use hydrocortisone cream for 10 days to break the cycle, but excessive use can cause skin atrophy and itching on withdrawal of the cream.

Follow-up

Review at regular intervals (1–3 months) once diagnosis is achieved to gauge the effect of therapies.

Haemorrhoids

Haemorrhoids are enlargements of the venous tissue in the rectum, which can cause symptoms by prolapsing or bleeding. Haemorrhoids are very common and are a very common cause of perianal bleeding. However, just because haemorrhoids are present does not mean they are the only cause of the perianal bleeding. Haemorrhoids can co-exist with cancers or other serious pathology and should not be assumed to be the cause of rectal bleeding, especially in those over 50. Haemorrhoids may be classified as follows.

- First degree: bleeding but no prolapse.
- Second degree: prolapse but reduce spontaneously.
- Third degree: prolapse and require manual reduction.
- Fourth degree: irreducibly prolapsed.

History

Take a general colorectal history. Commonly patients complain of prolapse and bleeding. The bleeding is bright red on the toilet paper or dripping into the pan. Pain is uncommon but can be present in up to 20%. Prolapse may be associated with mucoid discharge and perianal wetness.

Examination

Perform a general examination. External inspection of the anus may be normal or the piles may already be visible. Alternatively there may be skin tags visible, which are an indicator of previous episodes of prolapsed piles. Occasionally, a pea-sized blue swelling is present on the anal margin, which represents a thrombosed perianal haematoma, which is often confused with haemorrhoids. Ask the patient to strain down and the haemorrhoids may appear. Digital examination may be normal.

Investigations

Investigate with sigmoidoscopy to exclude higher carcinoma. Proctoscopy is the best way to demonstrate the haemorrhoids, which prolapse into the lumen of the scope. Often there is a history of bleeding but minimal to see on proctoscopy.

Treatment

Conservative measures include laxatives, bulk forming agents and advice to avoid straining at stool.

- Injection sclerotherapy: phenol in almond oil produces fibrosis. Use 3 ml injected at the root of each haemorrhoid. Repeat after 3–4 weeks. Useful for all primary piles and smaller second-degree piles. Contraindicated in third-degree piles, thrombosed piles or associated anal fissure. There is a small risk of pelvic sepsis or prostatitis if injection is misplaced.
- Rubber band ligation: bands are placed at the base of the piles, which strangulates a disc of tissue. It sloughs and leaves an ulcer, which scars and fixes the mucosa in place, preventing the mucosa from becoming engorged and prolapsing.
- Haemorrhoidectomy: used if failed to respond to injection sclerotherapy or rubber banding. Late complications include pain, fissure and fistula formation along the tracks of cutaneous wounds. Stenosis may develop by three weeks – treat with an anal dilator. Recent advances include the introduction of 'stapled haemorrhoidectomy', in which a circular stapler is introduced via the anus and fired, removing a circle of mucosa.

Thrombosed haemorrhoids need conservative treatment (ice, analgesia, bed rest) or immediate operation, which can be technically difficult and bloody.

Perianal haematoma
This is a bluish, pea-sized swelling at the anal margin. It can be managed conservatively with analgesia and ice, or incised and drained with instant relief of discomfort.

Summary of treatment options for haemorrhoids
- First degree: dietary modification.
- Second degree: rubber band ligation, sclerotherapy (haemorrhoidectomy).
- Third degree: rubber band ligation, sclerotherapy (haemorrhoidectomy).
- Fourth degree: haemorrhoidectomy.

Follow-up
Once diagnosis is made (and concurrent pathology is excluded) review at six-weekly intervals to gauge the effect of injection or banding. Discharge patients once they are symptom-free, with advice to avoid constipation and straining at stool, or book them for haemorrhoidectomy if not they are responding to repeated outpatient management.

Post-operative follow-up
Review to determine success of operation and to confirm healing. Complications include prolonged healing and anal stenosis. Anal stenosis can be treated with anal dilators. For prolonged healing, exclude any co-existing pathology or infection and allow 1–2 months before further EUA. Incontinence may occur due to anal stretching, loss of the anal cushions or overuse of laxatives. Most cases settle with conservative measures, but anal physiology studies may be required for persistent cases.

Anal fissure
Anal fissures are common. They represent up to 10% of referrals to colorectal clinics. They are longitudinal tears in the anoderm which are typically seen at 6 o'clock (posterior midline) but may be seen anteriorly (especially in women). They are often seen in association with a 'sentinel pile', a skin tag at the distal extreme of the fissure. Patients enter a vicious cycle in which pain causes fear of defaecation, leading to constipation and the passage of hard stool, which exacerbates the problem. Spasm of the internal sphincter (the white fibres of which are often visible in the base of a chronic fissure) reduces the blood supply to the anoderm (vessels penetrate the muscle and are occluded by sphincter spasm) further reducing the ability of the sphincter to heal.

Differential diagnosis
This includes atypical ulceration of the perianal margin, TB, syphilis (if suspected requires biopsy and culture of tissue). For gross fissures, suspect UC or Crohn's; if indurated suspect malignancy and send tissue for histology.

History
There is severe pain for 20–30 minutes after defaecation. Bleeding on paper and slight mucoid discharge. There may be history of proctocolitis or Crohn's.

Investigation
Usually no investigations are necessary but the following can be performed if atypical features are present: FBC and C-reactive protein for inflammatory bowel disease; serological tests for syphilis; rectal biopsy; biopsy of the ulcer edge with tissue for bacterial and viral cultures if infective cause suspected; and histology if there is any suspicion that the fissure is atypical and may in fact be a malignancy, Crohn's etc. Perform anal manometry if disordered defaecation is suspected.

Examination
There may be the sentinel pile – the perianal skin tag in the posterior midline. The distal extent of the fissure may just be visible as the perianal skin is gently distracted and the white, transverse fibres of the exposed internal sphincter in the base of a chronic fissure may be visible. Rectal examination is frequently not possible due to the pain.

Treatment
Most acute fissures heal spontaneously in 2 to 3 weeks with laxatives and fibre supplements. In the interim, 5% lignocaine cream applied well within the anal canal may offer symptomatic relief. Glyceryl trinitrate (GTN) ointment (0.2%) applied twice daily to the anal region decreases sphincter tone and enables healing in approximately 67% of patients. Topical diltiazem is an alternative, notably in those who cannot tolerate the headache frequently associated with GTN. For those who fail to heal, botulinum A toxin (Botox) can be injected either in the outpatients department or under sedation/GA. Initial healing rates of 70–96% have been reported, but the effect of the blockade wears off after about three months and recurrences do occur even after this time.

Surgery is required both to exclude more serious conditions (fissure biopsy) and to speed recovery. Operation consists of examination under anaesthetic (rectal examination, sigmoidoscopy and biopsy if indicated) and lateral internal anal sphincterotomy (healing rates of up to 85–95%, but incontinence to flatus in up to 35%). Uncontrolled manual anal dilatation (the four finger stretch) is no longer recommended due to the unacceptably high risk of sphincter injury.

Follow-up
Review at short intervals (1–4 weeks) to determine the success of conservative measures in relieving symptoms. Failure is an indication to consider surgery.

Post-operative follow-up
Review with histology if biopsy taken. Determine success of operation in relieving symptoms and confirm healing (may take 4–6 weeks). Continued pain or non-healing may require further EUA to reconsider diagnosis or further treatment, e.g. advancement skin flaps (V-Y advancement, rhomboid advancement flaps). Mild degrees of incontinence usually recover or respond to constipating agents.

Carcinoma of the anal canal and anus

Squamous cell carcinoma of the anus is rare: 1–2% of gastrointestinal malignancies, about 500 new cases per year in the UK. Differentials include anal fissure, simple papilla, anal condyloma, prolapsed haemorrhoids and Crohn's.

Adenocarcinoma of the rectum may spread down and invade the anal canal. Lesions tend to be softer and more mucoid, but are differentiated on the basis of biopsy and histology. Predisposing factors include human papillomavirus (HPV) infection, HIV and immunosupression.

History

Take a general colorectal history. Patients may complain of painful defaecation, rectal bleeding or bloody discharge and/or a lump. Occasionally they may complain of symptoms relating to a rectovaginal fistula. Patients presenting with inguinal lympha-denopathy should always have anal cancer excluded.

Examination

Perform a general examination. Anal carcinoma may present as a warty protuberance, flattened plaque or penetrating ulcer. Rectal examination may be difficult due to pain. Examine for the presence of enlarged inguinal nodes.

Investigations

All suspicious lesions need an examination under anaesthetic and biopsy. Make fine-needle aspiration of enlarged inguinal lymph nodes. Local staging is clinical, by MRI and/or endoanal ultrasound. The presence of distant metastases (affecting 40% of patients in the chest or abdomen) is diagnosed by CT scans.

Treatment

The primary treatment of anal cancer is chemoradiotherapy, but small lesions at the anal margin can be treated by local excision alone with equally good results. Inguinal lymph node involvement is seen in 10–25% of those with anal cancer and may be treated by radiotherapy, although some advocate radical groin dissection (histological proof of nodal involvement should be obtained before embarking on this). Surgery may be required in four main scenarios:
- residual disease
- complications of primary treatment
- incontinence or fistula after tumour resolution
- subsequent tumour recurrence (salvage abdominoperineal excision).

Follow-up

Follow up at short intervals (1–2 weeks) until diagnosis is achieved and treatment insti-gated. Anal cancer is increasingly being treated in regional centres in view of its relative rarity. Lymph nodes not thought to be involved should be examined every month for the first six months after treatment of the primary lesion, then every two months for the next 18 months. Suspicious lesions require fine-needle aspiration or lymph node dissection.

Post-operative follow-up

Review wide local excision – 55% survival at five years. If lymph nodes were involved at presentation it is 0% survival at five years. With delayed involvement of inguinal lymph nodes there is 60% survival at five years.

Lymph nodes not thought to be involved should be examined every month for the first six months after treatment of the primary lesion, then every two months for the next 18 months. Suspicious lesions require fine-needle aspiration or lymph node dissection.

Rare lesions of the anal region

✧ Basal cell carcinoma is a small raised and indurated lesion, occasionally ulcerated. It is usually only 1–2cm in diameter, and good results are obtained from wide local excision.
✧ Bowen's disease is a rare intraepidermal cancer of the anal region, usually diagnosed after biopsy of an unusual anal lesion. It is treated by wide local excision with or without skin grafting.

Other rare tumours of the anal canal include basiloid (cloacogenic) carcinoma and malignant melanoma. Malignant melanoma may mimic a perianal haematoma due to its colour, although amelanotic lesions can occur. Its prognosis is even worse than that at other sites so radial surgery is generally avoided.

Perianal papillomas (condyloma accuminata)

These represent one of the commonest sexually transmitted diseases, especially among homosexual men (of whom as many as 50–75% will harbour asymptomatic condylomas). It is caused by the human papilloma virus and is important because of the association with malignant change and the development of anal carcinoma. Differential diagnosis includes condyloma latum, molluscum contagiosum and hypertrophied anal papillae.

History

Take a general colorectal and sexual history. Symptoms include bleeding, discharge causing permanent wetness and pruritus ani.

Examination

Perform a general examination. Appearance may vary from a few pink spots to a confluent mass of sheet of warts.

Investigations

Proctoscopy and sigmoidoscopy may reveal papillae within the anal canal which also require eradication if treatment is to be successful.

Treatment

Principles of treatment include the complete eradication of all lesions and biopsy of lesions to detect malignant change.
✧ EUA and diathermy excision of perianal and intra-anal lesions.
✧ Podophyllin: requires multiple treatments. Can cause histological changes similar to carcinoma in situ, which reverse four weeks after treatment.
✧ Bichloroacetic acid: multiple, weekly treatments are required.

Follow-up

Review with histology to exclude carcinoma in situ and confirm healing. Recurrence requires further treatment. Carcinoma in situ requires further follow-up and repeated biopsies.

Pilonidal sinus disease

The name literally means 'nest of hairs'. This disorder is commonly referred to colorectal clinics although it is not strictly a disease involving the bowel. It is a disorder of the skin near the anus – the natal cleft – and it occurs in men and hirsute women. It is a disease of chronic inflammation involving the presence of hairs within sinuses in the skin. It can be confused with perianal fistula disease and in rare cases a congenital sinus originating from the spinal cord.

History

Take a general colorectal history, which is usually normal. The onset of the disease is after puberty and the presence in childhood should raise the possibility of a congenital spinal sinus. The disease can present either as an acute abscess or as chronic sinus periodically discharging pus. There may be a history of previous surgery in the area.

Examination

Perform a general examination, which is usually normal. Examination of the perianal area reveals usually one or more midline pits within the skin of the natal cleft. Some of these pits may have lateral extensions. Some sinuses may be inflamed and indurated. Pressing may produce some pus from the pits, or hairs may exude from them. There may be scars or unhealed wounds from previous surgery.

Investigations

Investigations are usually not required, apart from urinalysis to exclude glycosuria. Imaging such as CT or MRI may be required if a congenital spinal abnormality is suspected.

Treatment

Asymptomatic pits do not require treatment.

Acute abscess

If possible, repeated aspiration and antibiotics allow the disease to settle, enabling definitive surgery at a later date. The fewer operations that are performed, the better. If incision and drainage are required, the preferred approach is incisions away from the midline and definitive treatment of the sinus once the acute infection has resolved.

Chronic abscess

This usually requires a surgical procedure, but mild chronic disease may settle if the area can be maintained hairless by regular shaving or the use of depilatory creams. Brushing of the pits and injection with sclerosant has been attempted with variable success.

Surgery

A variety of surgical options exists. The choices include the following.
- Excision and packing (healing by secondary intent: often prolonged time to healing).
- Excision and midline closure (frequent wound breakdown).
- Pit excision and lateral drainage ('Bascom' procedure).
- Excision with asymmetric closure: aims to keep the wound out of the midline to allow better healing and is often combined with an approach that flattens the natal cleft to reduce recurrence.
- Complex plastic surgical reconstructions (including Z-plasties and myocutaneous flaps).

Follow-up

Review within weeks after an acute episode and arrange definitive treatment as soon as possible. If the disease is chronic, decide whether surgery is indicated.

Post-operative follow-up

Review with histology to confirm diagnosis and monitor healing. Healing can take a long time after incision and drainage or after definitive surgery using midline wounds. Aim to keep the area free of hair by regular shaving until and after healing occurs. The commonest complication is the chronic non-healing midline wound. This may be due to recurrent disease, but generally is due to the problems of healing at this site. Further lateral surgery may be indicated. For large wounds, plastic surgical procedures may be required.

Intestinal stomas

A stoma is a surgically constructed opening of the bowel (or urinary system) on to the skin of the abdomen. Stomas can be permanent or temporary. The aim with temporary stomas is to restore bowel continuity at a later date. End stomas are usually permanent and are one end of the bowel sutured to the skin. Loop stomas are usually temporary, where a loop of bowel is brought through the abdominal wall and the anterior wall is opened so that two orifices, proximal and distal, are visible, but only the proximal end discharges. Over time the distal orifice may shrink so that it is barely visible. The double-barrelled stoma is similar, except that two ends of bowel are brought out together, usually after the segment of bowel between has been resected. Double-barrelled stomas are usually temporary.

Ileostomies are constructed from the terminal ileum.

Complications of stomas

Many problems may arise with stomas and present to the outpatient clinic, but they can frequently be addressed by the stomatherapists by the use of different appliances.

One of the first considerations is to determine whether the stoma is temporary or permanent. If significant problems arise in a temporary stoma the correct management may be to bring forward the operation to restore bowel continuity. Most centres have experienced stoma care nurses – always involve them in the management decisions.

⋄ Constipation and diarrhoea: management may depend to a certain extent on the underlying disorder, but this can usually be treated with appropriate drugs.

⋄ Prolapse of stoma: a common problem, which often occurs when an originally dilated obstructed bowel returns to normal calibre. It is unsightly and uncomfortable but rarely dangerous, although ulceration and ischaemic changes at the apex can occur. If surgery is indicated it usually involves re-siting the stoma and excising redundant bowel.

⋄ Stenosis of stoma: a stoma should usually admit a gloved index finger easily. If not, dilators can be used but are seldom a long-term solution. Surgical re-siting is usually necessary.

⋄ Skin rashes: usually due to irritation of the skin because of a failure of the bag to fit snugly around the stoma. Occasionally it is caused by a contact dermatitis, and a change of appliance is required. Involve the stoma nurse for advice regarding appliances.

⋄ Parastomal hernia: weakness in the abdominal wall predisposes to hernia formation and a bulge underneath the stoma. If asymptomatic, this can be treated conservatively. If troublesome, surgical re-siting is required, but this can be a difficult procedure. Local repair has a high incidence of recurrence, but hernias also tend to occur in the new site and represent a generalised weakness of the abdominal wall. Laparoscopic repair using a prosthetic mesh is a potential solution to prevent the need for relocation of an otherwise acceptable stoma.

⋄ Bleeding stoma: may be due to lesions on the edge of the mucocutaneous junction, or lesions further up the gastrointestinal tract. Superficial granulations respond to silver nitrate cauterisation. Unusual lesions may need biopsy, especially if the primary surgery was for malignancy. More troublesome bleeding requires further investigation, including proctoscopy/sigmoidoscopy or flexible endoscopy down the stoma.

Vascular
Umar Sadat and David Cooper

TEN

Vascular surgery

Vascular surgery covers the management of a large and varied number of disorders affecting the arterial, venous and lymphatic systems. Most arterial disorders are caused by the effect of atherosclerosis. However, some, such as Raynaud's, are vasospastic in nature, while others, such as thoracic outlet syndrome, result from extrinsic compression. Arteries are also vulnerable to inflammation (vasculitis), connective tissue disorders and chronic degeneration (fibrodysplasia). Venous disorders are also very common, ranging from primary varicose veins to venous hypertension and ulceration. A cross-section of the common disorders referred to a vascular clinic will be described.

General vascular assessment

Most disorders seen by vascular surgeons are arterial and the result of atherosclerosis causing ischaemic symptoms of an end organ. However, atherosclerosis is very common. Evidence of arterial disease may be present without this being the primary cause of the patient's symptoms. In particular, symptoms affecting the lower limb may be due to musculoskeletal or neurological pathologies and not vascular disease, even though some element of vascular dysfunction is present. Once a vascular cause is established the nature, site and severity of the condition is assessed to determine the need and timing for interventional treatment.

The underlying cause of ischaemic symptoms is insufficient delivery of oxygen to the tissues, of which diseased arteries may be considered as just the final stage of a process. A general assessment of the patient is necessary to detect other conditions that may affect oxygen delivery such as anaemia, cardiovascular disease and/or respiratory disease.

Although the patient may have presented with symptoms specific to one body site, if vascular disease is identified this indicates general atherosclerosis, which affects every artery in the body. The most common causes of death of patients presenting with intermittent claudication are myocardial infarction and stroke. It may be possible to reduce the risk and improve the function of the peripheral vascular system by modification of risk factors such as smoking, lipids, control of hypertension, haemostatic and rheological variables and diabetic control.

Vascular history

A general history is taken initially, until a vascular cause becomes apparent. A vascular history consists of specific questions related to the presenting complaint and general questions related to general cardiovascular status, risk-factor analysis, family and drug history and so on. Specific questions will be covered in the relevant sections; general questions will be covered here.

Generalised atherosclerosis is an important cause of morbidity in patients undergoing peripheral vascular interventions. Therefore, a careful assessment of the cardiac status is important. Enquire regarding angina or previous myocardial infarction, cardiac valve disease, dysrhythmias and heart failure.

Aspirin 75–150 mg per day has been shown to decrease the cardiovascular risk of patients with peripheral vascular disease but must be avoided in patients with a history of oesophagitis or peptic ulceration, due to the risk of gastrointestinal bleeding.

Risk factors

Much can be done to improve the prognosis and symptoms of patients presenting with peripheral vascular disease through identification and modification of cardiovascular risk factors.

Hypertension

This is the most significant risk factor in strokes, heart failure and ischaemic heart disease. The majority (95%) of cases of hypertension are primary (no identifiable cause), but this is diagnosed by elimination of the uncommon secondary causes such as renal disease, endocrine disease, coarctation of the aorta and so on.

Smoking

Smoking is associated with a four times higher risk of peripheral vascular disease (PVD). The majority of patients with PVD will have a significant current or past smoking history. The amount and duration of tobacco use should be determined – this is often underestimated. Stopping smoking is the biggest single factor in improving the short- and long-term prognosis of all patients with PVD.

Diabetes mellitus

Suffering from diabetes mellitus is associated with a three times higher risk of PVD in men and a five times higher risk in women. Good diabetic monitoring in the form of blood glucose levels and foot care and neuropathy are important factors in the prevention of serious complications of PVD.

Obesity and diet

Obesity may have several effects on vascular disease. Losing weight reduces the load and therefore the work the muscles need to perform. Obesity usually indicates an unhealthy diet high in saturated fat and salt. Modification to a healthier diet and controlled weight loss may improve the long-term prognosis of these patients as well as helping to improve their current symptoms.

Serum lipids

A raised serum cholesterol increases the risk of developing PVD up to two times. Low-density lipoprotein (LDL) transports cholesterol from the liver to the peripheral tissues. High density lipoprotein (HDL) transports cholesterol from the peripheral tissues to the liver. High LDL levels and/or low HDL levels are associated with an increased risk of PVD. High serum triglyceride levels may also be associated with the development of PVD.

Haemostatic and rheological variables

Anaemia and polycythaemia may both make the symptoms of PVD worse and can be corrected.

Family history

Premature atherosclerosis may be due to an inherited disorder of lipid metabolism. Brothers of patients with abdominal aortic aneurysm (AAA) have a 50% chance of also being affected and should undergo an abdominal ultrasound scan.

Drug history

Drug history can give important clues to underlying medical conditions not previously mentioned by the patient. Also, some medications may exacerbate PVD, e.g. beta-blockers; while other medications may need to be stopped before vascular procedures, e.g. metformin prior to angiography.

Vascular examination

A general examination is performed. Examine for signs of anaemia or hyperlipidaemia. All peripheral pulses are palpated and the volume and character of each pulse is recorded – radial, brachial, axillary, subclavian, carotid, aortic, femoral, popliteal, dorsalis pedis and posterior tibial. The dorsalis pedis or posterior tibial pulse may be absent in 10% of normal individuals. The blood pressure is measured with the patient semi-reclined. Examine for radio-radial delay and radio-femoral delay. Listen for carotid, subclavian, aortic, iliac, femoral and popliteal artery bruits.

Examine the respiratory and cardiovascular systems. Examine the abdomen; in particular, palpate for any AAA. Remember, the abdominal aorta bifurcates at about the level of the umbilicus, therefore AAAs are palpated above this, iliac aneurysms below this. Auscultate for an aortic bruit – this may indicate aortic, renal or iliac stenotic disease. A machinery-type murmur associated with an aneurysm may indicate an aortocaval fistula, especially if associated with swelling of the legs.

In the legs, examine for limb swelling, ulceration or the presence of varicose veins. Port-wine stains or differing limb size may indicate underlying arteriovenous malformations. Examine for signs of ischaemia: relative skin temperatures, venous guttering, delayed (greater than 2 seconds) capillary return, red shiny skin on the toes or patches of infarction/gangrene on the toes.

Perform Buerger's test. Raise the legs and note the angle at which the soles of the feet turn pale. After a minute hang the legs down and note the time for the feet to develop a brick red colour and the veins to refill. A brick red colour is positive for ischaemia.

Investigation of vascular disorders

Laboratory investigations

Biochemistry

To screen for underlying renal disease, renovascular disease, diabetes mellitus.

Serum tests: include general biochemical screen, renal function, serum lipids (HDL, LDL, very low-density lipoprotein (VLDL), triglycerides).

Haematology

Test for anaemia, polycythaemia. Look at clotting and coagulopathies.

Immunology

Test for coagulopathies, protein C, protein S deficiencies, lupus anticoagulant. Auto-antibody screen for connective tissue disorders (CTD) and vasculitis.

Physiology/imaging techniques

Ultrasound

The predominant imaging technique used in vascular surgery is ultrasound, but there are many different types and applications.

Continuous wave Doppler (CWD)

CWD is the simplest form of ultrasound and is ideal for use by the doctor in the out-patient clinic to detect flow within blood vessels. The probe is the size of a pencil and the set is the size of a typical personal stereo. In the head of the probe are a transmitter and a receiver, which are continuously active. The probe is moved over the area where an artery is thought to be. When blood flow is detected the typical whoosh-whoosh sound becomes audible.

Ankle-brachial pressure index (ABPI)

In health, the systolic blood pressure at the ankle should be the same or slightly higher than that at the arm. Atherosclerosis usually affects the leg vessels and spares the arm vessels. To measure the ankle-brachial pressure a blood pressure cuff is placed on the upper arm and the radial pulse is detected at the wrist using the CWD. The cuff is then inflated until the CWD signal disappears. The cuff is deflated slowly until the signal returns and the pressure is noted. The procedure is then repeated for the lower limb, with the cuff applied just above the ankle and the probe placed on either the dorsalis pedis, posterior tibial and/or peroneal arteries. The pressure at which the signal returns is compared for the arm and the leg and expressed as a ratio – the ABPI. An ABPI of 0.9–1.0 is normal. Less than 0.9 indicates vascular disease, less than 0.5 indicates severe vascular disease.

ABPI is unreliable in the presence of incompressible arteries. In some patients the arteries are so calcified they are incompressible by the cuff and the patient appears to have a high ABPI because a CWD signal can always be detected at very high cuff pressures, even in the presence of obvious vascular disease. This commonly occurs in diabetic patients. In this instance an experienced vascular technologist may comment that the arterial signal sounds damped, based on the subjective interpretation of the quality of the audio signal. This can be investigated further by measurement of the toe pressure or by using the pole test.

Resting ABPI may miss mild cases of arterial disease or not provide sufficient evidence to convincingly exclude vascular disease in cases where symptoms may be caused by other disorders. Mild disease can be detected by repeating the ABPI after a period of exercise (*see* exercise testing).

Pole test

In some patients the arteries are so calcified they are incompressible by the cuff and the patient appears to have a high ABPI. This can be tested by detecting the arterial signal in the foot and then raising the foot until the signal disappears. The height at which the signal disappears is recorded – in health the signal should never disappear. The measurements on the pole have been calibrated so that the height in centimetres corresponds to the mmHg, e.g. less than 50 mmHg indicates severe ischaemia.

Toe-pressures measurement

This is an alternative method in patients with incompressible arteries. A small cuff is inflated around the big toe until the arterial signal in the digital arteries disappears. Smaller arteries in the digits are usually not affected by calcification and provide a more reliable toe-brachial pressure index (TBPI). TBPI less than 0.8 indicates ischaemia. Less than 30–35 mmHg absolute pressure measurement indicates critical ischaemia.

Treadmill exercise testing

This is particularly useful in detecting mild disease or excluding vascular disease in patients complaining of leg pain due to other pathology, e.g. arthritis. The commonest method utilises a treadmill. The resting ABPI is measured, then the patient walks on the treadmill at a pace of 3.5 km/h and a gradient of 10 degrees for 10 minutes or until the symptoms prevent further exertion. The ABPI is measured immediately on stopping the exercise. In the presence of vascular disease the ABPI falls after exercise. A normal ABPI after exercise that has precipitated the symptoms excludes a vascular cause.

Not all patients are capable of walking on a moving treadmill, especially those unsteady on their feet due to arthritis. An alternative method is to walk the patient along the corridor until symptoms are produced or to use an ankle flexion/extension.

Ankle flexion/extension exercise testing

This is useful in patients unable to use the treadmill. The patient sits reclined and repeatedly flexes and extends the ankle of the affected limb against a fixed resistance device, thereby exercising the calf muscle. The ABPI is measured before and after exercise and is interpreted in the same way as the treadmill exercise.

This technique is more sensitive than resting ABPI in detecting or excluding significant vascular disease. It is useful for patients who are unable to walk on the treadmill. However, the technique simulates rather than replicates the action of walking.

Colour Duplex ultrasonography

This is the combination of B-mode images and colour-coded pulsed Doppler information. It has become the dominant non-invasive investigation in vascular practice. Acoustic water-based gel is applied to the skin overlying the area of interest and the probe is applied. The depth and power of the signal is adjusted until the artery is visualised. Doppler waveforms are then sampled from different parts of the artery. Colour coding allows high velocity signals and turbulence within the artery to be identified, indicating the site of possible stenoses.

Diagnostic arterial angiography

Prior to the procedure the renal function is checked by measurement of serum urea, creatinine and electrolytes. A creatinine less than 125 µmol/l is acceptable, at 125–300 µmol/l stop all non-steroidal anti-inflammatory drugs (NSAIDs) and hydrate with intravenous fluids both before and after the procedure to ensure a good diuresis. Greater than 300 µmol/l requires a nephrology opinion prior to the procedure. Metformin is associated with a risk of lactic acidosis and renal failure and is therefore stopped 48 hours before angiography and restarted 48 hours after angiography if renal function has not deteriorated. Anticoagulation with warfarin is stopped and converted to intravenous heparin. Heparin is stopped four hours prior to the procedure and restarted two hours after the procedure. Warfarin is restarted the following day if there are no bleeding complications.

The most common portal of entry into the vascular system is the femoral artery (3–5Fr), although the axillary (3Fr) and brachial arteries (3Fr) can also be used. Under local anaesthesia the femoral artery is punctured using a hollow needle through which a floppy ended wire is passed. The needle is then removed and a plastic sheath is passed over the wire into the artery and an injection of contrast confirms the intraluminal position. A pigtail catheter is advanced into the aorta and contrast is injected. Radiographs are taken as the contrast is displaced through the distal vasculature, utilising arterial digital subtraction imaging. Repeated injections are often necessary to image the full length of both legs. At the end of the procedure the catheter is removed and direct pressure is applied for 10–20 minutes (sometimes longer) until the bleeding stops. The patient then remains supine on absolute bed-rest for two to four hours after the procedure and remains in hospital overnight for observation of the puncture wound, pulse and blood pressure and distal circulation.

The technique provides an accurate map of the arterial tree, identifying stenoses and occlusions. Diagnostic angiography can be combined with therapeutic balloon angioplasty/stenting for the treatment of stenoses and occlusions.

Complications include bleeding, trauma to the artery, haematoma, retroperitoneal haematoma, false aneurysm formation, embolisation, arterial dissection, acute limb-threatening ischaemia occasionally leading to limb loss, allergic reactions to the contrast and exacerbation of renal failure. All patients should be fully informed of these major complications before consenting to the procedure.

Digital subtraction angiography

Digital subtraction angiography (DSA) is a computerised technique for improving the image quality obtained at angiography. X-ray images are digitalised and the images of soft tissue and bone are suppressed while the images of contrast within the blood vessels are enhanced. The increased sensitivity has enabled the intravenous delivery of contrast to image the arterial system (IV-DSA). The venous circulation is cannulated and the cannula tip is placed in the right atrium. Contrast is then injected and digital images are generated of the limb in question. Larger volumes of contrast are need for IV-DSA compared to arterial DSA.

CT angiography

A computed tomography (CT) scan is performed with injection of intravenous contrast. The technique can be used with standard CT but is more sensitive when combined with spiral (helical) CT. Spiral CT consists of the patient moving through a continuous X-ray field. The digital images obtained are processed to enhance the images and generate 3-D reconstructions and superior imaging of vascular structures. CTA is useful for assessing the anatomy of large vessels, e.g. AAA, but is less sensitive for the assessment of small vessels.

Magnetic resonance imaging (MRI) angiograph

Either moving blood is used, as its own contrast, or contrast is given. For imaging of small vessels additional small coils are placed over the area concerned. Improved images can be obtained with the intravenous injection of gadolinium and T1 acquisition.

The technique is not applicable to patients with significant metal implants. Images are still not accurate enough for small vessels.

Ascending venography

A vein in the foot is cannulated and low osmolar contrast is injected with a tourniquet inflated at the ankle at sufficient pressure to prevent filling of the superficial veins and to direct the contrast into the deep veins. This is an invasive technique and cannot reliably identify reflux. Much of the information can be obtained by colour Duplex.

Descending venography

The common femoral vein is cannulated and contrast is injected. Reflux is induced by generating a standardised Valsalva manoeuvre by the patient blowing into a manometer device for 10 seconds with 60 degrees head-up tilt on the X-ray table. The technique was once used to demonstrate the extent of deep and superficial venous incompetence, but it is an invasive technique and most of the information can be obtained by colour Duplex.

Varicography

Contrast is injected directly into a varicose vein to demonstrate the distribution and connections with the deep venous system and to identify the origin of recurrent varicose veins. This invasive technique has been largely replaced by colour Duplex.

Contrast lymphangiography

A mixture of local anaesthetic and vital blue dye is injected subcutaneously into the first webspace. The dye is taken up by the lymphatics and outlines the main channels in the foot. One of these channels is cannulated and contrast is infused over a period of an hour. Serial X-rays of the leg, groin, pelvis, abdomen and chest are taken over the first few hours, at 24 hours or even several days later.

The technique provides anatomical detail of the lymphatics. It is useful for imaging the thoracic duct, lymph leaks in the pelvis, abdomen, and chest, and distinguishing reactive from malignant lymph nodes. It is an invasive technique, largely superseded by isotope lymphangiography.

Isotope lymphangiography

Radio-labelled technetium colloid is injected into the second or third web space of the toes. Gamma cameras track the progress of the marker.

This is a very specific method that can demonstrate such abnormalities as delayed transit, presence of collaterals, dermal backflow and reduced uptake in one or more groups of nodes.

Vascular disorders

Atherosclerotic disorders of the arteries

Atherosclerosis is the major cause of lower limb ischaemia, which is the condition most frequently seen in vascular surgical outpatients. The overwhelming majority of patients presenting with intermittent claudication or rest pain will be suffering from atherosclerosis. However, there are other causes of lower limb ischaemia, especially in younger patients, which may need to be considered. These include cystic adventitial disease, popliteal entrapment, fibromuscular dysplasia and Buerger's disease.

Intermittent claudication

Intermittent claudication occurs when stenosed arteries cannot supply sufficient blood to the exercising muscles during exercise. The patient describes cramp-like symptoms in the lower legs, most commonly the calf muscles, occurring at a predictable distance, which is quickly relieved by rest. Once the pain is relieved the patient may then describe the ability to walk further the second time before the pain returns. These symptoms need to be differentiated from other causes of pain in the legs when walking, such as arthritis or sciatica.

The decision to treat is based on the severity of the symptoms and the effect on the patient's lifestyle. Severity is not decided purely on the distance walked. A claudication distance of 400 yards may be an occasional inconvenience to a retired patient but may be job-threatening to a manual worker.

History

Take a general vascular history.

Calf claudication

This is commonly associated with femoral artery disease. A typical history of vascular calf claudication is pain in one or both calves that occurs after walking a certain distance and is relieved by rest. The distance tends to be constant but may be gradually getting less over weeks and months as the disease progresses. The pain is quickly relieved by rest (for one to two minutes).

Buttock claudication

This is commonly associated with aortoiliac disease. It is slightly different in character to calf claudication. Patients describe more aching and weakness or complain of their hip giving way. However, the pain is exacerbated by exercise and relieved by rest. Male patients with bilateral aortoiliac disease may admit to impotence on questioning.

Foot claudication

This is very rare and occurs only in patients with Buerger's disease and occlusive disease, which affects the distal arteries first and spreads proximally. Patients describe pain and numbness that affects the forefoot with exercise. This is often diagnosed as an orthopaedic pain and may have progressed to persistent rest pain by the time a vascular opinion is sought.

Other common causes of pain in the calf or leg
Arthritis

Arthritis of the knee or ankle may cause referred pain to the calf. Arthritis of the spine or hip may produce symptoms similar to buttock claudication.

However, arthritic symptoms tend to vary in severity from day to day or with weather conditions. The pain may occur at rest or start with exercise. The amount of exercise necessary to produce symptoms varies and the pain may persist for hours after the exercise stops.

Nocturnal cramp

Nocturnal cramp is pain in the calf that typically occurs in bed and wakes the patient, and it is relieved by massage of the calf or getting out of bed and walking around.

Spinal stenosis

There is usually a history of arthritis, and the condition is caused by osteophytes narrowing the spinal canal. The pain occurs on walking and is relieved by rest but especially by bending forward. However, this pain can also be precipitated by prolonged standing. There may be associated numbness and paraesthesia, especially around the perineum.

Chronic compartment syndrome

This often affects athletes with large calf muscles. The symptoms are similar to claudication but a large amount of exercise is required to produce the symptoms. Popliteal entrapment syndrome and cystic adventitial disease need excluding in young patients presenting with claudication.

If the symptoms are typical of vascular claudication, determine the distance walked before symptoms start. Determine how this affects the patient's lifestyle. If the walking distance is very small (less than 50 yards) ask about rest pain (pain in the toes at rest), especially at night in bed.

Risk factors

Smoking, diabetes mellitus, family history, cardiac history, hypertension, high-fat diet.

Examination

Palpate all the pulses and auscultate for bruits. Look for general stigmata of vascular insufficiency, e.g. loss of hair in the lower leg, atrophic skin and so on. Claudication is usually but not always associated with absent pulses – pulses may be present at rest but disappear with exercise. Try to determine the site of the arterial disease, e.g. an absent femoral pulse suggests iliac artery disease. Perform Buerger's test. Examine for evidence of distal embolisation, e.g. focal spots of skin infarction in an otherwise well-perfused foot (e.g. iliac artery disease).

Investigations

Perform a routine atherosclerotic screen – dipstick urinalysis, full blood count (FBC), urea and electrolytes (U&Es), serum lipids and electrocardiogram (ECG). Check ankle-brachial pressure index (less than 0.9 indicates underlying vascular disease). A treadmill test may reveal ankle pressure drop after exercise. Colour Duplex arterial scan can identify the site and length of stenoses/occlusions. Arteriogram identifies the site and nature of arterial disease, and is usually combined with angioplasty treatment.

Treatment
Mild claudication
Where mild claudication is not interfering with the patient's lifestyle, correct any underlying disorder such as hyperlipidaemia. Advise daily walks, losing weight and stopping smoking. Improve cardiac and respiratory function.

Moderate claudication
Where moderate claudication is affecting the patient's lifestyle but not severely so, treat as for mild disease but review earlier and proceed to active treatment if conservative measures fail. Some centres advocate a supervised exercise programme under the control of a physiotherapist. Results may be comparable to angioplasty without the risk of complications and they represent a non-interventional alternative.

Severe claudication
In cases severely affecting daily living, more active treatment is indicated. First choice is angiogram and angioplasty. If the patient is not suitable for angioplasty or angioplasty fails, consider for arterial bypass surgery (operations described under critical ischaemia).

Post-treatment follow-up
Mild claudication
Review in three months. If improved, discharge with advice. If stable or deteriorated, decide whether a further trial of conservative treatment is indicated. This is usually the case unless the symptoms have become severe.

Moderate claudication
Review in three months. Decide whether to continue conservative management or whether symptoms have become severe enough to merit angioplasty.

Severe claudication
Review after angiogram/plasty. Decide whether further angioplasty or surgical intervention is indicated.

Post-operative follow-up
Review after four to six weeks to determine the success of the procedure and detect any complications. Angioplasties for critical ischaemia have a re-occlusion rate of up to 40% in the first six months, but may have remained patent long enough to allow ulcer healing. A recurrence of severe symptoms or critical ischaemia requires urgent Duplex reassessment and reangioplasty or bypass if necessary. Complications include groin haematoma and false aneurysm formation. Both can be assessed by Duplex.

The post-operative follow-up of surgical procedures is described under critical ischaemia.

Critical ischaemia, rest pain, gangrene
Ischaemic rest pain occurs when not enough blood is reaching the foot to maintain the integrity of the foot even at rest. The pain starts at that part of the lower limb furthest away from the heart, i.e. the tip of the big toe, and spreads proximally. If ischaemia is not reversed then dry gangrene ensues. Gangrene also occurs when a small injury occurs in a critically ischaemic foot. Healing tissue requires up to 10 times the blood supply of normal tissue in order to heal. If this increase in blood supply does not occur then the tissue dies back to the point of adequate blood supply. In this way a small wound sustained to the tip of the big toe of a critically ischaemic foot can result in the whole leg turning gangrenous.

Ischaemic rest pain needs to be differentiated from other causes of pain in the foot at rest, e.g. arthritis of the toes or metatarsophalangeal joints. The site of the pain is important – it is very unusual for ischaemic rest pain to occur in the ankle without also affecting the toes.

History

Take a general and vascular history. Rest pain may first start at night when the foot is lifted on to the bed thereby losing the help of gravity to supply blood to the foot. Patients may describe attaining relief from the pain by dangling the foot over the side of the bed. Eventually, even with the leg dependent there is still not enough blood supply and the foot is painful all the time. Pain starts at the point furthest away from the heart and spreads proximally.

Other causes of constant lower limb pain
Embolisation

Distal embolisation (from an aortic or iliac lesion) may result in rest pain affecting the toes, but the foot appears well perfused and foot pulses may be palpable.

Arthritis

Arthritis also causes pain in the foot or ankle at rest, but tends to be localised to the joints or areas proximal to the toes. Metatarsalgia can occur at night and is relieved by standing, and can be confused with vascular night pain. However, metatarsalgia tends to run a fluctuating course, causing symptoms for several days or weeks with similar asymptomatic periods. Confusion can occur when the two conditions co-exist.

Painful peripheral neuritis

This condition tends to occur in diabetics and is characterised by a constant burning pain affecting both lower legs. The pain is worse at night when the legs become warm.

Reflex sympathetic dystrophy

This produces a burning pain similar to painful peripheral neuritis. The condition is ill-defined but there may be a history of preceding trauma that may be relatively minor. The limb becomes swollen and is initially warm and dry but later becomes cool, mottled and cyanotic. However, the arterial tree is normal.

Causalgia

This results from incomplete nerve injury and produces a similar constant burning pain.

Examination

Palpate all the pulses and listen for bruits. Look for signs of peripheral ischaemia – loss of hair, thin shiny skin or atrophic musculature. The foot may be oedematous from chronic dependency. Note that a critically ischaemic foot may actually appear erythematous with good capillary return. This appearance may prompt doctors to think that the foot is infected, when in fact the appearance is due to an inflammatory reaction to the underlying ischaemia. The appearance is similar to a positive Buerger's test.

Investigations

Peform a routine atherosclerotic screen of urinalysis and blood tests. Plain X-rays may be indicated if joint disease is suspected. On the ankle-brachial pressure index, a ratio of less than 0.9 indicates peripheral vascular disease; a ratio of less than 0.5 indicates severe ischaemia. Peripheral disease may exist in the presence of apparently normal ABPI, due to incompressible arteries. Colour Duplex scan of the leg arteries is a very useful non-invasive technique that is very reliable in identifying stenoses/occlusions when performed by an experienced operator. Diagnostic angiography may be combined with therapeutic angioplasty if this is appropriate for the lesion and the patient.

Treatment

It is usually too late for conservative therapy and some form of active intervention is indicated. Patients usually require admission for adequate pain relief, elevation of the limb to reduce tissue oedema and intravenous antibiotics if indicated. Improve cardiac and respiratory function. Different hospitals vary in their criteria for angioplasty or operative treatment. In unfit patients who would be high risk for a long surgical procedure, angioplasty is preferred if the lesion is suitable.

Operative treatment

Treatment depends on the site of the disease. As a general rule the most proximal lesion is corrected first, and ischaemic skin lesions have the best chance of healing if there is a continuous channel of blood into the pedal arch. Many different operations are available. Only the commonly performed procedures will be described.

Aortobifemoral bypass

Occlusive disease of the iliac arteries can be bypassed using a prosthetic bifurcated graft from the aorta to both femoral arteries. The patient must be fit enough to withstand clamping of the aorta. In unfit individuals an axillobifemoral graft is a less invasive alternative. It is unusual for gangrene or rest pain to be associated with aortoiliac occlusions alone.

Femoropopliteal bypass

Occlusive disease of the superficial femoral artery can be bypassed by using either a prosthetic graft or the patient's own vein. Vein has the better long-term patency but prosthetic graft to the above knee popliteal artery is acceptable, and patency of prosthetic grafts to the below popliteal artery is improved when a cuff of vein (Miller cuff) is interposed between the graft and the artery.

Femorodistal bypass

Bypass operations performed to the distal run-off vessels (posterior tibial, anterior tibial and peroneal) require autologous vein to be used to obtain reasonable long-term patency.

Chemical lumbar sympathectomy

This procedure is reserved for trying to achieve skin healing in very unfit individuals with extensive distal disease for whom neither angioplasty nor bypass is possible.

Follow-up

Investigations and treatment need to be performed and reviewed within days or weeks, depending on the severity. In the case of tissue loss or gangrene, admission to hospital for in-patient assessment is justified.

Post-operative follow-up

When angioplasty and/or arterial bypass operations have been performed for critical ischaemia, long-term regular follow-up is indicated to detect recurrence, progression of disease or complications developing in the graft.

Vein-graft surveillance

When autologous vein has been used to bypass occlusions in the leg arteries, many hospitals follow patients with regular Duplex ultrasound scans of the vein to detect subclinical stenoses rather than requiring regular attendance at clinic. Significant vein-graft stenoses are treated by urgent angioplasty or operative vein patch angioplasty. Patients are advised to seek urgent medical attention if the leg turns white, cold, numb or painful between scans, as the graft may have occluded and may be salvaged if operated on soon enough. Surveillance is performed on all patients for the first year and extended for a second year for grafts that are considered at risk. Thereafter patients are reviewed in the outpatient department (OPD) with Duplex scans at 6–12 months and discharged if symptom-free.

Complications

Complications include wound infections. Superficial infections should be treated aggressively with antibiotics and weekly review. Deeper infections may require in-patient treatment and intravenous antibiotics, especially if prosthetic grafts have been used. If the wound near an anastomosis becomes infected or opens up, in-patient therapy is mandatory as there is a real risk of secondary haemorrhage.

Wound haematomas and lymph collections can be managed conservatively provided they do not become infected. Limb swelling is normal after arterial bypass surgery and can be treated conservatively if deep-venous thrombosis (DVT) and cellulitis have been excluded.

Cystic adventitial disease

Cystic adventitial disease (CAD) is an uncommon cause of lower limb ischaemia in younger patients. The adventitia of the popliteal artery undergoes a degenerative process and develops a cyst. When the pressure of the contents of the cyst exceeds arterial pressure, the cyst may compress the artery, causing sudden-onset ischaemia.

The differential diagnosis includes popliteal aneurysm, popliteal entrapment and simple knee joint cysts. Exclude cardiac source for emboli, vasculitis and/or CTD.

History

Patients are usually young males and complain of claudication of recent onset. Symptoms may be severe due to the lack of collateral development. Patients may describe ischaemic neuropathy symptoms of burning, paraesthesia and cold.

Examination

There is usually a lack of atherosclerotic signs in other body sites. All pulses in the affected limb may be present at rest but foot pulses disappear on flexion of the knee. Palpation of the affected artery may simulate a popliteal aneurysm. A popliteal bruit may be audible. Later, if occlusion of the popliteal artery occurs, pulses are lost.

Investigations

Colour Duplex may demonstrate the compression of the artery and also identify the cyst and exclude a popliteal aneurysm. CT and MRI scans may better define the lesion in relation to other anatomical structures. Arteriography demonstrates a smooth localised stenosis behind the knee.

Treatment

Angioplasty tends *not* to be successful, because the walls are compliant and cyst content may embolise distally. Aspiration of cysts under CT scan control can be attempted but lesions tend to recur. Surgical evacuation of the cyst is effective treatment if the artery has not progressed to occlusion, when resection and interposition vein graft repair is required.

Follow-up
Review with results of investigations to confirm diagnosis.

Post-operative follow-up
Review after four to six weeks to confirm the success of the procedure. If aspiration has been performed, medium-term follow-up may be required to detect recurrence. Follow-up of bypass procedures is described under critical ischaemia.

Popliteal entrapment syndrome
Popliteal entrapment is an uncommon disorder but should be excluded in all young patients complaining of lower limb ischaemia. Its most common form is caused by compression of the artery by the medial head of the gastrocnemius muscle. Other forms are caused by abnormal strips of muscle or fibrous bands. Exclude cardiac emboli, vasculitis and/or CTD.

History
Most patients are young and active and describe typical symptoms of claudication associated with physical exercise. Patients may describe atypical features such as numbness of the foot, blanching, paraesthesia or pain on walking but not running. Enquire regarding cardiac abnormalities and arrythmias or possible vasculitic pathologies, CTD and the like.

Examination
Exclude cardiac or other sources of embolisation. There is usually a lack of atherosclerosis affecting other arteries. Pulses may be palpable at rest but disappear on dorsiflexion or forced plantar flexion of the foot. Later cases may have absent pulses due to popliteal occlusion. Alternatively, some patients may have post-stenotic aneurysmal degeneration of the popliteal artery.

Investigations
Perform FBC, plasma viscosity/erythrocyte sedimentation rate (PV/ESR) and autoantibody screen to investigate haematological or vasculitic causes. Consider echocardiogram to exclude cardiac source of emboli. Duplex ultrasound may demonstrate compression of the artery and identify aneurysmal dilatation. MRI scanning is being increasingly used to identify the soft tissue abnormalities in this condition. Angiography is used to confirm the diagnosis and exclude any arterial abnormality. In cases of occlusion, angiography defines the distal run-off vessels.

Treatment
All confirmed cases are treated surgically, with release of the constricting band or muscle and reconstruction of the artery if necessary.

Follow-up
Review with results (at one to three months), confirm diagnosis and plan treatment. Popliteal entrapment tends to be bilateral and symptoms may develop in the other limb with time.

Post-operative follow-up
Review to determine the success of the procedure and detect any complications. If a vein interposition graft has been used, the regular vein graft surveillance is appropriate to detect stenoses and prevent occlusion.

Carotid artery disease

The most common carotid conditions are transient ischaemic attacks (TIA) and strokes caused by carotid artery stenotic disease. Data from a number of randomised trials have identified that patients with embolic neurological symptoms originating from significant stenosis of the internal carotid artery benefit from carotid endarterectomy compared to medical therapy alone.

Carotid disease is primarily an embolic disease and the degree of stenosis is only an indirect marker of the severity of the atheroma. Increasingly, patients are assessed in TIA clinics by a multidisciplinary team consisting of a vascular surgeon, neurologist or stroke physician and a radiologist. Patients have their symptoms assessed, their arteries scanned and treatment arranged at the one visit. The medical opinion is particularly useful for patients with non-specific or non-hemispheric conditions, for which the differential diagnosis includes epilepsy, brain tumours, hypoglycaemia, migraine, cardiac arrythmias and vertebrobasilar ischaemia.

Other rare causes of stroke include systemic lupus erythematosus (SLE), polyarteritis nodosa (PAN), giant cell arteritis, migraine, brain tumours and fibromuscular dysplasia (FMD).

History

The classic embolic neurological event is the transient ischaemic attack (TIA). A TIA is a mini stroke (e.g. limb weakness, speech defects, facial weakness) which recovers completely within 24 hours. The symptoms affect the limbs on the opposite side to the stenosed artery. Amaurosis fugax (fleeting blindness) occurs when an embolus temporarily occludes the main stem or branch of the retinal artery causing temporary blindness. Amaurosis fugax consists of transient monocular blindness that occurs on the same side as the stenosed artery. All or part of the visual field may be lost, but usually the embolus breaks up and vision returns. Occasionally, loss of vision is permanent and complete (central retinal artery occlusion).

Patients with residual motor or visual defects may still be considered for endarterectomy if they have a good quality of life and/or if a further stroke would threaten their independence.

Non-specific or non-hemispheric symptoms such as blackouts, drop attacks, fainting, dizziness, double vision or vertigo are more suggestive of cardiac, neurological or ear, nose and throat (ENT) disease, and further investigation or referral to the relevant speciality should be considered. However, some of these symptoms may indicate vertebrobasilar ischaemia (VBI), which may have a primary vascular cause, and this should be excluded (*see* VBI section).

Examination

Perform a general and vascular examination. Listen for bruits over the carotid and subclavian arteries. Note that the absence of a carotid bruit does not exclude the presence of a severely stenosed carotid artery. Perform a general neurological examination and record any existing neurological deficits. Perform a cardiac examination. In particular examine for arrythmias, valve abnormalities and heart failure.

Investigations

Colour Duplex ultrasonography can determine the degree of stenosis and is reliable when performed by an experienced operator. Carotid angiogram is useful to confirm total carotid artery occlusion, which may be difficult to diagnose on colour Duplex, or to identify aortic arch, brachiocephalic or subclavian artery disease. Computed tomography angiography/magnetic resonance angiogram (CTA/MRA) scans are less invasive alternatives to carotid angiography. CT/MRI brain scans may be indicated to exclude neurological disease.

Treatment

All patients should receive the best medical therapy – aspirin, anti-hypertensives and lipid-lowering agents.

Symptomatic carotid stenosis

Male patients with carotid stenosis greater than 50% benefit from early surgery. Females benefit if stenosis is greater than 70%.

Asymptomatic carotid stenosis

Fit male patients under the age of 75 with carotid stenosis greater than 50–60% benefit from surgery. Female patients (and males over the age of 75) may benefit depending on co-morbidities and low surgical morbidity/mortality rates.

Follow-up

Investigations need to be performed and reviewed as soon as possible. For those patients confirmed to have a severe symptomatic carotid stenosis, carotid endarterectomy is most effective within two days of the onset of symptoms. In those patients with mild/moderate carotid stenoses, best medical therapy should be instituted and the patient reviewed either in the surgical or medical clinic to monitor effectiveness. For patients in whom carotid artery disease is excluded, consider referral for neurology, cardiac, ENT or ophthalmological opinion as indicated by the results of the assessment performed.

Post-operative follow-up

Patients are seen four to six weeks after operation to check on local complications related to the wound. In some centres a further Duplex scan is performed on the operated artery to identify restenosis or asymptomatic occlusion. Restenosis is usually due to intimal hyperplasia, which does not cause embolic symptoms. Other complications following CEA include cranial nerve lesions, infection (superficial and deep) and false aneurysm. Transient cranial lesions occur in up to a third of patients and usually resolve within 12 months. Superficial infection is treated aggressively with antibiotics, especially if prosthetic patch angioplasty was performed, and most resolve. Persistent and deep infections may require admission and intravenous antibiotics and repeated Duplex scanning to confirm the integrity of the patch angioplasty. There is a risk of potentially fatal secondary haemorrhage.

Vertebrobasilar ischaemia (VBI)

The symptoms of vertebrobasilar ischaemia are less common than those of carotid ischaemia, and the criteria for surgical treatment are less well defined. Symptoms of VBI may be embolic or haemodynamic and arise from disease of the vertebral artery itself or from the subclavian artery proximal to the origin of the vertebral artery. The cause of symptoms may not be primarily vascular, e.g. the vertebral arteries may be compressed by osteophytes associated with cervical spondylosis. Other neurological pathologies, orthostatic hypotension, cardiac arrhythmias, ENT and other non-vascular causes may need to be excluded.

History

Determine exactly the circumstances when symptoms occur, e.g. head turning. This may indicate the non-vascular causes outlined in the introduction.

Vertebrobasilar symptoms (TIAs)

At least three of the following symptoms occurring simultaneously are required for diagnosis of vertebrobasilar syndrome (isolated symptoms are less significant): unilateral or bilateral simultaneous motor/sensory deficits, ataxia, diplopia, dysarthria, dysphagia, bilateral homonymous hemianopia, vertigo, tinnitus, transient global amnesia. Drop attacks or loss of consciousness may be the result of embolisation, or, if they coincide with vigorous use of the arm, represent the subclavian steal syndrome. Enquire regarding other neurological, ENT or cardiac pathologies.

Examination

Listen for supraclavicular and carotid bruits. Examine the neck for tenderness and range of movement. Examine the arms for evidence of upper limb ischaemia. Examine for cardiac abnormalities.

Investigations

Colour Duplex of the carotid subclavian and vertebral arteries is sensitive enough to detect significant disease. Definitive identification of lesions requires angiography. CT brain scan may be required to exclude brain tumours producing similar symptoms. 24-hour ECG may be required to investigate cardiac arrythmias.

Treatment

Embolic symptoms are treated initially with correction of vascular risk factors and low-dose aspirin. If this does not work, anticoagulation may be necessary. For haemodynamic lesions, angioplasty of subclavian stenoses/occlusions may be undertaken.

Indications for surgery include severe (greater than 70%) stenoses of the vertebral artery, short occlusions of both vertebral artery origins or stenosis of one remaining or dominant artery causing symptoms. Surgical reconstruction of the vertebral artery is a specialised technique performed mainly for recognised embolic or haemodynamic disease and consists of carotid to vertebral artery bypass or transposition of the vertebral artery to the carotid.

Follow-up

Review within short intervals (1–6 weeks) with results of investigations until diagnosis is made. Decisions regarding treatment are made and patients are reviewed to confirm the effectiveness of the various therapies. Patients are discharged once serious causes have been excluded or symptoms have stabilised. Neurology, ENT or cardiac referrals may be indicated.

Post-operative follow-up

Review to determine the success of the procedure and detect any complications, e.g. graft occlusion and/or recurrence of symptoms.

Carotid artery aneurysm

Carotid artery aneurysm is rare, but more frequently affects the common carotid artery than the internal or external carotid arteries. Causes include atherosclerosis, trauma, mycotic and fibromuscular dysplasia (FMD). Most aneurysms are fusiform rather than saccular.

Differential diagnosis includes tortuous carotid artery, carotid body tumour, lymph nodes overlying the artery, branchial cyst and cystic hygroma.

History

Most patients present because they have noticed a pulsatile swelling in the neck. Most are asymptomatic, but some present with carotid territory TIAs or stroke. High aneurysms of the internal carotid artery can cause symptoms due to cranial nerve neuropraxia, e.g. dysphagia, hoarse voice, facial pain. There may be a history of trauma or of an infective episode suggesting possible mycotic aneurysm.

Examination
Common carotid artery (CCA) aneurysms present with a pulsatile swelling at the angle of the jaw; internal carotid artery (ICA) aneurysms present as a swelling in the posterior pharynx. Bruits may be audible. Perform a neurological examination and examine for cranial nerve lesions.

Investigations
Colour Duplex scan will usually confirm or exclude the diagnosis. Alternatively, angiography can be used. In difficult cases or where surgery is considered, a CT/MRI scan of the neck is useful to define the relation of the aneurysm to other structures.

Treatment
Most aneurysms require surgical repair. Fusiform aneurysms require excision and vein graft bypass. Saccular aneurysms can be treated by aneurysmectomy and patch angioplasty. Very high aneurysms at the skull base can be treated by endovascular embolisation after test occlusion or other investigations have confirmed adequate collateral flow around the circle of Willis.

Follow-up
Patients should be reviewed quickly with results (within one to four weeks) to confirm or exclude the diagnosis. The majority of pulsatile lumps turn out to be a prominent or tortuous but otherwise normal carotid artery and the patient can be reassured and discharged. In very tortuous arteries investigate for FMD, especially if the patient is also hypertensive (*see* renal artery stenosis section). Confirmed carotid aneurysms require prompt treatment. Other causes are managed appropriately.

Post-operative follow-up
Review to confirm the success of the operation and to detect complications. The complications are the same as for carotid endarterectomy. Patients can be discharged once healed and symptom-free.

Carotid body tumour (CBT)
The carotid body is derived from neural crest cells of the third branchial arch and is located behind and between the internal and external carotid arteries. The correct term for a tumour of this gland is a paraganglioma. When these occur, 5% are bilateral and 10% are malignant. Although not strictly a vascular condition, these lesions are often referred to vascular surgeons because treatment sometimes requires reconstruction of the carotid arteries. Some rare cases may be associated with phaeochromocytoma.

Differential diagnosis includes carotid artery aneurysm, lymph node mass, branchial cyst and cystic hygroma.

History
Patients commonly present because they have noticed a pulsatile swelling in the neck. Other symptoms include headache, neck pain, dizziness, hoarse voice and dysphagia caused by local invasion or cranial nerve compression. CBTs seldom cause cerebral ischaemia, but occasional symptoms of flushing, dizziness, arrythmias and hypertension are caused by neuroendocrine secretion by the tumour.

Examination

A mass in the neck may be palpable. This mass may feel pulsatile because of its close proximity to the carotid arteries but, unlike an aneurysm, is not expansile. Classically these tumours can be moved from side to side but not up or down. Perform a neurological examination, looking for cranial nerve lesions (IX, X, XI, XII). An indirect laryngoscopy may be required. Occasionally there may be a Horner's syndrome. Examine for neuroendocrine effects.

Investigations

Growth of the tumour tends to splay the carotid bifurcation, which can be detected by colour Duplex or angiography. The blood supply from the external carotid artery (ECA) and the very vascular nature of these tumours may also be demonstrated. A CT/MRI scan may be useful to define the relation of the tumour to other structures, to define its extent and to exclude bilateral disease. The Shamblin classification grades these tumours from I to III based on size, site and degree of difficulty. Grade III may require resection of ECA or ICA and vein graft repair.

Treatment

Tumours require surgical excision and sometimes carotid artery reconstruction. Some centres recommend pre-operative embolisation of the blood supply of the tumour to reduce vascularity.

Follow-up

Patients should be reviewed quickly with results (within one to four weeks) to confirm or exclude the diagnosis. The majority of pulsatile lumps turn out to be a prominent or tortuous but otherwise normal carotid artery, and the patient can be reassured and discharged. Confirmed CBTs require prompt treatment. Other causes are managed appropriately. Exclude phaeochromocytoma in hypertensives (urinary catecholamines).

Post-operative follow-up

Review with histology to confirm complete excision and exclude malignancy. Malignant lesions require oncology referral and long-term follow-up. The complications of operation are the same as for carotid endarterectomy. Patients can be discharged if unilateral benign disease is confirmed, wounds have healed and the patient is symptom-free.

Inflammatory (vasculitic) disorders of the arteries

Vasculitis is the term used to describe a group of conditions characterised by inflammation of the blood vessel wall. Vasculitis tends to present to the vascular surgeon as skin ischaemia of the lower limbs, which mimics large vessel disease or embolic phenomena. Suspicion is raised by finding a raised ESR, PV or C-reactive protein, and screening for autoantibodies is performed. However, arterial biopsy is required for a diagnosis in most cases and should be considered in all suspicious cases unless tissues are too ischaemic to support wound healing.

Buerger's disease (thromboangiitis obliterans)

This uncommon disorder can affect all races but is more common in the Middle and Far East. It occurs only in smokers and predominantly affects men, although women are increasingly affected. Buerger's is an inflammatory occlusive disease involving muscular medium-sized arteries of the extremities, which produces a granulomatous reaction with giant cells within the thrombus. Later the occluded artery becomes contracted, with the artery and vein bound tightly together by fibrous tissue. The disease affects the very distal arteries first and progresses proximally.

History

Smoking history is positive. Foot claudication is the characteristic symptom caused by involvement of the foot arteries. Calf claudication can occur with infrapopliteal disease. The majority of patients are male and most have three to four limbs affected. It is very rare to have a single limb affected, although upper limb symptoms may predominate and resemble Raynaud's. Initial symptoms include coldness, paraesthesia, skin colour changes, skin lesions, rest pain and intermittent claudication. *Note* – gangrene and ulceration may precede claudication.

Examination

Perform a general and vascular examination. Affected digits are purplish red, cold and damp. Venous filling in the foot is very slow. Gangrene and ulceration may be present. Proximal pulses are normal. In the acute phase there may be redness and tenderness of the skin over the affected vein/artery. There may be phlebitis migrans. There may be evidence of an underlying CTD in women.

Investigations

Perform a general atherosclerotic screen and PV/ESR and autoantibody screen. If tobacco is denied, measure cotinine levels in the urine (greater than 50 ng/ml indicates smoking). ABPI ankle pressures may be normal in the presence of disease affecting foot arteries only – compare ankle and toe pressures.

Arteriography tends to be diagnostic, showing multiple segmental occlusions of distal extremity arteries. Occlusions may be tapered or abrupt, with extensive reticular collaterals around each occlusion (corkscrew collaterals). The arterial walls are smooth, not irregular as in atherosclerosis. Biopsy of the artery provides a histological diagnosis.

Treatment

Correct positive risk factors. Advise stopping smoking and walking training for foot claudication to develop collaterals. To heal ulcers, intra-arterial prostaglandin E1 (PGE1) or prostacyclin (PGI2) infusions may be effective, as may sympathectomy. Hyperbaric oxygen therapy has also been proposed. Epidural analgesia for short periods (1–2 weeks) may be useful to allow pain-free time for healing to occur. Transcutaneous electric nerve stimulation (TENS) is an alternative for long-term analgesia. Surgical debridement and amputations are performed as appropriate.

Follow-up

Follow-up depends on severity and patient behaviour. If the patient stops smoking and the condition is mild, it tends to stabilise. Review at regular intervals (1–3 months) and discharge once stable. More severe cases need to be reviewed at shorter intervals to detect the need for in-patient therapy.

Post-operative follow-up

Review to determine the success of procedures. This usually consists of ensuring the healing of amputation sites.

Takayasu's disease (non-specific aorto-arteritis)

Takayasu's disease is an arteritis mainly affecting the aorta and its branches, causing segmental stenosis, occlusion, dilatation and aneurysm formation. It occurs all over the world, but is commonest in females from the Far East, usually under the age of 40. However, it can affect people of any age. Lesions are characterised by intimal proliferation and fibrosis of the medial and adventitial layers. Active lesions have a lymphoplastic infiltrate, Langhans and foreign body giant cells.

In the acute phase patients complain of non-specific fever, myalgia, arthralgia, weight loss and pain over the arteries. Pulses are present, blood pressure is elevated and there are bruits and early ischaemia.

In the late phase inflammation has settled, pulses are absent and symptoms of vascular insufficiency predominate.

✧ Type I affects the aortic arch.
✧ Type II affects the descending and abdominal aorta.
✧ Type III combines types I and II.
✧ Type IV is type II and pulmonary artery disease.

The most commonly affected vessels are subclavian, descending aorta, renal, carotid, mesenteric, ascending aorta and abdominal aorta.

History
General symptoms include dizziness, syncope, claudication, angina, stroke, myocardial infarction (MI) and upper or lower limb ischaemia, depending on which arteries are affected.

Examination
Pulses may be absent, especially the carotid and upper limbs. Hypertension may be present secondary to renal artery stenosis or coarctation of the aorta. This may result in congestive cardiac failure due to hypertension, aortic insufficiency or coronary ischaemia. Erythema nodosum and pyoderma gangrenosum may be present and associated with juvenile rheumatoid arthritis, sarcoid and inflammatory bowel disease.

Investigations
In the acute phase FBC may show anaemia and a leucocytosis, and the ESR is raised. An autoantibody screen should be performed to exclude CTD. Angiography is diagnostic and may show either variable lengths of narrowing of the aorta and other arteries progressing to segmental occlusion or arterial dilatation and fusiform and saccular aneurysm formation – or a combination of the two (the majority).

Treatment
Treat with long-term steroids, cyclophosphamide or methotrexate. Angioplasty is useful in the chronic stage, especially for renal artery stenosis.

Surgery should be avoided in the acute phase if possible. Bypass from and to arteries free of disease on angiography. Endarterectomy is seldom possible. Therefore carotid and vertebral disease is treated by bypass procedures taken from the ascending aorta.

Aneurysms are resected in younger patients.

Follow-up
Joint care with relevant physicians. All patients require long-term follow-up. The condition is monitored using serial Duplex scanning, angiography or MRI angiography.

Post-operative follow-up
Routine post-arterial surgery follow-up depending on procedure performed.

Polyarteritis nodosa
PAN is a systemic necrotising vasculitis affecting small and medium-sized muscular arteries. It is associated with hepatitis B and most frequently diagnosed in men between

the ages of 40 and 60, although any age can be affected. Damage to the blood vessel wall can result in aneurysm formation.

History
Symptoms depend on the artery affected. General symptoms include malaise, abdominal pain, weight loss, fever and myalgia. Gastrointestinal involvement is common and manifests as abdominal pain, nausea and vomiting. This can proceed to bowel perforation and haemorrhage.

Examination
Perform a general and vascular examination. Hypertension is a frequent finding due to renal artery involvement. Skin manifestations include nailfold infarcts, palpable purpura, and livedo reticularis. Aneurysm may be palpable. Mononeuritis multiplex commonly occurs, and other important sites to examine are the testes and retina.

Investigations
Urinalysis may reveal proteinuria with renal failure developing in two-thirds of patients. A FBC may reveal anaemia and the ESR may be elevated. Antineutrophil cytoplasmic antibody (ANCA) may be raised. Hepatitis B surface antigen and antibody should be determined in all patients.

Angiography shows the characteristic findings of saccular or fusiform aneurysms and arterial narrowing. Arterial biopsy may reveal a vasculitis, which is diagnostic when combined with the angiographic appearance.

Treatment
Treat with corticosteroids with cyclophosphamide if control is difficult. Angioplasty may be useful once the acute disease has settled.

Post-treatment follow-up
Follow up at regular intervals by relevant physician to determine the course of the disease. Long-term follow-up is required to detect late arterial complications.

Wegener's granulomatosis
This is a systemic necrotising vasculitis which preferentially affects the upper respiratory tract, lungs and kidneys. Cutaneous manifestations include cutaneous ulceration, subcutaneous nodules and palpable purpura.

Investigations include sinus radiographs or CT scans, which show mucosal thickening and sinus opacification of air-fluid levels, and the CXR is abnormal. Diagnosis is made through biopsy. Elevated c-ANCA levels are associated with Wegener's. Treatment is with immunosuppressant therapy and follow-up by relevant physicians.

Giant cell arteritis
This is a systemic granulomatous vasculitis that affects large and medium-sized blood vessels, commonly the cranial branches of the aorta and in particular the ophthalmic artery, causing sudden blindness. It occurs mainly in the over-fifties and is three to five times more common in women.

History
Fever, weight loss and fatigue may be the earliest symptoms, but these are often missed. Classically, patients present with severe headache. Jaw claudication is described in over half of patients, due to facial/maxillary artery involvement. Once blindness is complete it is permanent, but amaurosis fugax is reversible with steroid treatment.

Examination

Perform a general and vascular examination. Tenderness of the scalp over the superficial temporal artery region may be elicited. Examine for disease of the carotid, vertebral and subclavian arteries.

Investigations

Diagnosis is usually based on the clinical findings, a raised ESR (positive in 80%) and positive granulomatous histology from a temporal artery biopsy (negative in 50% due to skip pattern). Therefore, a negative biopsy in the presence of a strong clinical suspicion should still be treated with steroids. Exclude other causes of amaurosis fugax, e.g. Duplex of carotid arteries.

Treatment

High-dose steroids initially, gradually tailing down to a maintenance dose.

Post-treatment follow-up

Usually by physicians, with patients referred to vascular surgeons to perform the temporal artery biopsy.

Post-operative follow-up

Review with histology and confirm wound healing. Refer to relevant speciality for further management.

Cutaneous vasculitis

This typically occurs in the post-capillary venules, although capillaries and arterioles are also involved. Most patients have a single episode that is self-limiting and requires no special treatment. Patients with severe or recurrent episodes are investigated by skin biopsy and treated with steroids.

Idiopathic cutaneous vasculitis

This is the most common form. It produces symmetrical palpable purpura typically affecting the lower leg. Lesions occur in crops, appearing as a macular erythema progressing to purpura. The condition is distinguished from urticaria because lesions last longer than 24 hours. Biopsy of lesions shows leucocytoclastic vasculitis with endothelial swelling, often necrosis, haemorrhage, fibrin deposition and infiltration with polymorphonuclear neutrophils.

Necrotising vasculitis

This form is associated with infections, drugs or CTD. Infections are often viruses affecting the upper respiratory tract, e.g. Henoch-Schönlein purpura. The commonest drugs are penicillin and sulphonamides. Diuretics and NSAIDs can also cause it. Histology shows a leucocytoclastic vasculitis.

Cutaneous vasculitis as a manifestation of systemic disease

The most common disease is SLE. Other diseases are Churg-Straus and Behçet's disease.

Non-atherosclerotic, non-inflammatory disorders of the arteries
Arterial fibrodysplasias

Fibrodysplasia describes a group of disorders of unknown aetiology that are neither inflammatory nor atherosclerotic, and which result in stenoses, occlusions and aneurysms.

Variations of the disorders include intimal fibroplasia, medial hyperplasia, medial fibroplasia and perimedial dysplasia. The most important of these conditions is renal artery fibrodysplasia, which affects 0.5% of the population and is the second most common surgically correctable cause of hypertension.

The pathogenesis is unclear, but the underlying cause may represent mural ischaemia from inadequate vaso-vasorum blood flow.

Intimal fibrodysplasia

Primary intimal fibrodysplasia presents in children and young adults as a focal smooth stenosis or web in otherwise normal arteries and may represent residual or persistent neonatal intimal cushions.

Medial hyperplasia

This is hyperplasia of the media causing a stenosis but without accompanying fibrosis. This is rare, affects mainly females, age range 40–50s, and presents as a focal stenosis in the main renal artery.

Medial fibroplasia

This represents 85% of dysplastic renovascular disease. Two forms are recognised: peripheral, which is confined to outer media; and diffuse, which affects the whole media. It tends to progress from the periphery. Compact fibrous tissue replaces smooth muscle and ground substance. Adventitial tissues are not involved but the internal elastic lamina fragments.

Perimedial dysplasia

Perimedial dysplasia represents 10% of renal artery dysplasias and may co-exist with medial fibrodysplasia. It produces focal or multiple stenoses of the main artery but without aneurysmal formation. Microscopically there are collections of amorphous tissue in the adventitia.

Renal artery fibrodysplasia

See renal artery stenosis section.

Carotid and vertebral artery fibrodysplasia

Intimal and medial fibrodysplasia affect these arteries and both are associated with elongation, kinking and coiling of the arteries. Medial fibrodysplasia almost totally occurs in females, at a mean age of 55. ICA and vertebral artery (VA) disease co-exist with renal artery fibrodysplasia in 50% of cases and intracranial aneurysm in 25%.

Carotid artery

It affects the mid-carotid artery adjacent to the 2–3 cervical vertebrae, but involvement of the ICA origin is rare (unlike atherosclerosis). It produces serial stenoses, which are often bilateral.

Vertebral artery

The lower part of the vertebral artery is affected more than the upper segments. Multiple stenoses and aneurysms are produced, but not the 'string of beads' appearance seen on angiography in renal artery fibrodysplasia.

History

Take a general and vascular history. These lesions may be incidental asymptomatic findings or may present with TIAs, stroke, rupture or acute dissection affecting the relevant vascular territory. Patients may complain of a pulsatile mass in the neck. A history of hypertension raises the possibility of renal artery stenosis.

Examination
Perform a general and vascular examination. Examine the carotid, vertebral and subclavian arteries for bruits. The finding of a pulsatile mass in the neck often raises the suspicion of an aneurysm or carotid body tumour, but usually is due to coiling and kinking of the artery. However, fusiform aneurysmal dilatation can occur with FMD.

Investigations
Colour Duplex helps to identify the coiled and elongated artery or aneurysm formation. Carotid body tumour can be excluded. Angiography is indicated to define the disease and identify intracranial aneurysms and renal artery stenosis. If hypertension is a feature, angiographic examination of the renal arteries is particularly indicated.

Treatment
Treatment is indicated for symptomatic disease and includes resection and interposition vein bypass. Angioplasty is indicated for non-embolic, non-aneurysmal stenotic disease.

Follow-up
Review with results of investigations and decide on a treatment plan. The finding of intracranial aneurysms is referred for a neurosurgical opinion. Renal artery stenosis is treated as appropriate (see renal artery stenosis section).

Post-operative follow-up
Review after 4–6 weeks to determine the success of the operation. Complications are similar to those for carotid endarterectomy. Long-term follow-up with annual Duplex scans to detect FMD in the contralateral side and other arteries should be considered.

Iliac, femoral, popliteal and tibial artery fibrodysplasia
FMD can affect any of these arteries, but is rare. It most commonly affects the external iliac artery, producing serial stenoses with intervening mural aneurysms affecting the proximal third of this vessel. It affects females in the 50–60s age range. There is associated renal artery disease in 1–6%. Management consists of excluding renal artery disease and treatment of the stenoses by angioplasty or bypass surgery.

Subclavian, axillary and brachial artery fibrodysplasia
Smooth focal or long tubular stenoses produce symptoms of arm ischaemia. It is difficult to differentiate from Takayasu's. Once again, these lesions are rare and tend to respond to angioplasty.

Splanchnic artery fibrodysplasia
This has origins of coeliac, SMA and IMA stenoses and occasional aneurysms, e.g. splenic artery aneurysm. Stenoses caused by FMD may be a rare cause of intestinal ischaemia, which respond well to angioplasty. FMD is one of the causes of splenic artery aneurysms, which occur particularly in multiparous young women and can cause fatal rupture during pregnancy. Therefore these aneurysms should be repaired when detected.

Aneurysmal disorders of the arteries
A true aneurysm is an abnormal dilatation of an artery that affects all three layers of the

wall of the artery. It is considered significant if it causes symptoms if or the dilatation exceeds twice its normal diameter. The cause of 90% of aneurysms is degenerative secondary to atherosclerosis. Aneurysms can be associated with other disease processes including FMD, SLE, Takayasu's, giant cell arteritis, PAN, Behçet's, Marfan's, and Erhler's Danlos. Aneurysms can also arise as a result of systemic infection (mycotic aneurysms) or dissection of the wall of the artery or they can be secondary to trauma including post-stenotic.

False aneurysms occur secondary to an escape of blood from the artery, which is contained only by the adventitia and usually occurs secondary to cannulation of the artery followed by inadequate compression.

It is useful to consider true aneurysms as peripheral, visceral and central, based on the site and behaviour of the aneurysms.

✧ Peripheral aneurysms affecting the limb arteries seldom rupture but commonly embolise or thrombose, causing distal ischaemia.
✧ Visceral artery aneurysms seldom embolise but are prone to rupture.
✧ Central aneurysms such as thoraco-abdominal and abdominal aortic and iliac aneurysms can both embolise distally, causing ischaemia, and/or rupture.

Central aneurysms
Thoraco-abdominal aneurysms (TAA)

Thoraco-abdominal aneurysms are classified as types I–IV.

✧ Type I affects the descending thoracic aorta and abdominal aorta to just above the renal arteries.
✧ Type II affects all the descending thoracic and abdominal aorta and can include the ascending thoracic aorta.
✧ Type III affects most of the descending thoracic aorta and all the abdominal aorta.
✧ Type IV affects all the abdominal aorta from the diaphragm.

The aetiology of thoraco-abdominal aneurysms includes medial degenerative disease, aortic dissection, atherosclerosis, aortitis, infection and trauma.

These aneurysms can present with complications associated with compression or erosion of neighbouring structures such as nerves or viscera in the chest or abdomen.

Surgical repair of these aneurysms is a major surgical undertaking, which only the fittest patients are likely to survive.

History

Many patients are asymptomatic, but if symptoms are present they may include pain in the chest or abdomen secondary to expansion or compression. Compression of the trachea or bronchus can cause cough, wheeze or evidence of chest infection. Compression of the oesophagus can cause dysphagia. Compression of liver or bile ducts may cause jaundice. Vagus nerve traction may present as a hoarse voice. Thrombosis of spinal arteries may present with paraplegia.

Assess cardiorespiratory fitness to undergo surgery, e.g. exercise tolerance, angina, shortness of breath (SOB) and so on.

Examination

Examine for evidence of atherosclerosis and aneurysmal disease. Assess cardiorespiratory fitness.

Investigations

A CT scan with intravenous contrast is required to determine the extent of aneurysm and whether it is suitable for endovascular repair. Angiogram is performed if there is evidence of visceral, renal or limb stenotic disease. Lung function tests and cardiac assessment (e.g. echocardiogram) are obtained together with an anaesthetic opinion. Liaison with cardiothoracic surgeons for all thoraco-abdominal aneurysms other than type IV is indicated.

Treatment
Treatment involves correction of risk factors and improvement of cardiorespiratory function. Patients who are suitable undergo operation, consisting of either open or endovascular repair. Hybrid procedures consist of both open and endovascular surgery.

Follow-up
Review with results to classify the extent of the aneurysm and assess the fitness of the patient to withstand surgery. Liaise with cardiothoracic surgeons if indicated.

Post-operative follow-up
Review to determine the success of the operation. This will usually have been apparent before the patient was discharged from hospital. Major complications include paraplegia, limb loss and death.

Abdominal aortic aneurysm (AAA)
The commonest site of the abdominal aorta to be affected by aneurysmal disease is below the renal arteries, and it may involve the iliac arteries. Aneurysms affecting the aorta above the renal arteries (suprarenal, supracoeliac) require much more complex surgery to repair and may require referral to a tertiary centre (*see* thoraco-abdominal aneurysm repair). Once an AAA ruptures the operative mortality is approximately 50%, therefore the aim of surgery is to operate before rupture occurs, when the mortality is approximately 5%. However, not all aneurysms rupture and a number of patients will die of other causes without the aneurysm ever causing any symptoms. Recent research has identified that once an AAA reaches 5.5cm diameter, elective surgery should be considered. Surgery should also be performed on smaller aneurysms that become symptomatic.

History
Take a general and vascular history. The majority of AAAs are asymptomatic and are detected on routine clinical examination, on USS of the abdomen performed by another speciality, e.g. urology, or on an aneurysm screening programme. Patients may present having noticed a pulsatile swelling in the abdomen. Symptoms such as backache or abdominal pain may indicate a rapidly enlarging aorta, which requires urgent assessment. Assess cardiorespiratory fitness, e.g. angina and exercise tolerance. Enquire regarding family history, especially brothers.

Examination
Perform a general and vascular examination with the aim of confirming the diagnosis, detecting aneurysms or stenotic disease affecting other arteries and determining the general cardiorespiratory fitness of the patient should surgery prove to be necessary.

Investigations
Perform a general atherosclerotic screen of urinalysis and blood tests. USS is usually adequate to confirm the diagnosis of AAA and gives an accurate estimate of the diameter. USS should also confirm the AAA arises below the renal arteries and whether it extends to involve the iliac arteries. A CT scan with intravenous contrast is performed to determine suitability for endovascular repair (EVAR). Angiography is performed if the patient has evidence of stenotic/occlusive disease of leg arteries, which may require

bypass, or evidence of renal artery stenosis meeting the criteria for revascularisation. Investigations performed prior to surgery include lung function tests, cardiac assessment (e.g. echocardiogram) and an anaesthetic opinion.

Treatment

Correct risk factors and optimise cardiorespiratory function. Asymptomatic AAA greater than 5.5cm diameter should undergo operative repair. Smaller aneurysms are considered for surgery if they are symptomatic.

Open aneurysm repair

This is the established operation, performed via a large midline or transverse abdominal incision. The aorta is clamped above and below the aneurysm, and the aorta is replaced with an artificial graft. Clamping the aorta puts a major strain on the heart and lungs, which is why a pre-operative assessment is necessary, and care in the intensive care unit is necessary post-operatively.

Endovascular aneurysm repair (EVAR)

This involves stenting of the AAA via delivery systems inserted through the femoral arteries. EVAR is currently being performed in designated centres and its major advantage is that its less invasive approach is associated with a lower 30-day peri-operative mortality rate – but at a cost of increased rate of reintervention (40%), lifelong surveillance and no improvement in long-term survival over open repair.

Follow-up

Asymptomatic aneurysms less than 5.5cm in diameter undergo USS at regular intervals to detect any increase in size. Initially this should be every three months, increased to six months or even yearly if the aneurysm appears stable and not increasing in size. Smaller aneurysms that become symptomatic should be repaired. Aneurysms approaching 5.5cm are scanned more frequently again or undergo a CT scan with contrast as there is some evidence that USS may underestimate the aortic diameter compared to CT. All patients are counselled as to the nature of the disease and advised that any abdominal or back pain should be considered secondary to a leaking AAA requiring urgent admission to hospital.

Post-operative follow-up

Open repair

At first visit confirm wound healing and return to normal activity. Most complications of aneurysm surgery occur immediately after surgery, e.g. distal embolisation causing trash foot, ischaemic toes etc; renal failure; or ischaemic bowel. Long-term complications include graft infection, indicated by non-specific general malaise and loss of appetite. An urgent CT scan is performed and infection is suspected if fluid or even air is detected around the graft. Graft infection may result in false aneurysm formation or even an aorto-enteric fistula, which may present with haematemesis or rectal bleeding. All must be investigated urgently as an in-patient. Other complications may result from adhesions causing intermittent bowel obstruction. Impotence may result from damage to the autonomic nerves on the anterior surface of the aorta. Anastomotic stenoses may develop resulting in ischaemic symptoms. Incisional hernias are not uncommon.

Endovascular repair

A CT scan is performed at three months to check for complete repair on the aneurysm and yearly thereafter. 'Endoleak' is the term given to incomplete sealing and it is classified from type I to IV.

✧ Type I represents a leak from one of the ends of the stent graft and requires urgent repair.
✧ Type II represents backbleeding from the IMA or lumbar arteries. Usually these can be monitored, and as long as the AAA does not increase in size, no intervention is required.
✧ Type III represents a leak from a join where two stents have been placed together and requires urgent action.
✧ Type IV is a breach in the stent material and requires urgent repair.

Other complications include occlusion of a limb or the whole graft, which presents either urgently with acute ischaemia or as chronic ischaemia causing claudication/rest pain.

Buttock claudication can occur because one limb of the stent graft has covered the internal iliac artery, either intentionally or unintentionally.

Deterioration in renal function can occur due to a renal artery being covered by the stent.

Iliac artery aneurysm

Iliac artery aneurysm tends to refer to aneurysm of the common and/or internal iliac arteries. The external iliac artery is seldom aneurysmal. Common iliac artery aneurysms often occur in conjunction with AAA, and the two are repaired together using a bifurcated graft. Occasionally common iliac aneurysms occur in isolation, or are associated with a small AAA, and merit repair because they have reached a size at risk of rupture or are associated with distal embolisation. Internal iliac aneurysms are less common but may also rupture or embolise. Repair of these aneurysms is important because the blood supply to the bowel has to be considered.

History

Like AAAs, the majority of iliac aneurysms are asymptomatic and are detected on routine clinical examination or on USS. The patient may have noticed a pulsatile swelling in the abdomen. Symptoms such as backache or abdominal pain may indicate a rapidly enlarging aneurysm that requires urgent assessment. Iliac artery aneurysms may give rise to embolisation, and the patient presents with distal limb ischaemia. Internal iliac aneurysms may compress structures in the pelvis, such as nerves, producing symptoms of sciatica or obturator neuralgia.

Examination

Perform a general and vascular examination with the aim of confirming the diagnosis, detecting aneurysms or stenotic disease affecting other arteries and determining the general cardiorespiratory fitness of the patient should surgery prove to be necessary. The aorta bifurcates at the level of the umbilicus so an iliac aneurysm is palpable below the umbilicus.

Investigations

Perform a general atherosclerotic screen of urinalysis and blood tests. USS is usually adequate to confirm the diagnosis and give an accurate estimate of size. CT scan with contrast defines the extent of the aneurysm and its relationship to surrounding structures and suitability for endovascular repair. In some cases it is possible to repair an iliac aneurysm without clamping the aorta, but all patients should be prepared for theatre assuming that the aorta will have to be clamped. Therefore, lung function tests, cardiac assessment and an anaesthetic opinion are obtained.

Treatment

The normal diameter of the common iliac artery is 1.0–1.5cm. Any aneurysm greater than 3cm or any symptomatic aneurysm should be considered for operative repair.

Isolated common iliac aneurysm (normal diameter 1–1.5cm)

Endovascular stenting or open repair with Dacron inlay graft.

Common iliac aneurysm and co-existing AAA

Bifurcated aortic aneurysm repair.

Internal iliac aneurysm (normal diameter 0.75–1.0cm)

If the contralateral internal iliac artery is normal, ligate the aneurysmal internal iliac. If both internal iliac arteries are aneurysmal, ligate one and use polytetrafluoroethylene (PTFE) or vein to revascularise the other.

External iliac aneurysm (normal diameter 1–1.5cm)

Seldom aneurysmal.

Follow-up

Review with investigations and decide on need and fitness for surgery.

Post-operative follow-up

Follow-up and complications are the same as for AAA.

Peripheral artery aneurysm

A peripheral artery is aneurysmal when it is two times the normal diameter. When the underlying cause is atherosclerosis, a number of arteries are commonly affected together, e.g. femoral and popliteal arteries. Other causes include trauma, congenital, FND, arteritis and infection (mycotic). When infection is the cause, the aneurysm often arises suddenly and is related to a systemic infective episode, e.g. *Salmonella* infection. The main complication of peripheral aneurysm is not rupture (although this can occur) but thrombosis or embolisation resulting in ischaemia.

True aneurysm is a dilatation of all three layers of the vessel wall; false aneurysm results from bleeding from the lumen underneath the adventitia, resulting in expansion of just the adventitia. False aneurysms commonly affect the femoral artery and are caused by cannulation of the artery, e.g. angiogram followed by inadequate compression.

History

Try to identify an underlying cause from those listed above. Determine whether the aneurysm is asymptomatic or symptomatic. False aneurysm will usually have been preceded by some trauma or puncture of the artery, most commonly by the performance of an angiogram. Symptoms may consist of pain due to expansion or pressure on adjacent structures, distal embolisation or ischaemia.

Examination

Perform a general and vascular examination. Palpate all peripheral arteries and pulses to detect co-existing aneurysm or evidence of arterial occlusion and distal ischaemia. Palpate for co-existing iliac or AAA. True aneurysms are pulsatile and expansile. False aneurysms are pulsatile but not expansile.

Investigations

Duplex USS is the primary investigation, which will confirm the diagnosis, differentiate between true and false aneurysms and provide an accurate estimate of the size and extent of the aneurysm. Also scan the aorta to exclude co-existent AAA disease. Blood cultures are indicated if mycotic aneurysm is suspected.

Treatment
Common femoral aneurysm (normal diameter 1–1.5cm)
Open repair with Dacron or PTFE inlay graft.

Superficial femoral artery aneurysm (normal diameter 0.75–1.0cm)
Focal aneurysm affecting one segment of artery; or fusiform aneurysmal disease affecting the whole length of the artery. For focal disease, open repair with PTFE or Dacron inlay graft. For fusiform disease, bypass the whole length of the artery using vein or PTFE with ligation of the superficial femoral artery (SFA) proximally and distally.

Popliteal artery aneurysm (normal diameter 0.5–1.0cm)
Saccular or fusiform extending into SFA. Saccular or fusiform bypass using vein or PTFE with proximal and distal ligation of the aneurysm.

Carotid artery aneurysm
Open repair and vein bypass (*see* carotid aneurysm section).

Subclavian/axillary artery aneurysm
Open repair and PTFE graft, often associated with a cervical rib or band, which will also need treatment.

Follow-up
Review with results of investigations and decide on those patients suitable for surgery.

Post-operative follow-up
Review to determine the success of the operation and to detect any complications. Complications are specific to the procedure. Vein grafts are entered into the vein graft surveillance programme with regular Duplex scans to detect developing stenoses.
Otherwise discharge when all wounds have healed and patient is symptom-free.

Visceral artery aneurysms
Visceral artery aneurysms are very rare, but are associated with a high mortality rate if they rupture. Therefore most are repaired. Causes include infection (mycotic), fibromuscular dysplasia or atherosclerosis. Urgent angiography is indicated for symptomatic or large aneurysms, and prompt surgical repair in patients suitable for surgery. In patients unfit for surgery endovascular embolisation may be successful.

Vasospastic disorders of the arteries
Raynaud's phenomenon
Most commonly, Raynaud's describes an abnormal arterial vasospasm in response to cold, usually affecting the fingers. Classically the fingers turn white and numb on exposure to cold, the static blood becomes deoxygenated producing a blue colour, then the vasospasm is released and a reactive hyperaemia occurs and the fingers turn bright red. Two forms are recognised.

Raynaud's disease (primary)
This is the more common form and has no underlying disease. The symptoms are usually mild and seldom produce tissue loss.

Raynaud's syndrome (secondary)

This form has an underlying disease, although Raynaud's symptoms may precede the systemic illness by 20 years. The symptoms are usually more severe and associated with ulceration and tissue loss.

There are numerous variations to the classic description. Triphasic colour change is not necessary; for diagnosis; blanching and reactive hyperaemia are sufficient. Vasospasm can be provoked not only by cold but also by emotion, hormones, trauma, chemicals, vibration and tobacco exposure. Vasospasm does not just affect the fingers – toes are also commonly affected and the vasospasm can be systemic, affecting the nose, ear-lobes, cerebral and coronary arteries, lung vessels (producing pulmonary fibrosis) and oesophagus (producing dysphagia).

Venous spasm produces intense venous congestion and purple colour change and has the same primary and secondary forms as Raynaud's. Acrocyanosis is the term for venous vasospasm and venous infarcts are commonly known as chillblains.

Underlying disorders

Immunological

Systemic sclerosis (90%), SLE, mixed connective tissue disease, dermatomyositis/poly-myositis, rheumatoid arthritis, cryoglobulinaemia, Sjogren's.

Occupational

Vinyl chloride workers, ammunition workers, outside workers, frozen food packers. Vibration white finger.

Obstructive

Thoracic outlet, Buerger's.

Drugs

Ergotamines, betablockers, cytotoxics, cyclosporin.

Other

Malignancy, endocrine (hypothyroidism), uraemia, hepatitis B, reflex sympathetic dystrophy, A-V fistula.

History

A history of blanching is usually adequate for diagnosis. Recent onset, especially in childhood or middle age, is suggestive of secondary Raynaud's. Determine the provoking factors. Enquire about underlying disorders according to the list above. Raynaud's is usually bilateral. Raynaud's affecting just one hand is suspicious of a local traumatic or obstructive cause, e.g. cervical rib. Confusion can also be caused by Buerger's disease, predominantly affecting the upper limbs.

Examination

Perform a general and vascular examination. In primary Raynaud's the fingers are usually normal to inspection and all pulses are present and normal. In severe and secondary Raynaud's there may be scars on the finger pulps from previous ulcers or ulcers may be present. Look for evidence of secondary infection. Examine for any underlying causes. Absent pulses may suggest an atherosclerotic cause, Buerger's disease or a mechanical cause such as thoracic outlet compression syndrome. Use an ophthalmoscope on high power to examine the skin proximal to the nailfold. Normally, capillary vessels underneath the skin are not visible. If they are, this is evidence of significant ischaemia usually associated with secondary Raynaud's.

Investigations

The diagnosis of Raynaud's is mainly clinical. Some centres define Raynaud's as a drop in systolic finger pressure on cooling the hand under controlled laboratory conditions, but the results are not totally sensitive and specific. The most important investigations are to exclude a secondary cause.

Take FBC, TFTs (hypothyroidism), ESR/PV and urinalysis for renal disease in CTD or diabetes. Use CXR to detect lung fibrosis or malignancy, thoracic inlet views to detect a cervical rib. Upper limb Duplex is useful to exclude major arterial disease. Immunological tests include autoantibody screen for RhF, antinuclear antibodies (ANA) for SLE, anticentromere for localised systemic sclerosis (SS) and antitopoisomerase for diffuse SS. These investigations may need to be repeated every few years if the symptoms persist or deteriorate.

Treatment

General measures include stopping smoking, changing occupation, changing medications and stopping the contraceptive pill if there is a clear link. Heated gloves and socks or chemical handwarmers may be advised. Advise regarding The Raynaud's and Scleroderma Association, Alsager, Cheshire for practical advice and support.

Mild to moderate primary Raynaud's will often respond to a combination of these general measures to control the symptoms. If the symptoms are still affecting lifestyle or employment, or secondary Raynaud's is present, drug therapy may be necessary.

Drugs

Nifedipine retard 10 mg once a day taken at bedtime is effective and taken at this time minimises the headache and dizziness that can occur. The dose can be gradually increased to 20 mg bd/tds if tolerated. It is not licensed for use in pregnancy, so inform patient of this. Amlodipine, diltiazem and isradipine are also useful second-line drugs.

Inositol nicotinate (Hexopal) 4 g/day may take three months to have any effect.

Naftidrofuryl oxalate (Praxilene) 200 mg tds may decrease frequency and severity of attacks.

In-patient treatment

Iloprost infusion, a stable prostocyclin analogue, may be given intravenously for six hours for 3–5 days per treatment. This may terminate a prolonged attack and reduce the frequency of further attacks.

Sympathetomy

Lumbar sympathetomy is effective for the lower limb, not for the upper limb.

Treat any infection or ulcers aggressively with antibiotics. *Note* – usual signs of infection are often absent. Severe ulceration or gangrene may require surgical debridement or amputation.

Treatment of underlying connective tissue disorder may be needed.

Follow-up

After the first consultation, patients should be reviewed at short intervals (1–4 weeks) until secondary causes are excluded. Mild/moderate disease can be reviewed at longer intervals (1–6 months) to give a chance for treatment to become effective; or be reviewed only in winter when symptoms occur. Severe cases tend to have symptoms all year round and may need to be reviewed at shorter intervals with open appointments to attend the clinic if an attack fails to resolve quickly.

Post-operative follow-up

This is usually confined to reviewing the results of lower limb sympathectomy and/or amputations of digits. For amputations, wound healing can be prolonged and the normal signs of wound infection may not be present. Treat early with antibiotics based on culture and sensitivities.

Disorders of the venous system

By far the commonest venous disorder presenting to the vascular clinic is primary varicose veins. However, certain vascular malformations may present with dilated veins in the leg, e.g. arteriovenous fistulas or venous malformations. The Klippel-Trenaunay syndrome presents with a dilated varicose vein running down the outside of the leg, but is associated with hypoplasia of the deep veins. Dilated superficial veins may be secondary collateral veins in the presence of damaged, occluded or absent deep veins.

Chronic superficial and/or deep venous incompetence may present as varicose veins, leg swelling or venous eczema/ulceration.

Primary varicose veins

Varicose veins are dilated superficial veins in the leg caused by incompetent valves allowing high-pressure blood to reflux from the deep veins into the superficial veins. In the long term (years) this may lead to venous stasis, ankle oedema, lipodermatosclerosis and eventually ulceration. Most varicose veins referred to the vascular clinic consist of primary varicose veins affecting the long or short saphenous systems. However, up to 20% of patients present with recurrent varicose veins arising from previous varicose vein treatment. Other patients may present with dilated superficial veins that are not varicose, or they are worried about the cosmetic appearance of thread veins with or without associated varicose veins. Occasionally, visible veins are either normal or caused by some congenital abnormality or underlying pathology for which varicose vein surgery would be inappropriate.

History

Take a general vascular history. Most patients will describe the presence of these veins for several years. In females their appearance may coincide with pregnancy. Exclude previous deep vein thrombosis or conditions that may have led to this, e.g. long bone fractures, prolonged bed rest, plaster of Paris use. Determine the symptoms caused by the veins. Patients may complain of local tenderness in the region of a prominent vein or general symptoms of discomfort, aching or throbbing. There may be a history of acute haemorrhage from a prominent vein or episodes of superficial thrombophlebitis. Alternatively there may be no symptoms and the main concern is cosmetic.

Examination

Examine the patient standing and determine whether the varicose veins affect the long saphenous (medial side of thigh and calf) or short saphenous system (mainly lateral calf and originating from the popliteal fossa – but not all). Determine the site of incompetence using the tourniquet. Occasionally there is a communicating vein between the two systems. Examine for signs of venous stasis: oedema or lipodermatosclerosis spreading from the medial malleolus.

The presence of venous stasis should prompt investigations to exclude deep venous incompetence. Examine for the presence and extent of thread veins. Thrombophlebitis may result in firm, tender cord-like veins caused by thrombosis and fibrosis surrounded by erythema.

Investigations

For straightforward long saphenous varicose veins, no further investigation is necessary prior to treatment. Continuous wave Doppler examination may be helpful in experienced hands, but, where available, colour Duplex ultrasonography is preferable for confirming the site of incompetence, identifying short saphenous reflux and excluding deep venous reflux. Varicography is the more invasive alternative.

Treatment

Conservative treatment consists of compression hosiery (class II compression stockings), but most patients opt for operative therapy unless they are a high operative risk.

Isolated long saphenous vein reflux

This is usually treated operatively with a Trendelenburg tie, stripping of the vein to the knee and lower leg avulsions. In young, fit patients this can be performed as a day-case providing the patient meets the day-case criteria. Newer local anaesthetic techniques include endovenous laser ablation (EVLA) and VNUS® Closure. Ultrasound-guided foam sclerotherapy is an outpatient technique and represents a non-operative alternative.

Isolated short saphenous vein reflux

This is treated by short saphenous ligation in the popliteal fossa. However, the sapheno-popliteal junction is variable and can originate from the mid-posterior thigh. Therefore, pre-operative Duplex marking of the junction is recommended. Combined long and short saphenous vein reflux can be treated during the same operation but requires turning of the patient halfway though the operation. Bilateral long saphenous incompetence can be treated simultaneously but is usually considered inappropriate for day-case surgery.

Co-existing superficial and deep venous reflux

This condition usually precludes superficial surgery. This is because in the presence of deep venous reflux, superficial surgery is ineffective and may impair the venous circulation of the limb. Surgery may be indicated if ambulatory venous pressure measurements indicate that superficial vein occlusion improves venous refilling time or the superficial veins are causing specific symptoms, e.g. bleeding.

Co-existing venous and occlusive arterial disease

The arterial disease is treated first.

Threadveins

Most patients can be treated by sclerotherapy.

Follow-up

Most of these problems are routine and there is no urgency for investigations unless deep-venous thrombosis is suspected.

For those patients who have undergone EVLA, VNUS® or sclerotherapy, late complications include local skin ulceration due to extravasation of sclerosant (slow to heal but no specific treatment). Superficial thrombophlebitis is caused by a clot in the vein due to inadequate compression. The clot can be aspirated under local anaesthetic. If there is an allergic skin rash to the bandage put a cotton stocking under the bandage. Nerve damage is usually transitory. Skin staining mostly fades with time.

Post-operative follow-up

Patients are usually reviewed at 4–6 weeks after operation. Common complications are usually related to the wound. Deep vein thrombosis is no more common than after other operations. Patients may be concerned about prominent residual or 'missed' veins. The best course of action is reassurance and review in 6–12 months time rather than to proceed immediately to further surgery. By that time the residual veins may not be such a concern, or further veins may have become prominent, which would have been missed by immediate re-operation. Repeat the Duplex scan and treat appropriately according to findings. Residual veins not associated with reflux can be treated by avulsions under local anaesthetic or sclerotherapy.

Complications of varicose vein surgery include bruising in the groin or along the track of the treated long saphenous vein. A cord of thrombus may be palpable along the line of the stripped vein. Both will usually resolve.

There may be small areas of skin paraesthesia in relation to the groin wound or avulsion site due to damage to cutaneous nerves. Once again, this should resolve if mild. Saphenous neuritis is caused by damage to the great saphenous nerve. This can cause distressing pain, tingling, and paraesthesia in the distribution of the great saphenous nerve. Referral to the pain clinic may be required in some cases.

Tattooing of the skin can occur if incisions are made through ink marks placed pre-operatively to mark the vein. Plastic surgical referral may be necessary for severe tattooing.

Avulsions at certain sites should be avoided to remove the risk of damage to other structures, e.g. around the neck of the fibula to avoid the common peroneal nerve, the posterior tibial vessels behind the medial malleolus and the sural nerve in the medial line of the posterior calf.

Superficial thrombophlebitis

Thrombophlebitis is inflammation of a vein due to thrombosis. It can occur in normal or varicose veins.

When thrombophlebitis occurs in normal veins it may indicate an underlying condition such as thrombophilia or occult malignancy, and patients should be investigated to exclude these.

When thrombophlebitis occurs in varicose veins it is usually as the result of stasis, but all patients with thrombophlebitis are at increased risk of DVT (25% association) and this should be excluded.

Patients who have thrombophlebitis extending to the saphenofemoral junction may have a tongue of thrombus protruding into the femoral vein and are at risk of pulmonary embolus.

History

Patients complain of tender inflammation over the superficial limb veins. There may be a history of varicose veins and/or DVT. Enquire regarding symptoms of systemic disease. Enquire about a family history of thromboses.

Examination

Perform a general and vascular examination. Examine for the presence of varicose veins and limb swelling. The skin overlying the affected vein is red, inflamed and tender and may appear infected (but is not). The vein may be palpable as a firm thrombosed cord underneath the skin. Determine the extent of the thrombophlebitis.

Investigations

The diagnosis is essentially clinical. Duplex will define the extent of the thrombus and exclude protrusion of the thrombus through the saphenofemoral junction (SFJ) and a DVT.

FBC, PV/ESR and thrombophilia screen are performed to investigate underlying causes.

Depending on the result of the history and examination, appropriate investigations are performed to exclude underlying malignancy.

Treatment

Uncomplicated thrombophlebitis is treated with analgesia, NSAIDs and compression. DVT is treated with anticoagulation. Varicose veins are treated appropriately once inflammation has subsided. Extensive thrombophlebitis extending to the SFJ is treated by immediate ligation of the SFJ and anticoagulation, e.g. low molecular weight heparin or warfarin, is considered. Underlying causes are treated as appropriate. Females with thrombophlebitis should stop the contraceptive pill and be counselled regarding their increased risk of DVT.

Follow-up

If extensive thrombophlebitis or DVT is suspected, admit for further investigation and anticoagulation as an in-patient. Otherwise, review promptly (1–4 weeks) with results of investigations. Refer to relevant speciality if an underlying cause is found. Advise regarding increased risk of DVT.

Post-operative follow-up

As for varicose veins.

Recurrent varicose veins

Approximately 20% of patients presenting to the vascular clinic with varicose veins have had previous treatment and complain that the varicosities have returned.

Usually these patients can be separated into three groups.

- ⟡ Persistent veins: varicose veins that were not adequately removed at the original operation and have never gone away.
- ⟡ New varicose veins: varicose veins developing in a system, e.g. short saphenous vein (SSV) not part of the original operation.
- ⟡ True recurrent varicose veins: varicosities have recurred in the same system that was originally operated on. Recurrence may be due to inadequate saphenofemoral/ saphenopopliteal junction disconnection, a residual untreated mid-thigh perforator vein or new growth of veins reconnecting the saphenofemoral/saphenopopliteal system.

History

Determine the nature of the original surgery. Assess the symptoms caused by the recurrent veins.

Examination

Perform a general examination of the distribution of the varicose veins, including tourniquet tests.

Investigations

Colour Duplex scan to define the source of recurrence and plan surgery.

Treatment

As with primary varicose veins, treatment is either conservative with compression hosiery or active with sclerotherapy or surgery. Reflux arising from a non-operated venous system is treated by the relevant procedure.

Follow-up

Review with the results of investigations and decide on appropriate therapy. There is usually no urgency unless ulceration is present.

Post-operative follow-up

Review to assess the success of surgery and detect any complications of surgery.

Chronic venous insufficiency

Chronic venous insufficiency occurs when the venous return is impaired by reflux, obstruction and calf muscle pump failure. Sustained venous hypertension leads to oedema and leg swelling; eczema, especially around the medial malleolus; lipdermatosclerosis and eventually ulceration. Swelling initially consists of oedema fluid but eventually results in subcutaneous fibrosis and induration.

History

Take a general and vascular history. Previous history of deep vein thrombosis, leg swelling, prolonged immobilisation, plaster of Paris use or long-bone fractures may suggest deep venous incompetence, while the presence of varicose veins, past or present, may suggest a superficial venous cause.

Symptoms associated with chronic venous hypertension include pruritis, aching pain and limb swelling. Occasionally the patient may complain of venous claudication, which consists of a bursting calf pain on walking a certain distance, not relieved purely by rest but also requiring elevation of the limb.

Examination

Perform a general and vascular examination. Examine for the presence of varicose veins, limb swelling, lipodermatosclerosis (LDS), ulceration and co-existent arterial disease.

Investigations

Colour Duplex scanning is useful to identify both superficial and deep venous reflux and may identify scarred, thickened or obstructed deep veins. In the absence of reliable Duplex, ascending venography is useful to identify scarred, thickened or obstructed deep veins, while descending venography is useful to identify deep and superficial reflux. The resting and post-exercise venous pressure and refilling time at the ankle can be measured directly by ambulatory venous pressure measurements. ABPI or arterial Duplex scans are performed to exclude co-existing arterial disease, especially if compression therapy is considered. Compression in the presence of arterial disease can result in critical ischaemia, gangrene and limb loss.

Treatment

Treatment is conservative. Bed rest with the legs elevated reduces the venous pressure at the ankle to 12–15 mmHg and is useful for reducing leg swelling in grossly swollen legs prior to compression therapy.

Graduated compression bandaging (Charing Cross four-layer) generates compression of approximately 40 mmHg at the ankle and 18 mmHg at the knee and is used to heal venous ulcers in the absence of arterial disease.

Compression stockings are used to prevent ulceration in non-ulcerated or healed legs with deep venous incompetence. Class I stockings generate less than 25 mmHg pressure at the ankle; class II generate 25–35 mmHg; class III generate 35–45 mmHg and class IV generate 45–60 mmHg. Below-knee stockings class II are adequate for most patients, but compliance can be a problem due to difficulties putting the stockings on or discomfort in hot weather. Non-compliance is greater for class III–IV and full-leg stockings.

Surgical treatment is indicated for patients with isolated superficial venous incompetence. This is sufficient to heal ulcers with or without compression therapy.

Surgical options for deep venous outflow obstruction include Palma's procedure for iliac vein stenosis/occlusion or thigh vein bypass for thigh vein occlusion. These procedures are rarely performed.

Follow-up

Review with results of investigations and decide on appropriate treatment. Venous ulcers undergoing compression are reviewed (1–3 months) until healing is underway, and the patient can be discharged with advice to progress to compression stockings once the ulcer is completely healed and four-layer bandaging is no longer necessary. Patients prescribed compression stockings may be reviewed once to confirm compliance and improvement in symptoms, then discharged with advice as to lifelong use.

Post-operative follow-up

Review to determine the success of the operation and to detect complications of varicose vein surgery (*see* primary varicose veins section). Patients can be discharged once they are symptom-free and wounds have healed.

Leg ulceration

The commonest cause of leg ulceration is venous disease, and up to a quarter of these patients will have co-existing arterial insufficiency. Approximately 10% of ulcers are due to pure arterial insufficiency. Other causes include diabetes mellitus and rheumatoid arthritis.

⋄ Venous ulceration: the cause of venous ulceration is sustained venous hypertension, which can be due to superficial and/or deep venous incompetence. Venous hypertension causes the typical leathery skin of lipodermatosclerosis around the medial malleolus, which eventually leads to venous ulceration. Venous stasis ulceration can occur in the presence of normal veins, due to the non-function of the calf muscle pump secondary to arthritis of the ankle, or severe arthritis in other lower limb joints limiting mobility and contraction of the calf muscles.

⋄ Arterial ulceration: arterial insufficiency can produce ulceration anywhere on the lower limb. These ulcers usually result from some minor trauma to the skin. Healing skin requires up to 10 times the blood supply of ordinary skin. If the diseased arterial system cannot supply this extra blood the wound never heals and an ulcer develops.

⋄ Neuropathic ulceration usually occurs on the sole of the foot or over pressure points. The absence of sensation means the patient is not aware that something is pressing or rubbing on the foot until an ulcer is produced. This is most commonly seen with diabetic neuropathy.

⋄ Vasculitic ulceration: a vasculitis disease produces small infarctions of the vessels supplying the skin, resulting in areas of the skin dying and producing ulcers. Initially these start as a number of small ulcers with surrounding vasculitic skin changes, but eventually the ulcers may coalesce to form a larger ulcer. There is usually a known vasculitis process, e.g. rheumatoid arthritis.

⋄ Infective ulcers: primary infective ulcers are rare in the UK. More common is secondary infection of existing ulcers.

⋄ Neoplastic ulcers: primary skin cancers forming ulcers on the leg are uncommon. However, long-standing ulcers from other causes may turn malignant (Marjolin's ulcer).

⋄ Mixed pathology: often ulceration may have more than one cause and all underlying causes need to be addressed, e.g. mixed arterial and venous ulcers.

History

Take a general and vascular history. A history of claudication or rest pain suggests an arterial cause. Note any risk factors for venous disease, as outlined for chronic venous insufficiency.

Symptoms associated with chronic venous hypertension include pruritis, aching pain and limb swelling. Occasionally the patient may complain of venous claudication, which consists of a bursting calf pain on walking a certain distance, that is not relieved purely by rest but also requires elevation of the limb.

Ulcers occurring over the pressure points of the foot in diabetics or patients with other neurological conditions suggest a neuropathic cause, but there may also be co-existing arterial or venous disease. History of a skin rash progressing to multiple small ulcers suggests a vasculitic cause. Ulcers presenting for several years that start to deteriorate may indicate neoplastic change.

Examination

Perform a general and vascular examination. Varicose veins and absent pulses are noted. An ulcer occurring in an area of lipodermatosclerosis, with or without visible varicose veins or leg swelling, suggests a venous cause. Examine the distribution of any visible veins. A pale ulcer in a leg with no pulses suggests an ischaemic cause. Ulcers occurring on the sole of the foot or over the pressure points suggest a neuropathic cause. An ulcer with a raised exophytic edge suggests possible malignant change. Arthritis limiting movement of the ankle joint may be associated with venous stasis ulcers.

Investigations

Do a general atherosclerosis screen, FBC, U&Es, immunology and plasma viscosity. Obtain Duplex USS of the superficial and deep venous systems of the leg and ABPI of the ankle arteries with arterial Duplex scan or arteriography if abnormal. X-rays of ulcers occurring over bones and joints are performed to exclude underlying osteomyelitis. Microbiological swabs are taken of ulcers thought to be infected. A bluish-green discharge suggests possible *Pseudomonas aeruginosa* infection. Potentially malignant or vasculitic ulcers undergo biopsy for histology.

Treatment

Treatment consists of treatment of the ulcer and treatment of the underlying cause. Generally ulcers are treated with non-adherent dressings while the underlying cause is corrected. Infected ulcers with spreading cellulitis are treated with systemic antibiotics (flucloxacillin, cefuroxime) guided by the results of microbiological assessment. Infected ulcers not associated with spreading cellulitis can be treated with topical antibiotics or activated charcoal dressings, but their use may be associated with allergic skin reactions. *Pseudomonas* infection responds to silver sulphadiazine cream or combined activated charcoal and silver sulphadiazine preparations applied daily for 1–2 weeks. Ulcers are then re-swabbed.

Chronic ulcers

Chronic ulcers covered in adherent slough or eschar should be surgically debrided back to bleeding tissue to speed healing. Generally, topical desloughing agents are slow and inefficient.

Venous ulcers

Varicose veins in the presence of competent deep veins are treated by standard varicose vein surgery. If superficial venous incompetence co-exists with deep venous incompetence, superficial vein surgery is unlikely to improve the situation. Ulcers associated with deep venous incompetence in the absence of arterial disease are treated by compression bandaging (Charing Cross four-layer). Compression bandaging is changed at twice-weekly to weekly intervals or when there is strike-through. Copious exudate not controlled by this regime may require admission for bed rest and leg elevation. Valvuloplasty, or valve transposition for deep venous incompetence, are still experimental procedures.

Patients with venous stasis ulcers with normal veins but arthritis of the ankle limiting function of the calf muscle pump are referred to the physiotherapy department to try to improve mobility at this joint.

Venous outflow obstruction

Surgical options include Palma's procedure for iliac vein stenosis/occlusion or thigh vein bypass for thigh vein occlusion – rarely performed procedures.

Arterial ulcers

These ulcers will not improve unless the blood supply to the limb is improved. This is achieved by either angioplasty or vascular bypass surgery.

Mixed arterial-venous ulcers

Correct the arterial problem first. Once normal ankle pressures are restored, venous surgery can be performed, or use three-layer compression bandaging under close surveillance to detect an ischaemia.

Neuropathic ulcers

There is usually joint management with diabetologists, who arrange pressure-relieving footwear and so on. Arterial insufficiency can co-exist with neuropathic ulceration and should be corrected if this might impair ulcer healing.

Skin grafting: split skin or full-thickness pinch grafts can be used to speed up ulcer healing, but they are most successful if venous reflux has been corrected and there is no infection.

Follow-up

Infected ulcers are reviewed at regular intervals (1–4 weeks) until the infection is under control. Occasionally admission for intravenous antibiotics is required.

Chronic venous ulceration is reviewed at longer intervals (1–3 months) until healing is well established. Patients can then be discharged with an open appointment when complete healing is anticipated. Patients are prescribed two pairs of compression stockings to wear every day to prevent ulcer recurrence once healing is achieved. Patients are instructed in the correct fitting of compression stockings. Usually class II stockings are preferred, but if these are too tight or difficult for an old person to put on, class I are acceptable.

Neuropathic ulcers are generally followed up in the diabetic foot clinic.

Post-operative follow-up

Arterial ulcers are reviewed at regular intervals (2–6 weeks) after any procedure to improve the blood supply, until healing is established. Deterioration in the ulcer after a period of healing may indicate the artery has re-occluded and this should be investigated.

Venous ulcers treated by surgery should heal within 1–6 months if surgery has been effective, irrespective of whether compression bandaging is also employed. Failure to improve after this time should prompt investigation with a Duplex ultrasound scan to confirm adequate surgery. Further surgery is performed if indicated.

The swollen limb

This most commonly refers to lower limb swelling, although upper limb swelling also occurs. The cause of swelling is generally due to tumour, overgrowth of normal tissue or oedema. The aetiology of the swollen limb can be classified according to whether one or both legs are swollen; and whether the onset is acute or chronic, primary or secondary.

The rarer causes develop in childhood and include congenital conditions such as primary lymphoedema, gigantism and arteriovenous fistulae.

In adulthood the general causes of bilateral limb swelling include heart failure, liver failure, renal failure, hypoproteinaemia, fluid overload, myxoedema and lymphoedema.

Sudden-onset single limb swelling may be due to trauma, deep vein thrombosis, cellulitis, allergy or rheumatoid.

Chronic limb swelling in the adult may be venous: varicose veins; deep venous incompetence; intrinsic and extrinsic obstruction to venous return, e.g. pregnancy, pelvic tumours; inferior vena cava (IVC) obstruction; and postphlebitic limb. Other causes include aortocaval fistula, popliteal or femoral aneurysm, lymphoedema, vascular malformations, paralysis – failure of calf muscle pump, and chronic dependency of the limb due to immobility.

Acquired secondary causes include filiariasis, malignant involvement, surgical block dissection, radiotherapy, trauma, cellulitis, chronic inflammatory eczema and rheumatoid arthritis.

History

Take a general and vascular history. The onset of the swelling is important. Swelling present from birth, even though it is now getting worse, suggests one of the congenital causes. Sudden-onset, single limb swelling suggests one of the acute causes or lymphoedema. Bilateral swelling may indicate a general cause or lymphoedema.

Take a venous history regarding previous venous pathology. Assess the patient's mobility – one of the commonest causes of limb swelling in the elderly is chronic immobility, sitting in a chair all day with dependent legs. Enquire about periods of infection or cellulitis, previous malignancy and radiotherapy.

Examination

Perform a general and vascular examination. Is one leg affected or both? In younger patients look for skin staining or soft tissue or bony overgrowth, which may suggest a vascular malformation or tumour. Examine for dilated veins and determine their pattern. Examine for the typical lipodermatosclerosis of chronic venous insufficiency. Lymphoedema starts with toes and makes them square – inability to pinch a fold of skin at the base of the second toe is known as Stemmer's sign. It then spreads up the legs and can produce huge limbs. Chronic lymphoedematous limbs display the typical furry lichenification. Assess the mobility of the patient. Examine for the signs of a DVT or cellulitis.

Investigation

History and examination should indicate the affected system. Investigations are then directed to confirming the diagnosis. Duplex ultrasound is the standard investigation of most venous causes, although venography may be helpful. Duplex can also identify the typical 'honeycomb' appearance in the subcutaneous tissues of lymphoedema. Lymphangiography may be used to demonstrate hypoplasia or blockage of more proximal lymphatics. Ultrasound is also useful to identify or exclude pelvic masses, although CT/MRI is more specific.

Treatment

Treatment is appropriate for the underlying cause. The management of chronic lymphoedema consists of specialised massage and compression bandaging techniques. Class I or II compression hosiery can be used to keep swelling under control once arterial disease has been excluded. Repeated episodes of cellulitis progressively destroy more lymphatic channels, so long-term flucloxacillin is indicated to reduce infective episodes. Tissue reduction and mesenteric bridge operations for lymphoedema are specialised operations (*see* lymphoedema section).

Follow-up

Review with results of investigations and assess the effect of treatment. Acute cases may require hospital admission for investigation. More chronic cases can be reviewed at longer intervals (1–3 months). Once the condition has stabilised patients can be discharged or given an open appointment to return if deterioration occurs.

Lymphoedema

The primary causes of lymphoedema may be familial or non-familial and present at different ages. Lymphoedema congenita occurs before one year of age (Milroy's); praecox occurs before 35 years; tarda occurs in those older than 35.

Secondary lymphoedema occurs due to a blockage of primarily normal lymphatics by malignant disease, surgery, radiotherapy, and infection (parasitic, pyogenic – beta haemolytic *Streptococcus*, *Staphylococcus aureus*, TB).

Lymphoedema can also be classified according to the mechanism of lymphoedema as follows.

✧ Obliterative: the lymphatics are progressively obliterated from distal to proximal. Represents 80% of lymphoedema cases, predominantly affects females.
✧ Proximal obstructive: lymphatic obstruction is caused by disease in the abdominal, pelvic or inguinal lymph nodes. Usually unilateral.
✧ Lymphatic valvular incompetence and hyperplasia: the lymphatic equivalent of varicose veins.

History

The history is one of slow progressive swelling of the limb or limbs, starting at the toes and spreading proximally. There may be an episode of trauma or infection that precipitates the swelling, which persists despite healing of the original condition. Decrease in swelling overnight suggests a reversible cause. Enquire about possible secondary causes. Enquire about recurrent episodes of cellulitis.

Examination

Lymphoedema swelling tends to be uniform, non-inflamed and non-pigmented, and it pits on pressure in the early stages. The toes are affected early and become square. Later there may be hyperkeratosis of the toes and skin fissuring secondary to fungal infection. Chylous vesicles may appear on the pretibial area, but ulceration in pure lymphoedema is rare. Examine for evidence of secondary causes and chest, abdominal and pelvic pathology.

Investigation

The diagnosis of lymphoedema is mainly clinical. Colour Duplex is often performed to exclude venous disorders. The diagnosis can be confirmed and the type of lymphoedema classified using isotope or contrast lymphangiography. CT/MRI scan can be used to exclude pelvic and abdominal disease and can also demonstrate the typical honeycomb appearance of the lymphatic tissue in the tissues of the affected limb.

Treatment

The aims of treatment are to decrease limb swelling and weight, decrease the risk of infection and improve function. Lymphoedema can be reduced by regular massage (manual lymphatic drainage – MLD), compression bandaging, exercise and breathing exercises. Diuretics are useful as a short-term treatment only. Improvement in leg swelling can be maintained by compression stockings, but note that lymphoedema compression stockings are different to venous compression stockings. Recurrent episodes of cellulitis are treated by long-term prophylactic flucloxacillin to prevent further damage to lymphatic channels. Secondary fungal infections are treated with diethylcarbamazine. The legs are washed daily and the feet protected with well-fitting, comfortable shoes.

Indications for surgical therapy include gross lymphoedema, inability to walk or work, lymphorrhagia and recurrent lymphangitis. Generally, debulking operations are indicated for obliterative causes and bypass procedures for proximal obstruction. These procedures are rarely performed these days and the mainstay of therapy is MLD.

Follow-up

Follow up at regular intervals to review the results of investigations, monitor the effectiveness of treatment and detect complications. Once a long-term management plan has been instituted and is controlling symptoms the patient can be discharged with advice to return if deterioration occurs.

Post-operative follow-up

Review to determine the success of the procedure and to detect complications.

The diabetic foot

The feet of diabetic patients are prone to the development of infection, ulceration and gangrene due to a combination of neuropathy, peripheral arterial disease and arthropathy. Sensory neuropathy reduces the sensation of the feet and makes then more prone to minor injury, which leads to the development of ulcers. Autonomic neuropathy leads to dry skin, prone to injury. Motor neuropathy leads to muscle imbalance and increased shear stresses on the skin, which can also cause ulceration. This also leads to joint and gait abnormalities, which increase shear stress on the skin and decrease the efficiency of the ankle joint and the calf muscle pump, decreasing the efficiency of the venous circulation in the leg, which also predisposes the limb to ulceration. Peripheral arterial disease renders the tissues more prone to ulceration, and once ulceration has occurred healing is delayed or prevented until the blood supply to the area can be improved.

Assessment of diabetic foot problems requires a multidisciplinary approach involving a diabetologist, vascular surgeon, orthopaedic surgeon, orthoptist and chiropodist.

History

Take a general and vascular history. Assess the diabetic control. Assess the neurological system – symptoms of central neuropathy include fainting spells, dizziness, nausea, vomiting of retained foods and impotence. Symptoms of peripheral neuropathy include motor weakness, dry feet, numbness or loss of sensation in the feet, hyperaesthesia (burning feet) or pain in the legs. Vascular symptoms include claudication, although rest pain or ulceration may be the first symptom in diabetics. Ask about previous ulcers and healing. Ask about other vascular causes of ulceration, e.g. venous incompetence.

Examination

Perform a general examination. Assess the characteristics of the ulcer. Assess the neurological, vascular and orthopaedic systems.

✧   The ulcer: site, size, character, neuropathic. Vascular or mixed, simple or complicated.

❖ Neuropathy: usually a glove and stocking pattern. Examine the lower limb for decreased sensation to light touch (cotton wool), sharp and blunt, vibration (tuning fork on the big toe or malleoli), temperature (coldness of tuning fork on the skin).

❖ Vascular: perform a general vascular examination.

❖ Orthopaedic: observe the patient walking for abnormalities of gait. Examine the foot for evidence of muscle imbalance, e.g. pes cavus, hallux valgus. Examine the joints of the lower limb for swelling, tenderness, range of movement, crepitus.

Investigations

Carry out more quantitative tests for neuropathy: nerve conduction studies, thesiometer, Semmes-Weinstein fibres. Arterial ABPI are performed. If the arteries are incompressible ABPI is unreliable, although arterial stenoses may be suspected from the detection of abnormal waveforms. Toe-pressures and/or the toe-pole test are alternative tests. Arterial colour Duplex scans are required and/or angiography with magnified foot views. Take X-rays of joints and bones underlying ulcers for evidence of osteomyelitis. Make tests of diabetic control. Venous Duplex if indicated. Microbiology swabs of ulcers. Take biopsy if long-standing, to exclude Marjolin's or vasculitis.

Treatment

Treat complicated ulcers with antibiotics; clean the ulcer; advise bed rest and limb elevation; and perform debridement.

For simple ulcers, if predominantly neuropathic, advise bed rest, remove callus around ulcer, use total contact plaster, moulded insoles and surgical shoes, silicon implants.

Diabetic arthropathy is similar to Charcot's. It needs correct footwear and surgery to stabilise the foot.

For neuropathy, improve diabetic control. Advise bed rest, remove callus around ulcer, use total contact plaster, moulded insoles and surgical shoes, silicon implants.

Vascular ulcers may need angioplasty or bypass, including popliteal-pedal bypass, or amputations.

Follow-up

Multidisciplinary diabetic foot clinic to assess results of investigations and monitor the effect of treatment.

Post-operative follow-up

Standard vascular follow-up, depending on procedure performed.

Vascular lesions of the upper limb

The same arterial, venous and lymphatic pathologies can occur in the upper limb as in the lower limb. However, the frequency and pattern of disease tends to be different. Also, the anatomy of how blood vessels leave the chest and how nerves leave the neck to pass over the first rib and under the clavicle to enter the arm plays an important role in the development of pathology in this region – the thoracic outlet syndrome.

Atherosclerosis is less common in the vessels of the arm, but when it does occur it tends to affect the aortic arch and the brachiocephalic and subclavian arteries proximal to the origin of the vertebral artery. Because of the origin of the vertebral artery, stenotic or embolic disease of the brachiocephalic and subclavian arteries may present with symptoms of vertebrobasilar ischaemia (VBI) rather than arm ischaemia.

Venous thrombosis and obstruction can occur as a result of thoracic outlet obstruction and present with a swollen cyanotic arm, but this is uncommon. Iatrogenic causes are much more common, such as subclavian vein cannulation. Lymphoedema and other causes of a swollen arm can occur and the underlying pathologies are similar to the lower limb.

Arterial lesions of the upper limb

Atherosclerosis occurs less frequently in the arm than in the leg, but is still the commonest cause of ischaemia, though not the commonest cause of ischaemic-like symptoms (*see* thoracic outlet compression syndrome (TOCS)).

Atherosclerosis affects the aortic arch and the brachiocephalic and subclavian artery proximal to the origin of the vertebral artery, and it may give rise to ischaemic and embolic symptoms in the arm. The source of emboli to the upper limb may be the arterial lesions, but is more commonly the heart, originating from atrial fibrillation or mural thrombus associated with myocardial infarction. Emboli can present with an acutely ischaemic arm, or chronic microembolisation may present to the outpatients with a Raynaud's-type picture affecting the one hand. Untreated, this may eventually lead to occlusion of the radial and ulnar arteries. Emboli originating from the subclavian and brachiocephalic arteries may also cause vertebrobasilar transient ischaemic attacks (TIA).

Occlusions of the proximal subclavian artery may also cause haemodynamic vertebro-basilar symptoms – the subclavian steal syndrome.

Non-atherosclerotic disorders of the arteries of the arm include Takayasu's and giant cell arteritis and Buergers. Irradiation of the chest and/or axilla for malignancy, e.g. breast cancer, may result in long strictures of the subclavian, axillary and brachial arteries.

Localised arterial lesions distal to the origin of the vertebral artery are most commonly due to compression resulting from TOCS. This may result in occlusion of the subclavian artery causing chronic arm ischaemia or in aneurysm formation causing neurogenic compression and distal embolisation.

History

Take a general and vascular history. History of general atherosclerosis affecting the heart and the lower limbs suggests atherosclerosis as the cause of the arm symptoms. A history of cardiac arrhythmias or recent myocardial infarct may suggest a cardiac source of emboli. Patients may present with symptoms related to the arm, but also enquire about vertebrobasilar symptoms.

- Arm symptoms include forearm fatigue, cold hand, rest pain in the hand and history of embolisation: episodes of a pale, cold, painful, weak hand. Symptoms may be similar to Raynaud's but are unilateral. Symptoms may be constant, with pain, paraesthesia, weakness and coldness, or intermittent with claudication, swelling and colour change.
- Vertebrobasilar symptoms (TIAs): isolated symptoms are of limited significance. At least three or more of the following symptoms are required for a diagnosis of VBI: unilateral or bilateral simultaneous motor/sensory deficits, ataxia, diplopia, dysarthria, dysphagia, bilateral homonymous hemianopia, vertigo, tinnitus, transient global amnesia. Drop attacks or loss of consciousness may be the result of embolisation, or if they coincide with vigorous use of the arm, may represent the subclavian steal syndrome.

Examination

Perform a general cardiovascular examination. Examine the hands for evidence of ischaemia and embolisation, e.g. splinter haemorrhages, skin infarcts. Examine for muscle wasting. Note the rate and rhythm of the pulse. Examine for radial-radial delay. Palpate all the pulses and listen for bruits. Examine the supraclavicular fossae for the presence of cervical ribs or subclavian aneurysms. Perform Roos' test. Perform a neurological examination of the arms. Perform a musculoskeletal examination of the neck and shoulder. Perform Tinel's and Phalen's test for carpal tunnel syndrome.

Investigations

Compare the blood pressure in both arms using the Doppler. Repeat the measurements with the cuff at the upper arm, upper forearm and lower forearm to detect segmental occlusions of the brachial and forearm arteries. A pressure drop greater than 15 mmHg is significant, but it may require exercise to produce it. Listen with the Doppler over the thenar and hypothenar eminences for arterial signals from the plantar arch.

Take colour Duplex of the subclavian, axillary and brachial arteries in different positions to detect stenoses, occlusions, aneurysms or compression. If vertebrobasilar symptoms are present this should be combined with insonation of the carotid and vertebral arteries. Visualisation of the brachiocephalic and proximal subclavian arteries is difficult with colour Duplex, but disease in these segments may be associated with damped waveforms more distally. Arch aortogram and selective brachiocephalic/subclavian angiogram is necessary to define the lesions and determine the distal run-off vessels.

CXR, cervical spine and thoracic inlet views are required if thoracic outlet syndrome is suspected, and these will define bony lesions, e.g. cervical ribs. MRI scan may detect fibrous bands.

If a cardiac source of emboli is suspected, ECG and cardiac enzymes can be performed. An echocardiogram may be indicated on the advice of a cardiologist.

If an arterial and cardiac lesion is excluded, suspect neurogenic TOCS and investigate as appropriate (*see* TOCS section).

Treatment

Embolisation to the arm or vertebrobasilar circulation is treated with aspirin initially and anticoagulation if this fails to control the symptoms.

Stenoses of the brachiocephalic and subclavian arteries can be treated with angioplasty alone or combined with stenting. This treatment is also suitable for stenoses secondary to arteritis or irradiation.

Lesions unable to be treated endovascularly may be considered for surgical repair. Surgery consists of thoracic and extrathoracic procedures. Extrathoracic procedures tend to be preferred because they are less invasive, e.g. subclavian-carotid transposition, carotid-subclavian bypass, axillo-axillary bypass.

Disease distal to the vertebral origin requires vein bypass. Severe multi-segment disease responds poorly to bypass and may respond better to upper thoracic sympathectomy or intermittent prostocyclin infusions.

Subclavian artery stenosis, occlusion or aneurysm associated with thoracic outlet syndrome requires resection of the constricting rib or band and repair or bypass of the arterial defect.

Follow-up

If embolisation is suspected, admit the patient for in-patient investigation or start antiembolic therapy and review at short intervals (1–3 weeks) with the results of investigations until the source is identified or serious causes excluded and symptoms controlled. Similarly, severe symptoms of ischaemia should be promptly investigated until an arterial lesion has been excluded or confirmed.

Post-operative follow-up

Review after operation or endovascular treatment to determine the success of the procedure. Detect any residual neurogenic symptoms and treat as appropriate.

Thoracic outlet compression syndrome (TOCS)

The arteries, veins and nerves of the upper limb pass through a narrow space over the first rib, between the sternomastoid and scalene muscles and under the clavicle to supply the arm. In some patients this space is very narrow and these structures can be compressed, resulting in the symptoms and signs of the TOCS.

In most patients (95%), symptoms are caused by compression of the nerves of the upper or lower brachial plexus. In 5% of patients the subclavian artery and/or vein is compressed. However, lesions of the subclavian artery may be limb threatening and should be excluded in every case.

The causes of TOCS include cervical ribs, abnormal scaleneus anterior or medius muscles, fibromuscular bands, abnormal first rib, callus or exostoses from the clavicle or first rib, and neoplasms near the thoracic outlet.

Conditions that may cause similar symptoms in the arm and need to be excluded include cervical spondylosis, cervical disc herniation, cervical spinal cord and plexus lesions, shoulder joint and capsule abnormalities, ulnar nerve compression at the elbow, median nerve compression (carpal tunnel syndrome), multiple sclerosis, motor neurone disease and cardiac angina.

History

Most patients describe symptoms of pain, paraesthesia, weakness, coldness, numbness, claudication, swelling or colour change. Symptoms may have occurred spontaneously or have been precipitated by trauma or physical overactivity, e.g. painting the ceiling. Symptoms may be worse during physical activity of the arm, e.g. carrying the shopping, or occur when the arms are elevated, e.g. hanging out the washing. Symptoms may become constant in long-standing cases.

- ✧ Upper plexus symptoms (C5, 6, 7) are suggested by pain in the neck, shoulder-tip, upper chest, supra-scapular area, outside of upper arm, volar surface of thumb and index finger.
- ✧ Lower plexus symptoms (C8, T1) are suggested by pain in the back of the neck and adjacent scapular area, axilla, medial side of arm, ring and little fingers.

Colour change, numbness and paraesthesia can simulate Raynaud's but represent chronic microembolisation from an arterial lesion. Other arterial symptoms include arm claudication, arm fatigue and weakness with exercise.

Venous symptoms include limb swelling and cyanotic colour change, heaviness accentuated by exercise and relieved by rest. Elevation of the arm may aggravate the symptoms by increasing the compression of the subclavian vein at the thoracic outlet.

Ulnar nerve compression at the elbow produces symptoms in the ulnar nerve distribution distal to this point. Median nerve compression at the wrist, which is called carpal tunnel syndrome, affects the median nerve in the hand only.

Lateral cervical disc prolapse tends to press on one nerve root, causing burning pain in the relevant dermatome and muscle weakness and decreased reflexes in the relevant myotome. Simultaneous pressure on half the spinal cord may cause Brown-Séquard syndrome.

Intraforaminal osteophytes occurring with cervical spondylosis can effect and cause symptoms in several nerve roots without an associated Brown-Séquard syndrome.

Examination

Examine the hands for evidence of ischaemia and embolisation, e.g. splinter haemorrhages, skin infarcts. Note the rate and rhythm of the pulse. Examine for radial-radial delay. Palpate all the pulses and listen for bruits. Examine the supraclavicular fossae for the presence of cervical ribs or subclavian aneurysms. Examine for arterial lesions as described above.

Examine for muscle wasting of the arm and hand and perform a neurological examination. Examine for muscle tone and motor weakness, reflexes and loss of sensation to pin prick and light touch. Perform Tinel's and Phalen's test for carpal tunnel syndrome.

Perform Roos' test. The arms are raised to the level of the shoulders, 90 degrees abducted, and externally rotated – like a soldier surrendering. The hands are then repeatedly clenched and unclenched for 1–2 minutes. Patients with TOCS can seldom complete more than 30–40 seconds before pain forces them to stop. The hand may also go pale and become hyperaemic when the position is released.

Perform a musculoskeletal examination of the neck and shoulder. Palpate for tenderness and restricted movement, which may indicate cervical spondylosis, disc prolapse or shoulder joint lesions, e.g. rotator cuff injuries.

A cyanotic, swollen arm with prominent venous collaterals suggests venous TOCS.

Investigations

Investigate arterial lesions as described above. Usually colour Duplex scan is sufficient to investigate both arterial and venous TOCS; however, arteriograms and venograms may be necessary.

CXR, cervical spine and thoracic inlet views are required if thoracic outlet syndrome is suspected, and these will define bony lesions, e.g. cervical ribs. MRI scan may detect fibrous bands.

Nerve conduction studies, electromyography and other neurophysiological tests are often normal in TOCS, but are useful to exclude other neurological causes, e.g. spinal cord lesions, ulnar and median nerve lesions.

Ultimately the diagnosis of neurogenic TOCS is clinical, after exclusion of other pathologies by the investigations described.

Treatment

In the absence of arterial and venous lesions the initial management of neurogenic TOCS is conservative, with analgesia, NSAIDs and physiotherapy to strengthen the neck and shoulder girdle.

Embolic symptoms are treated with aspirin or anticoagulation initially, or with treatment of the embolic source.

Surgery is reserved for cases where conservative measures have failed to relieve symptoms, there is impaired function of the limb or there are associated arterial or venous lesions.

- ✧ The transaxillary approach is used if lower brachial plexus symptoms predominate, for resection of the first rib and if there is no cervical rib or arterial or venous compression.
- ✧ The supraclavicular approach is used for excision of a cervical rib. It is used if upper brachial plexus symptoms predominate; if there are lesions of the subclavian artery or vein which need correction; or if fibrous bands or scalene muscle requires division. If the first rib requires resection then a second infraclavicular incision is required to access the anterior part of the rib.

Follow-up

The presence of arterial or venous lesions requires review at short intervals (1–4 weeks) until the lesion is defined and the symptoms are stabilised. Neurogenic TOCS can be reviewed at longer intervals (1–6 months) with the results of investigations and to assess the effect of physiotherapy.

Post-operative follow-up

Patients are reviewed to assess the success of the procedure and to detect complications. Initial complications include traction injuries to the brachial plexus or phrenic and long thoracic nerves, and these will resolve within six months. Injuries may also occur to the subclavian vessels and the thoracic duct.

Twenty per cent of patients develop recurrent TOCS within 18 months of the original procedure. If severe, re-operation is required, performing whichever procedure was not performed at the first operation, consistent with symptoms and physical signs.

Renal artery stenosis

Renal artery stenosis (RAS) is a potentially curable cause of hypertension and deteriorating renal function. There are two main disease processes: atherosclerosis and fibromuscular dysplasia (FMD). Other less common causes include Takayasu's arteritis, renal artery aneurysm, arteriovenous malformation, neurofibromatosis and Marfan's syndrome. Atherosclerosis tends to be associated with an atherosclerotic aorta and effects mainly the ostia of the renal arteries. FMD is more common in women and affects the more distal renal artery and its branches. FMD is a particularly common cause of renovascular hypertension in children.

History

Patients may be referred with hypertension that is difficult to control, often requiring 3–4 antihypertensive agents. There may be episodes of flash pulmonary oedema, or they are referred because of deteriorating renal function, especially after starting an ACE inhibitor. In renal artery stenosis, contraction of the efferent glomerular arteriole is a protective mechanism maintaining glomerular filtration. ACE inhibitors prevent this and renal function deteriorates.

Examination

Perform a general and vascular examination. Measure the blood pressure. Evidence of general atherosclerosis suggests this as the cause of renal artery stenosis. There may be absent pulses and audible abdominal and flank bruits.

Investigation

Dipstick urine and perform routine haematology, biochemistry and serum lipids testing. Perform abdominal USS to measure the length of the kidneys – less than 8–9cm indicates an irretrievable loss of renal parenchyma, and correction of the renal artery stenosis is pointless. Duplex of the renal arteries may identify stenoses, but is difficult due to bowel gas.

Captopril renography is performed before and after a dose of ACE inhibitor. The second renogram is worse than the first in the presence of RAS. This is sensitive only for stenoses greater than 50% and does not differentiate between FMD and atherosclerosis.

Contrast arterial angiography is the gold standard, using lateral and oblique views to define the RAS. FMD gives the classical string of beads appearance of alternating stenoses and microaneurysm formation. Angiography also demonstrates ostial disease and atherosclerotic aorta. Ask for lateral views of SMA and coeliac arteries as well, in case extra-anatomical bypass is to be considered. Angiography will also demonstrate renal artery aneurysms.

Treatment

This includes treatment of hypertension, hyperlipidaemia and renal failure.

Angioplasty

Angioplasty is the treatment of choice for FMD. Recurrent and renal artery branch lesions also respond well. Angioplasty is less successful for atherosclerosis, and the main indication is to try and preserve existing renal function. For atherosclerotic RAS causing hypertension, the most suitable cases for angioplasty consist of a unilateral stenosis with a normal contralateral kidney. If hypertension has caused nephrosclerosis in the non-stenosed kidney there will be improvement in the hypertension.

Surgical treatment
Nephrectomy is indicated for a small, scarred kidney producing significant amounts of renin (renal vein renin ratio >1.5) causing hypertension, with a normal kidney on the contralateral side.

Revascularisation
Revascularisation procedures are particularly appropriate where there is co-existing aortic disease or angioplasty has failed and for bilateral RAS caused by atherosclerosis. Surgery is the first-choice option for the solitary failing kidney.

Branch renal artery disease
FMD, renal artery aneurysm, dissection, diffuse atheroma and arteritis usually require removal of the kidney, bench surgery to correct the abnormality and reimplantation (autotransplantation).

Follow-up
Review with results of investigations and decide whether and which intervention is indicated.

Post-operative follow-up
Long-term follow-up is required to detect recurrent disease causing deterioration in renal function or hypertension so that secondary procedures can be instituted. Follow-up may be performed by the relevant physician and referred back when required.

Intestinal ischaemia
Intestinal ischaemia is most commonly encountered as an acute emergency caused by mesenteric artery embolism or thrombosis or by mesenteric venous thrombosis. Both conditions are associated with high mortality despite prompt surgical intervention. In the outpatient clinic, patients may be referred for investigation of symptoms attributed to chronic mesenteric ischaemia.

The blood supply of the intestinal tract is particularly rich in collaterals. Therefore, mesenteric ischaemia only occurs if two out of the three main intestinal arteries are occluded or severely stenosed. Isolated mesenteric artery disease is unlikely to result in mesenteric ischaemia unless previous abdominal surgery has been performed and the collateral pathways have been disrupted. The most important artery for intestinal blood supply is the SMA. Therefore, isolated stenosis of the coeliac or IMA rarely causes intestinal ischaemia.

History
Take a general, gastrointestinal and vascular history. Typically, patients describe a constant history of severe epigastric or periumbilical pain developing 30–45 minutes after food every time they eat. The pain is increasing in severity but the patient may have learned to reduce the pain by eating smaller meals, inducing vomiting before the 30–45 minutes or avoiding eating completely. There is usually a history of severe weight loss. There may be other symptoms of atherosclerosis, e.g. claudication, angina. There may be a history of extensive investigation for gastrointestinal or psychiatric disease.

Examination

Perform a general, gastrointestinal and cardiovascular examination. There may be evidence of severe weight loss and generalised atherosclerosis. Abdominal bruits may be audible.

Investigation

Carry out a routine atherosclerotic screen, haematology, biochemistry including LFTs, and serum lipids. Exclude more common causes of abdominal pain and weight loss, e.g. carcinoma of the tail of the pancreas – CT or MRI scan is recommended if not previously performed.

Duplex ultrasonography may identify mesenteric stenoses but examination is difficult and a negative result does not exclude disease.

Mesenteric angiography with lateral aortic views is the gold standard. This may reveal ostial occlusions, stenoses and disease of the aorta, renal arteries and other branches.

MRI scans and spiral CT angiography may also demonstrate disease.

Treatment

Consider if diagnosis is confirmed. Medical management consists of correction of pain, fluid and electrolyte disturbances and malnourishment. Consider parenteral nutrition until lesions can be treated.

Definitive treatment consists of angioplasty or surgery. Angioplasty of ostial lesions tends to be difficult because of co-existent aortic disease. Complications of angioplasty carry a high mortality and some centres recommend that angioplasty is reserved for patients unfit for surgery.

Surgery is indicated in otherwise fit patients or after failed angioplasty. Procedures consist of transaortic endarterectomy, mesenteric artery bypass or reimplantation of the SMA. Occasionally, a median arcuate band from the crura of the diaphragm compresses the coeliac artery and SMA. Release of this band relieves the stenosis. However, for revascularisation procedures always revascularise the SMA and revascularise more than one mesenteric artery if possible. Prolonged parenteral nutrition may be required in the post-operative period.

Follow-up

Review at short intervals (1–6 weeks) with the results of investigation until cancer is excluded and the mesenteric ischaemia is confirmed or excluded. Institute medical therapy prior to definitive treatment.

Post-operative follow-up

Most patients will spend a long time in hospital after any procedure so the success or otherwise of the procedure will be determined during this period. Long-term follow-up with regular Duplex scans is indicated to detect recurrent disease, for which angiogram and angioplasty may be appropriate. Redo surgery may be indicated for graft occlusion.

Vascular malformations

In contrast to common terminology, 'vascular malformations' refers to arterial and venous abnormalities that have normal endothelial turnover, are present from birth, but may not cause symptoms until later in life. Haemangiomas occur in infants, develop after birth, demonstrate endothelial hyperplasia and tend to resolve spontaneously, although this may not be complete.

Vascular malformations may be classified as high flow lesions or low flow lesions. High flow lesions consist of arteriovenous malformations. Low flow lesions may be capillary, venous, lymphatic or mixed malformations, but there is no arteriovenous shunting.

Acquired arterial and venous abnormalities may result from trauma or iatrogenic procedures. Certain malignant tumours may mimic the features of a vascular malformation and must be excluded. The tumours include angiosarcomas and renal and thyroid metastases.

Objectives

Differentiate vascular malformation from haemangioma; exclude malignant tumour; classify vascular malformation into high flow and low flow; treat lesions conservatively or with intervention.

History

Patients may describe a lesion that has been present from birth but may have become symptomatic or increased in size at puberty, pregnancy or after an episode of trauma. Patients with high flow lesions may complain of pain, excessive sweating over the lesion and even ulceration and bleeding. Extremities may be painful due to ischaemia caused by arteriovenous shunting proximal to their blood supply.

Patients with low flow lesions also complain of pain. For capillary lesions, pain may be a predominant symptom, with little skin staining or swelling evident, though local hyperhidrosis is common. Large venous lesions may cause pain due to engorgement and episodes of spontaneous thrombosis. Pain may be worse after exercise and last for days. Limb soft tissue and skeletal overgrowth is common, as is overlying eczema and ulceration.

Lymphatic lesions are associated with deformity and exudation of fluid and are prone to cellulitis.

For acquired vascular malformations there may be a history of trauma or iatrogenic injury.

Examination

Perform a general and vascular examination. Assess the cardiac status. Note that examination may be normal despite the presence of a significant lesion. A small cutaneous discoloration may indicate a large underlying malformation. If a mass is present, examine it for size, consistency, tenderness and pulsation bruits. Venous lesions tend to be soft and easily compressible with rapid refilling, and they engorge with dependency. Calcified phleboliths may be palpable with the lesions. Lymphatic lesions may transilluminate.

High flow lesions tend to be firm, pulsatile and poorly compressible.

Examine for limb length and soft tissue and skeletal hypertrophy, e.g. the Parkes-Weber limb. Tissue in such a limb does not pit on pressure, tends to be warmer than the contralateral limb and may be associated with a machinery-type murmur. Such a limb may demonstrate Branham's sign – inflation of a tourniquet above arterial pressure proximal to the high flow lesions is associated with slowing of the pulse, indicating a significant arteriovenous shunt.

Traumatic lesions may be associated with scars.

Investigation

Duplex is a useful first-line investigation for differentiating high flow from low flow lesions. MRI scan or spiral CT is then used to define the extent of the lesion and identify any suspicious characteristics. X-rays may be useful to define bony lesions, and biopsy for histology may be required to exclude malignancy.

For those lesions where intervention is considered appropriate, angiography for high flow lesions, or venography for low flow lesions, is useful to delineate the lesions and plan appropriate treatment.

Treatment

Treatment is multidisciplinary, involving a vascular surgeon, vascular radiologist, cardiologist, plastic surgeon, orthopaedic surgeon and sometimes a maxillofacial surgeon. Half of all lesions can be managed satisfactorily with compression hosiery and analgesia as required. In addition, small superficial arteriovenous malformations may be cured by surgical excision. For larger lesions not suitable for conservative treatment because of site or size, or for symptoms not controlled by conservative measures, further intervention consists of embolisation or surgical treatment.

✧ High flow lesions tend to be treated by repeated bouts of arterial or direct puncture embolisation to control symptoms over many years. Those lesions thought to be suitable for surgical excision can be pre-treated with embolisation to decrease intra-operative vascularity and blood loss.

✧ Low flow lesions are treated by direct puncture sclerotherapy under imaging control and either local or general anaesthetic. This tends to control the lesion rather than cure it and may need to be reviewed at regular intervals.

Bony and tissue overgrowth abnormalities are treated by the plastic and orthopaedic surgeons.

Follow-up

Patients are reviewed at short intervals (1–4 weeks) with the results of investigations until malignant tumours are excluded and the extent of the lesions is defined. Patients considered suitable for conservative therapy are reviewed at regular intervals (1–6 months) until the symptoms and condition are stable. They are then discharged or given an open appointment.

Post-operative follow-up

Complications of embolisation include inadvertent embolisation of other arteries, passage of emboli into the venous circulation and the post-embolisation syndrome of pyrexia, leucocytosis and malaise. Most of these complications occur while the patient is an in-patient, but post-embolisation syndrome may last for weeks. Infarction of overlying skin is not uncommon but usually resolves.

Lesions are seldom cured by therapeutic procedures, e.g. embolisation, and need to be repeated if and when the symptoms return as the lesion enlarges again. Therefore, long-term follow-up with repeated Duplex ultrasound to monitor the size of the lesions is advised.

Amputation

Unfortunately, treatment of vascular disease is not always successful or in the patient's best interest. Amputation of a gangrenous, ulcerated or critically ischaemic limb becomes the only way to relieve the patient's symptoms and sometimes to save his or her life. Although the original treatment may not have been successful, it is important to maintain a positive outlook for the overall well-being and to approach each amputation as an interesting challenge.

Goals of surgery

The aim of amputation is to achieve the most distal level consistent with the causal condition and a well-healed non-sensitive stump.

The goals of surgery are: firstly, ablation and secondly, reconstruction.

Many factors have to be taken into account when considering the level of amputation and the procedure to be performed. Is the patient likely to walk with a prosthesis? Can the knee joint be preserved?

Other considerations include the pathology, anatomy of the proposed level of amputation, surgery, prosthesis and personal factors (age, sex, occupation and so on).

Phases

Amputation can be divided into three phases: pre-operative, operative and post-operative.

✧ The pre-operative stage involves counselling, time to accept the decision (*see* breaking bad news), limb fitting service, talking to a prosthetist and a rehabilitation plan.
✧ The operative stage involves antibiotics, DVT prophylaxis, anaesthesia: local anaesthesia (LA) – sciatic, femoral block. Regional – spinal, epidural. GA. Perform the correct procedure with good surgical technique.
✧ The post-operative stage involves pain relief (oedema, infection, DVT, medical problems). Physiotherapy – early mobilisation – between bars, on crutches, pneumatic post-amputation mobility (PPAM) aid after 7–10 days. Children and young adults get immediate post-operative fitting. Exercise for balance, control of prosthesis, strength, donning and doffing, toilet, stairs, home. Removal of sutures at three weeks.

Complications

Complications include non-healing, pain (acute, chronic), phantom limb pain, protrusion of the bone end and inability to mobilise.

Non-healing is the most frustrating and demoralising complication for the patient. Factors affecting healing are:

✧ tissue blood flow – pulses, arteriogram, cellulitis
✧ poor nutritional status
✧ infection, diabetes, medical conditions
✧ suboptimal surgical technique
✧ poor post-operative stump management.

Limb amputation operations

Below knee transtibial amputation

✧ Advantages: preserves knee joint, better mobility.
✧ Disadvantages: non-healing.
✧ Transection level: 12–15cm measured from the joint line, the shortest length to preserve the tibial tubercle.
✧ Techniques: long posterior (Burgess) flap, sagittal – equal medial and lateral, skew flap. All myofasciocutaneous flaps.

Above knee transfemoral

✧ Advantages: healing.
✧ Disadvantages: poor mobilisation.
✧ Transection level: as long as possible.
✧ Techniques: anterior-posterior flaps, long medial-sagittal flaps.

Through knee and Gritti-Stokes amputation

✧ Advantages: long stump, less traumatic, better for bilateral amputations, suitable for hemiparesis with risk of hip and knee contractions.
✧ Disadvantages: non-healing.
✧ Techniques: knee disarticulation – end weight-bearing but bulky stump.

For Gritti-Stokes, remove the end of the femur and articular surface of the patella. The cut surface of the patella is then fixed to the cut surface of the end of the femur. Non-end weight-bearing stump.

Non-union between the patella and the end of the femur is the main problem.

Hip disarticulation, transiliac and sacroiliac amputations are more specialised techniques.

Syme ankle disarticulation

✧ Advantages: stump tolerates end pressure, long lever, ability to walk without prosthesis, good for trauma and congenital deformities.
✧ Disadvantages: non-healing in vascular and diabetic patients, for women it is less cosmetic.
✧ Technique: disarticulate calcaneum and talus and remove end of tibia. Bring up heel skin pad over end of stump.

Partial foot amputations

✧ Distal toe.
✧ Whole toe: racquet incision.
✧ Transmetatarsal: two levels head or base of metatarsal but always through cancellous bone.

Amputations of arm, wrist and fingers are less commonly performed.

Lumps and bumps

Miles Banwell and Michael Irwin

ELEVEN

Skin lesions

The skin consists of epidermis, dermis and adnexal structures, which include hair follicles, sebaceous glands and eccrine and apocrine sweat glands.

Benign and malignant lesions can arise from any of these elements.

Benign lesions of the epidermis
Skin tags (squamous papillomas)
History
Skin tags are common (found in 25% of adults), particularly in obese patients. They begin in the second decade, increasing in frequency up to the fifth decade. The axilla, neck and inguinal regions are most affected. The skin tags can catch on clothing or jewellery.

Examination
The squamous papilloma appears as a small non-inflamed tag of skin. It is skin-coloured, oval and mobile, with no deep fixation or induration of the base. A short broad-to-narrow stalk lengthens and narrows as it grows. It rarely exceeds 1cm diameter.

Investigations
None.

Treatment
Excision biopsy.

Post-operative follow-up
Review with histology and check wound healing.

Common wart
The common wart is caused by the papillomavirus. It may occur anywhere on the body but is commonly found on the hands and feet.

History
Occurs as slow-growing lesions, usually in the second decade of life. Painful if on the soles of the feet (verrucas), or may catch and bleed.

Examination
Appears as exophytic growth or hard, tender, black area on the sole of the foot.

Investigations
None.

Treatment
Cryotherapy, curettage, topical preparations (40% salicylic acid or 5-fluorouracil (5FU)), laser ablation. May regress spontaneously.

Post-treatment follow-up
Rarely indicated.

Seborrhoeic keratosis

This is associated with old age.

History

Painless, pigmented warty plaques that are unsightly and may catch on clothing and bleed.

Examination

Appears as a 'stuck-on' brown warty plaque, often with variegated pigment and truncal predominance. The plaque may grow quite large (to 1–2cm in diameter). Has a greasy texture.

Investigations

None.

Treatment

Treat by curettage or excision. Other modalities include cryotherapy or topical trichloroacetic acid.

Post-treatment follow-up

Review with histology and discharge.

Keratoacanthoma (molluscum sebaceum)

Benign, rapidly growing, self-healing skin tumour. Currently regarded as well-differentiated, low-grade squamous cell carcinoma (SCC) and managed as such.

History

Found from fifth decade onwards, more commonly in males than females (by a 3:1 ratio), and typically on the face or dorsum of the hand. It has a rapid six-week growth phase, then involutes over the next six months. Usually painless, but may catch and bleed.

Examination

Appears as a globular tumour, with keratin plug/horn and radial symmetry.

Investigations

Excision biopsy.

Treatment

Excision. May require reconstruction, depending on size and position.

Post-operative follow-up

Review with histology.

Pre-malignant lesions of the epidermis
Actinic and solar keratosis

These are pre-malignant lesions. They usually occur on skin chronically exposed to sunlight (face and hands). Approximately 5% become squamous cell cancers.

History

Occur from middle age onwards. The patient presents with erythematous macules and papules with coarse adherent whitish scales. They are slow-growing lesions, not usually associated with pain or bleeding.

Examination

The patient has erythematous, rough or scaly macules or papules, which may be ulcerated. Examine lymph node fields.

Investigations

An excision biopsy is often indicated; especially in immunosuppressed (e.g. renal transplant) patients, as these have a higher conversion rate to SCC.

Treatment

Cryotherapy, topical 5FU, excision. Less commonly, topical immune modulator (imiquimod) or photodynamic therapy (PDT) is required.

Post-treatment follow-up

Long-term follow-up is required to detect recurrence or new lesions in the same or other areas.

Bowen's disease (intraepidermal SCC in situ)

The principal aetiology is sun damage. Bowen's disease of glans penis is termed erythroplasia of Queyrat. Bowen's disease of the nipple is associated with underlying ductal carcinoma.

History

Bowen's disease is a slow-growing, red, scaly plaque that may irritate and occasionally bleed.

Examination

Examination shows a well-defined red hyperkeratotic plaque. There is clear potential for invasive transformation. Ulceration suggests invasion.

Investigations

Skin biopsy under local anaesthetic. It is critical to exclude an underlying malignancy (e.g. in the breast).

Treatment

Cryotherapy, 5FU, PDT, excision.

Post-treatment follow-up

No long-term follow-up is required once adequately treated.

Malignant lesions of the epidermis
Basal cell carcinoma (rodent ulcer) (BCC)

This is the most common skin cancer in white races. It is locally invasive, and metastasis is extremely rare.

History

A slow-growing skin lesion that gradually ulcerates and may bleed. It is not painful unless advanced.

Examination

Basal cell carcinomas are usually found on skin chronically exposed to sunlight and in areas rich in pilosebaceous follicles. Hence more than 90% are found on the face. The lesion is characterised by a pinkish colour, pearly edges and telangiectasia. There are many subtypes, which may be broadly grouped as: localised (e.g. nodular/nodulocystic), superficial, or infiltrative (e.g. morphoeic). Superficial BCCs are less easy to diagnose clinically as they may simply present as a persistent erythematous macule. Infiltrative (morphoeic) lesions tend to 'ghost' under the skin.

Investigations
Incision/excision biopsy if the diagnosis is uncertain. Uncommonly, in advanced lesions, morbidity arises from invasion into underlying structures – nares/sinuses/external auditory meatus/orbit/brain – and therefore may require magnetic resonance imaging or computed tomography (MRI/CT). Gorlin's syndrome (autosomal dominant inheritance) comprises lifelong multiple BCCs, palmar pits and jaw cysts.

Treatment
Surgical excision with a 2–3mm margin. A wider margin (5mm) is required if the border is indistinct or for larger lesions. For superficial BCCs, consider dermatology referral for topical 5FU, topical imiquimod or PDT. Recurrent or infiltrative BCCs in anatomically sensitive areas may require Mohs micrographic surgery. Also consider radiotherapy, particularly in elderly patients.

Post-operative follow-up
Review with histology and discharge if excision is complete. Incomplete excision generally requires further excision. Long-term follow-up is required for multiple recurrences or in lesions narrowly excised in anatomical areas at high risk of deeper invasion.

Squamous cell carcinoma (SCC)
This is the second most common skin cancer in white races, yet its incidence is still only one-quarter that of BCC's. Associated factors include exposure to sunlight, Bowen's disease, chronic ulcers and burns (Marjolin's). SCCs are prone to local recurrence (if well differentiated there is a 7% risk, if poorly differentiated there is a 28% risk) and metastases (there are lymph node metastases at presentation in 2–3%). Increased metastatic potential is determined by location (sun exposed, e.g. lip and ear), diameter (greater than 2cm), depth of invasion (greater than 4mm thick), poor differentiation and perineural invasion and host immunosuppression.

Differential diagnosis includes keratoacanthoma, basal cell carcinoma, Bowen's disease, actinic keratosis, malignant melanoma, pyogenic granuloma and traumatised seborrhoeic keratosis. Keratoacanthoma is now regarded as well-differentiated, low-grade SCC.

History
Patients describe a quickly growing lump that ulcerates and bleeds.

Examination
The edge of the ulcer is often raised and everted. Examine for regional lymphadenopathy.

Investigations
Diagnosis is confirmed by biopsy.

Treatment
Wide local excision (5–10mm margin). Carry out therapeutic lymph node dissection if indicated. Treatment should be co-ordinated through the local skin cancer multidisciplinary team (MDT). Radiotherapy may be considered by the MDT if there is a close margin or if the condition is recurrent or inoperable.

Post-operative follow-up

Discuss within the forum of the local MDT. Review with histology to confirm the diagnosis and that there was complete excision. Incomplete excision generally requires further surgery. Long-term follow-up by a plastic surgeon/dermatologist is indicated if high-risk lesions are found, as determined by histological thickness, if they are poorly differentiated or in a difficult anatomic site.

Benign lesions of the dermis
Dermatofibroma (fibrous histiocytoma)
History

This is a usually slow-growing, irritating, brownish nodular lesion. Approximately 20% are preceded by trauma or insect bite.

Examination

Dermatofibroma presents as a well-circumscribed reddish-brown nodule, which is firm to palpation due to abundant fibrous stroma. It usually occurs on the legs, and is typically less than 1cm in diameter.

Treatment

Excision biopsy.

Post-operative follow-up

Review with histology.

Hypertrophic scar

This is an abnormal scar limited by the initial boundary of the incision or wound. Proposed aetiologies include increased wound tension, infection and delayed healing. There is higher risk with an anatomical site (sternum, shoulders, deltoid). Hypertrophic scars often regress spontaneously as they mature.

History

The scar develops within weeks of a wound healing and shows some degree of improvement with time. There is little in the way of familial history.

Examination

It presents as a raised, thickened, pinky-red, often irritating scar confined to an injury site.

Investigations

None.

Treatment

The first treatment is time (expectant). Otherwise, topical silicone gels/silicone sheets or pressure garments (for at least six months). Finally, re-excision should be considered only if the aetiology is clear. There is otherwise a high risk of recurrence. Liaise with plastic surgery.

Keloid scar

This is an abnormal scar that develops months after injury, shows no regression and may get worse between six and twelve months. It is more common in black African races, and it has a familial tendency. Common sites include the face and earlobes (from piercing), as well as those anatomical sites prone to hypertrophic scarring (*see* above). Original wounds are often trivial and not under tension.

History
Exuberant scar formation progressing beyond six months. Itchy, hard and often painful. There may have been a similar reaction in previous wound scars.

Examination
It presents as a heaped-up, exuberant, overgrown scar. It is defined by firm scar tissue that extends beyond the boundaries of the incision or wound. By contrast, a hypertrophic scar does not extend beyond these boundaries.

Investigations
None.

Treatment
These are generally referred to plastic surgeons for management. Intralesional steroid, pressure garments or topical silicone may be indicated. Excision surgery is a last resort and should be performed only in conjunction with other modalities, such as steroid injection, pressure splints or radiotherapy.

Post-treatment follow-up
The response rates for all treatments are variable and follow-up depends on the treatment modality. There is a high chance of recurrence, whichever is chosen.

Malignant lesions of the dermis
Metastatic carcinoma
This is the most common in tumours of the breast, lung and bowel.

History
There are small, hard, painless nodules in the skin, which may or may not be related to the site of a previous tumour or irradiation.

Examination
Small hard nodules are found in an area adjacent to a previous surgical scar or radiotherapy field. If arising in independent areas, exclude undiagnosed underlying primary malignancy.

Investigations
Incision/excision biopsy.

Treatment
Excision, if possible. Defects from larger lesions may require plastic surgical reconstruction. Otherwise, consider adjuvant therapies as appropriate. Ensure adequate ongoing management of primary cancer.

Post-operative follow-up
Confirm diagnosis with histology and arrange appropriate therapy as indicated for primary tumour.

Pigmented skin lesions

Most suspicious pigmented lesions are referred to a dermatology or plastic surgery clinic for excision if malignancy is suspected. However, knowledge of these lesions is necessary for the general surgeon as they may be referred as simple skin lesions for day-case excision without the appreciation that they may be malignant, especially if not pigmented.

Melanocytes are specialised cells located at the basal layer of the epidermis. They synthesise melanin and store it in vesicles called melanosomes. Melanosomes are distributed to surrounding cells. Melanin production is stimulated by sunlight and a pituitary hormone, melanocyte-stimulating hormone (MSH). All races have approximately the same number of melanocytes, but the baseline activity of these cells varies.

Naevus cells are melanocytes that have entered the dermis and have a distinct phenotype. They are more spherical, have fewer dendritic processes and display aggregation in nests.

Benign pigmented lesions

Benign pigmented lesions may be subdivided into those containing melanocytes (melanocytic naevi) and those containing naevus cells (naevocellular naevi).

Melanocytic naevi

- ✧ Simple lentigo is a benign melanocytic naevus of the epidermis characterised by a tan or brown macule with slightly irregular borders.
- ✧ Blue naevus is a benign melanocytic naevus of the dermis. It appears as a round area of blue-black discolouration deeper in the skin.

Naevocellular naevi

- ✧ Benign naevocellular naevi include congenital (giant hairy naevus or non-giant hairy naevus), acquired (junctional, compound, intradermal) or special (spitz, dysplastic, halo) forms.
- ✧ Congenital naevus is histologically similar to a compound naevus, containing junctional and intradermal components. It may be disfiguring, causing great parental anxiety and concern. It appears as dark brown papules of variable size, and can be very large and often hairy (giant hairy naevus). There is 1–2% malignant transformation, mainly within the first five years of life. Sacral lesions are associated with spina bifida or meningocoele. Treatment is by serial excision, also dermabrasion, curettage and laser treatment.
- ✧ Junctional naevus is formed by nests of naevus cells clustered at the epidermal-dermal junction. It is a deeply pigmented macule with a well-defined border. It is often found on the trunk. It typically appears in the first and second decades. It progresses to compound or intradermal naevus with age.
- ✧ Intradermal naevus is formed by nests of naevus cells clustered within the dermis. It appears as a flesh-coloured or light tan dome-shaped papule. It is often found on the face or neck. It typically appears in the second and third decades.
- ✧ Compound naevus contains junctional and intradermal components. It appears as a dark brown papule with well-defined regular borders. It is often found on the trunk. It typically arises up to early adulthood.
- ✧ Dysplastic (atypical) naevus has an irregular outline, variegated pigmentation and a diameter greater than 5mm. It is often multiple (dysplastic naevus syndrome). There is a 5–10% risk of malignant change to superficial spreading melanoma.

Treatment

Excision biopsy if recent changes create suspicion of melanoma (*see* below).

Post-operative follow-up

Follow up with a histology review. For dysplastic naevi, re-excision with wider margins (up to 5mm) may be indicated.

Malignant pigmented lesions

There are a number of pigmented malignant skin lesions (e.g. pigmented BCC). However, by far the most important to exclude is malignant melanoma, due to its high metastatic potential and unpredictability. Absence of pigment does not exclude melanoma. A diagnosis of amelanotic malignant melanoma should always be considered.

Malignant melanoma

Malignant melanoma is a malignant tumour of epidermal melanocytes. There are four main subtypes.

- ✧ Superficial spreading melanoma is the commonest type of melanoma (60%). It has a flat, irregular border, heavy and irregular pigmentation and a raised surface. Ulceration indicates invasion. There is equal incidence in males and females, particularly in sun-exposed areas – backs in men, lower legs in women. Radial growth occurs prior to vertical growth.
- ✧ Nodular melanoma is the second most common melanoma (20%). It has early vertical growth and therefore a poorer prognosis. It is typically uniformly black, but may be amelanotic.
- ✧ Melanoma arising in lentigo maligna accounts for 5–10% of all melanomas. The precursor lesion is lentigo maligna (Hutchinson's freckle), which equates to melanoma in situ (radial growth only), 40% of which will become invasive.
- ✧ Acral lentiginous melanoma accounts for 2–8% of all melanomas in Caucasians, and 40–60% in dark-skinned races. It arises on palms, soles, mucocutaneous junctions and subungually. In subungual melanoma the great toe is the most common location, then the thumb. A biopsy is needed to distinguish it from pigmented naevus of the nail matrix. It is treated by amputation of the affected digit.
- ✧ Secondary melanoma (primary not identified) has a lymph node disease as its main presentation (primary lesion regressed). Non-lymph node metastatic sites include skin, brain, lung, bone, spinal cord and adrenals. Abdominal obstruction or intersusception is a possible presentation of metastasis.

Treatment objectives

These are to exclude melanoma and to stage and treat melanoma in the context of the regional melanoma MDT meeting.

History

Most patients present because they have noticed a new mole or a change in an existing mole. National Institute for Health and Clinical Excellence (NICE) suspected cancer referral guidelines (2005) detail three 'major' suspicious features of a mole: change in size, irregular shape and irregular colour. There are four 'minor' features: largest diameter greater than 6mm, inflammation, oozing and change in sensation. Major features score two points, minor features one point; and a total of three points should trigger referral to the local melanoma service for excision biopsy.

Examination

Examine the lesion for suspicious features (above). Check for satellite nodules, in-transit metastases, palpable regional nodes, lymphoedema and hepatomegaly.

Investigations

All suspicious pigmented lesions, which are not obviously benign on clinical examination, require full thickness excision biopsy for histological confirmation. At this stage ensure a minimal (2mm) margin until the histological diagnosis is certain. A cuff of subdermal fat should be included in the biopsy to allow accurate histological analysis of depth of invasion. Orientate the excision biopsy ellipse on limbs in a longitudinal axis to facilitate future wide local excision. Histological analysis of the depth of invasion provides useful prognostic information. The Breslow thickness (BT) classification measures the depth of invasion from the stratum granulosum of the epidermis to the deepest part of the tumour.

Melanoma staging is based on the tumour, node and metastasis (TNM) system, with modifications from the American Joint Committee on Cancer (2001). Invasion of less than 1.0mm carries a good prognosis. Invasion greater than 2.0mm carries a high risk of metastases. Other histological features associated with poor prognoses include ulceration, mitotic activity, neurovascular invasion and microscopic satellites.

Treatment

Treatment must be in accordance with NICE cancer service guidelines. Early referral to the local melanoma service is mandatory, with referral prior to excision biopsy if there is a high clinical index of suspicion. There must be immediate referral to the regional melanoma MDT following the excision biopsy diagnosis. Subsequent management will include wide local excision down to fascia, with margins determined by BT (1cm if BT less than 1mm, 2cm if BT greater than 1mm). Therapeutic regional lymphadenectomy is undertaken for nodal metastases and local control. Sentinel node biopsy remains controversial and is undertaken only in selected centres in the context of clinical trials. Chemotherapy, radiotherapy and immunotherapy, as guided by the oncologist in the context of clinical trials, should be considered.

Post-operative follow-up

Undertaken by plastic surgery, dermatology and oncology.

Vascular skin lesions
Campbell de Morgan spots (cherry angiomata)

These are small (1–3mm) bright red spots found on sun-exposed skin in older patients. They are an arteriovenous (AV) fistula of a dermal capillary. They are benign and require no treatment.

Pyogenic granuloma

This is a rapid-growing benign vascular nodule, consisting of proliferating capillaries in a loose stroma of connective tissue. Differential diagnosis includes amelanotic melanoma, glomus tumour and Kaposi's sarcoma.

History

There is usually a history of trauma at the site followed by a rapidly growing lesion, which may bleed.

Examination

It presents as a dark red nodule of exuberant granulation tissue which may have ulcerated. Common sites are fingers, upper chest, lip and toes.

Investigations
Excision biopsy to exclude malignancy.

Treatment
The condition often recurs after cautery, as proliferating vessels extend deep into the dermis. Hence, it generally requires excision biopsy.

Post-operative follow-up
Review with histology and discharge.

Port wine stain
Port wine stain is usually present at birth (0.3% of live births). It is classified as a capillary vascular malformation. It appears as a deep reddish-blue discolouration of the skin; mostly on the face (cranial nerve V distribution), rarely on the trunk and extremities. It grows in proportion to the child and persists lifelong. Two-thirds of patients develop hyperplastic skin changes (cobblestoning) by adulthood. The most well-known syndromic association is Sturge-Weber syndrome (ophthalmic CNV1 distribution) characterised by intracranial lesions causing intractable epilepsy. Others include Klippel-Trenauney syndrome (extremity distribution) and Cobb syndrome (truncal distribution). Treatment is by cosmetic camouflage or argon/pulsed-dye laser therapy. However, laser therapy shows no benefit in 20%, and the condition may recur in 50% after four years.

Strawberry naevus
Strawberry naevus is a red, soft, compressible, fleshy lesion arising on the head and neck within or just after the first two weeks of life. It is classified as a capillary haemangioma. It is relatively common. Multiple haemangiomas may be associated with internal hae-mangiomas of major organs. There is a cycle of proliferation (strawberry phase) and involution. Lesions tend to grow for six to eight months and then the majority regress with time. Typically, 50% of lesions will have regressed by age five. Therefore, treatment generally is non-operative and observation only is required. However, urgent treatment is required for periorbital haemangiomas if they are obstructing visual fields (there is a risk of deprivation amblyopia). If they are symptomatic (bleeding) or in an anatomically difficult site, then refer for plastic surgery. Excision, pulsed-dye laser or intralesional steroid injection may all be considered. Regressed lesions may leave a redundant skin fold requiring excision.

Spider naevus (acquired telangiectasia)
This is a small red lesion (angioma) consisting of a central feeding arteriole with radiating capillaries. It blanches on pressure. The presence of up to five is normal. It is common in pregnancy but disappears in puerperium. Large numbers are associated with cirrhosis of the liver. It also occurs in hyperthyroidism, carcinoid, post-irradiation, post-topical steroid use, systemic lupus erythematosus (SLE) scleroderma and dermatomyositis. It may be treated with pulsed-dye laser treatment.

Glomus tumour (angioneuromyoma)
Glomus bodies are small arteriovenous anastomoses involved in thermoregulation. Tumours are associated with nerve and muscle and classically occur in fingers and toes, particularly in the nail bed, where they cause nail ridging. They are dark bluish-red, cold intolerant and exquisitely tender due to association with nerves. Treatment is by surgical excision.

Kaposi's sarcoma

This is a malignant tumour of endothelial cells and perivascular connective tissue cells. It may occur in immunosuppressed patients and is commonly seen in AIDS patients (50%).

History

Patient complains of a slightly tender raised nodule. There may be a history of immunosuppression.

Examination

Examination finds a raised purplish nodule, which may be single or multiple.

Investigations

Excision biopsy.

Treatment

Excision biopsy. Local radiotherapy or cytotoxic therapy may be indicated for multiple lesions. Ensure aetiological factors are investigated and managed (e.g. immunosuppression).

Post-operative follow-up

Refer to the appropriate speciality: dermatology, plastics, or infectious diseases.

Lesions of skin appendages

Epidermoid cyst (sebaceous cyst)

These arise due to blockage of the duct of a sebaceous gland. Sebaceous glands are common on the scalp, face, neck and back.

History

An epidermoid cyst appears as a slow-growing lump, which occasionally discharges or becomes infected and inflamed.

Examination

Examination finds a soft/firm spherical lump with a central punctum on the skin surface. It arises within the dermis and often extends deeper, but it is tethered to the epidermis. It may discharge through the punctum.

Investigations

None.

Treatment

Treat by surgical excision. If the cyst is acutely infected, allow to settle first with antibiotics. An abscess may require incision and drainage. At excision, failure to remove the cyst wall completely may result in recurrence.

Post-operative follow-up

Review with histology and confirm wound healing. Wound infection is common, especially if the cyst ruptures during excision. It usually responds to antibiotics.

Dermoid cyst

Dermoid cysts may be congenital or acquired. Congenital cysts are usually present in young children. They are most common at the embryological fusion lines of the head and neck (inclusion cysts), usually at the outer angle of the eyebrow (external angular dermoid). Acquired cysts are a complication of trauma, where a piece of epidermis is translocated into deeper tissue (implantation cyst). They are commonly seen following hand injuries.

History

There is a firm subcutaneous lump arising at a site of trauma or previous surgery. Alternatively, a soft slow-growing lump, with no history of trauma and typically at the eyebrow, is noticed in early childhood.

Examination

Examination finds a firm discrete lump under the skin, located at embryological fusion lines (congenital) or associated with a previous scar (acquired).

Investigations

Excision biopsy. Congenital cysts are referred to paediatric surgery/plastics for work-up (CT/MRI is indicated for deep extension).

Treatment

Excision biopsy.

Post-operative follow-up

None.

Pilonidal sinus

Pilonidal sinus is a chronic infection of the skin caused by penetration of hairs into the skin and subcutaneous tissues. A sinus is formed that leads to a cavity filled with hair and granulation tissue. Common sites include the natal cleft, between the fingers (hairdressers) or occasionally the umbilicus or axilla.

Differential diagnosis includes perianal fistula, hidradenitis suppurativa and simple boils.

History

Pilonidal sinus is seen as a chronically discharging skin infection that fails to clear despite courses of antibiotics. There may be repeated episodes of inflammation and discharge.

Examination

Perform a general examination. Depending on the site, there will usually be evidence of one or more sinuses, and hairs may be visible within these. There is usually evidence of chronic inflammation or discharging sinus.

Investigations

Microbiology, blood sugar, urine dipstick.

Treatment

Treat conservatively with careful wound toilet and shaving of surrounding hair. Use antibiotics in acute phases, incision and drainage for acute abscesses. Surgical excision may be required for chronic disease; and it may require plastic surgical reconstruction. Consider laser depilation to prevent recurrence.

Post-operative follow-up

Review with histology and to confirm healing.

Hidradenitis suppurativa

This is a chronic indolent disease of skin and subcutaneous tissue in apocrine gland-bearing areas, characterised by recurrent deep abscesses in axillae, groins, perineum and perianal areas. *Staphylococcus aureus* is the usual organism, but occasionally coliforms are cultured.

Differential diagnosis includes folliculitis, carbuncle, cellulitis or, in the perianal area, pilonidal sinus or perianal fistula.

History

There is recurrent inflammation and infection that fails to respond to repeat courses of antibiotics. It is most common in young adult females.

Examination

There is an involved area of skin that is indurated and fibrotic, with evidence of chronic inflammation. Chronically discharging sinuses may be present.

Investigations

Microbiology.

Treatment

Non-surgical treatment should include advice on weight loss and stopping smoking (both are strong risk factors). Encourage careful personal hygiene and antiseptic washes (chlorhexidine). Consider dermatology referral for advice on long-term antibiotics (clindamycin) and antiandrogens (cyproterone acetate) in females. Abscesses require incision and drainage. In severe disease, excision of the affected hair/gland bearing skin may be indicated. Healing is by secondary intention or primary closure for small defects. Alternatively, larger defects are reconstructed with split skin grafts or a local flap (plastic surgery).

Post-treatment follow-up

Review at regular intervals (1–3 months) to monitor the effect of conservative therapy and decide if surgical intervention is indicated.

Subcutaneous lesions

Lipoma

A lipoma is a soft benign tumour of adipose tissue. Lipomas usually occur singly, but may be multiple. They are commonly subcutaneous, but can be intramuscular. Lipomas are normally painless. If the tumour is tender, then it is more likely to be an angiolipoma. Rarely, liposarcomatous change can occur in a benign lipoma. There is a higher index of suspicion for malignant change if the lesion is large, rapidly growing or painful.

History

Appears as a slow-growing lump under the skin; is usually asymptomatic.

Examination

Examination finds a lump in the subcutaneous tissue not attached to the dermis. It is often lobulated. The absence of a punctum helps differentiate it from an epidermoid cyst. The contraction of the underlying muscle helps to distinguish between subcutaneous and intramuscular locations.

Investigations

There are usually none. If diagnosis is uncertain or there are unusual features, ultrasound (USS) or CT/MRI scan is indicated. Consider FNA cytology if the lesion is suspicious.

Treatment

Most lipomas can be excised (shelled out) under local anaesthetic. Large or intramuscular lipomas require general anaesthetic excision. Liposuction may be considered with larger lesions to minimise scarring, but it is associated with a higher recurrence rate.

Post-treatment follow-up

None, unless reviewing with result of investigations or to assess wound healing following large lipoma removal.

Neurofibroma

A neurofibroma is a benign tumour arising from neural tissue and supporting stromal cells. It is a soft fleshy tumour, which is either sessile or pedunculated. Neurofibromatosis (von Recklinghausen's disease) patients have multiple tumours, arising throughout life. It is a disfiguring condition that causes great distress to sufferers. It is commonly caused by autosomal dominant inheritance following sporadic mutation. Type 1 neurofibromatosis is associated with mainly cutaneous features, and type 2 neurofibromatosis is associated with central nervous system (CNS) tumours (neurofibromas). Occasionally, malignant change to neurofibrosarcoma occurs (with increase in size and pain).

History

A single lump or, more commonly, multiple soft cutaneous lumps over the body. Otherwise asymptomatic, although it may become traumatised, leading to inflammation or infection. There may be a positive family history.

Examination

There are usually several fleshy lesions, which may be tender to palpation. Neurofibromatosis is associated with café-au-lait patches and axillary freckles.

Investigation

Excision biopsy to confirm the diagnosis.

Treatment

Treatment is by excision if symptomatic or if there is suspicion of neurofibrosarcomatous change. Delayed healing is common.

Post-operative follow-up

Review with histology and confirm wound healing. Discharge with advice or refer to clinical genetics.

Disorders of the nails
Ingrowing toenail (onychocryptosis)

Ingrowing toenail is a common condition, mainly in young people. It usually affects the lateral edge of the great toenail. A sharp edge of the nail traumatises the nail bed causing pain, ulceration, infection and a granulation tissue response, which exacerbates the condition.

History

There is a history of pain, recurrent inflammation and infection at the side of the nail.

Examination

The condition most commonly affects the lateral side of the great toe but can affect both sides or other toes. The affected skin at the side of the nail is inflamed, boggy and swollen, with onycholysis and creeping over-granulation.

Investigations

Usually none. Microbiology, including fungal scrapings, if diagnosis unclear.

Treatment

Mild cases may respond to antibiotics and chiropody.

Other cases require surgical treatment. Surgical procedures include simple nail avulsion, wedge excision and phenolisation, and Zadek's procedure (total excision of the germinal matrix).

Post-treatment follow-up

Follow up at regular intervals (1–3 months) if using conservative management. Proceed to surgery if such management fails.

Post-operative follow-up

Review to determine wound healing. Complications include infection, prolonged wound healing and recurrence.

Onychogryphosis

This is a 'rams horn' deformity of the toenail, usually affecting the big toes of elderly people.

History

Patients complain of increasing thickening and deformity of the nail, which is difficult to cut and interferes with footwear.

Examination

The nail is thickened, yellow and hooked. Aetiology includes trauma and fungal infections.

Investigations

Microbiology (fungal scrapings).

Treatment

Initial treatment is chiropody. Otherwise removal of the nail or Zadek's procedure.

Post-operative follow-up

Review to confirm healing. Complications are the same as for ingrowing toenail.

Subungal exostosis

This is a bony lump arising from the distal phalanx, which grows underneath the nail. It usually affects the great toe.

History

A young patient complains of pain and deformity of the toenail. The nail may have failed to respond to treatment for ingrowing toenail.

Examination
The toenail appears to be pushed up by a lesion arising underneath the nail bed.

Investigations
An X-ray of the toe reveals the bony exostosis.

Treatment
Consider plastic or orthopaedic surgery referral for removal of the nail and excision of the bony nodule, with careful nail bed preservation.

Post-operative follow-up
Review with histology before discharge.

Groin lumps
One of the most common presentations in general surgery is with a lump in the groin. The differential diagnosis is large but in practical terms the main distinction is between hernias and other causes. Differential diagnosis of a lump in the groin:
- skin and soft tissues
  - sebaceous cyst
  - lipoma
- hernias
  - inguinal
  - femoral
- vascular
  - femoral artery aneurysm
  - sapheno varix
- lymphadenopathy
  - generalised versus localised
- renal/urogenital system
  - ectopic or maldescended testis
  - transplanted kidney.

Inguinal hernias
History
There may be a sudden onset related to abdominal straining. There is a reducible lump, which may be increasing in size.

Examination
There is a reducible lump in the groin arising from above the inguinal ligament (usually above and medial to the pubic tubercle). There is an expansile cough impulse. Direct hernias appear medial to the deep ring.

Investigations
None, or USS.

Treatment
Conservative if unfit for surgery, but most are repaired surgically.

Post-treatment follow-up
None, or review with results of investigations.

Post-operative follow-up

Review to confirm successful repair and wound healing at around six weeks.

Femoral hernias

History

There may be sudden onset related to abdominal straining, typically in the female. There is a reducible lump, which may be increasing in size.

Examination

Examination finds a reducible lump in the groin arising below the medial end of the inguinal ligament (below and lateral to the pubic tubercle).

Investigations

None, or USS.

Treatment

Surgical repair.

Post-operative follow-up

Review to confirm successful repair and wound healing at six weeks.

Lymph node mass

Enlarged lymph nodes in the groin can be a great source of diagnostic confusion.

The femoral canal normally contains a lymph node, which if enlarged can be mistaken for a femoral hernia. Lymph nodes overlying the femoral artery may transmit the pulsation and resemble a femoral artery aneurysm.

If enlarged lymph nodes are recognised, their management is the same as lymph nodes elsewhere in the body.

The objective is to determine whether the enlargement is localised or whether it is part of a generalised lymphadenopathy. If it is localised, *examine the whole drainage area* for a cause, i.e. infective, neoplastic.

History

Ask about local symptoms for the drainage area of that group of lymph nodes, e.g. leg, perineum, anus, scrotum, lower abdomen or back. Ask about other lumps elsewhere on the body. General symptoms include weight loss and night sweats.

Examination

Examine the lump, noting size, consistency and so on. Determine whether the lump is isolated or part of a general enlargement. Perform a general examination of all lymph node sites including the liver and spleen. Perform a thorough examination of the drainage area of the lymph node for a possible infective or neoplastic cause of lymph node enlargement. Include a rectal examination for possible anal tumour.

Investigations

Excision biopsy of the enlarged lymph node is not the first investigation. Laboratory tests include FBC and blood film, plasma viscosity/erythrocyte sedimentation rate (PV/ESR) and Monospot/Paul Bunnel (for glandular fever). Perform fine-needle aspiration of non-pulsatile lumps for cytology, and use microbiology, including Ziehl-Neelsen (ZN) stain and TB culture. Use USS to exclude other causes. Perform an excision biopsy for lymphoma.

Treatment

Treatment depends on the results of investigations.

In children and young people, once *lymphoma is excluded*, the cause is *usually infective* and will settle. Similarly, the management of TB lymphadenopathy is the relevant chemotherapy.

In cases related to generalised lymphadenopathy, e.g. lymphoma/leukaemia or glandular fever, the management is of the underlying condition. Local causes may include SCC, melanoma, genital infection/neoplasm or an infective lesion on a leg.

Follow-up

Review at short intervals until cancer is excluded. Determine whether excision biopsy is necessary.

Post-operative follow-up

Review with histology and confirm wound healing. Treat any underlying condition appropriately.

Possible complications include damage to surrounding structures, lymphocoele, infected lymphocoele and non-healing. Non-healing is particularly associated with TB or neoplastic causes and responds to treatment of the underlying condition.

Lipoma

(*see* above)

Sebaceous cyst

(*see* above)

Hydrocoele of the cord

Usually, the hydrocoeles are confined to the scrotum. Isolated hydrocoeles can occur in the spermatic cord and present with lumps in the inguinal canal.

History

There is a slow-growing, non-reducible lump in the groin.

Examination

Examination finds a non-reducible lump in the groin that does not arise from the deep inguinal ring. The lump is usually mobile, has *no expansile cough impulse* and may be made to transilluminate. The lump moves down with traction on the ipsilateral testis.

Investigations

None, or USS and/or FNA.

Treatment

Aspiration or surgical excision.

Follow-up

None, or review with results of investigations (at four to eight weeks).

Post-operative follow-up

Review with histology and to confirm wound healing (at four to six weeks). Complications are similar to those for inguinal hernia.

Undescended/maldescended testis

Undescended testes are seldom palpable in the groin except in the thinnest of individuals, but maldescended testes may lie in an abnormal position after emerging through the external inguinal ring.

History

There is a tender lump in the groin, upper thigh or lower abdomen. There is an absent testicle on one side of the scrotum. Ask whether the testicle has always been absent or has been noticed in the scrotum at some time. Maldescended testes are usually asymptomatic. If symptoms occur it may be that the testicle is now diseased.

Examination

Examination reveals an absent testis in the scrotum. There is a testicle-like lump in one of the above sites.

Investigations

None, or USS to identify testicular internal architecture.

Treatment

If the patient is pre-pubertal, replace in the scrotum if the testis is normal to inspection at operation. After puberty, orchidectomy is performed, as the testis is unlikely to function and carries an increased risk of tumour formation.

Follow-up

Review with results of investigations (at four to eight weeks).

Post-operative follow-up

Review with histology (if orchidectomy performed) and confirm wound healing. Complications are similar to those for inguinal hernia or hydrocoele repair.

Sapheno varix

A sapheno varix may be best described as a venous aneurysm of the long saphenous vein just before its junction with the femoral vein in the groin.

History

There is a soft lump in the groin which disappears on lying down. Usually there is a history of varicose veins.

Examination

Examination finds a soft reducible lump in the groin arising below the middle of the inguinal ligament. The lump disappears on lying down. Varicose veins are usually visible in the affected leg.

Investigations

None, or venous Duplex scan.

Treatment

Varicose vein operation.

Post-treatment follow-up

Review with results of investigations (at one to three months)

Post-operative follow-up
Review to determine the success of the operation and to confirm wound healing. Complications are those described for varicose vein operation.

Femoral artery aneurysm
True femoral aneurysms involve *all three layers* of the artery wall and often occur in conjunction with abdominal aortic or popliteal aneurysms, which may also require treatment. False femoral aneurysms usually occur after arterial injury or cannulation of the femoral artery. Blood escapes from the lumen of the artery but is 'contained' by the adventitia of the artery to produce a swelling that transmits a pulsation.

History
True femoral aneurysms usually present with a history of a gradually increasing firm pulsatile lump in the groin. Femoral aneurysms may embolise and block off distal arteries, so ask about claudication, rest pain or blue toes. If there is a history of recent injury or cannulation, e.g. cardiac angiography, then consider false femoral aneurysm as the cause.

Examination
Look for a pulsatile lump in the groin that does not reduce or disappear when the patient is lying down. A true aneurysm is expansile in three directions at once (medial, lateral, anterior). A false aneurysm has only transmitted pulsation.

Examine all other arteries for aneurysmal disease. Examine for evidence of distal embolisation and peripheral ischaemia.

Investigations
Duplex ultrasound of aorta, iliac, femoral and popliteal arteries.

Treatment
Surgical repair of both forms of aneurysm.

Follow-up
Review with investigations (at one to three months)

Post-operative follow-up
Review to confirm graft function and wound healing.

Scrotal lumps/testicular swellings
Although disorders of the testes and scrotum are increasingly being referred to urologists, they are still a common problem in general surgery clinics.

By definition, scrotal lumps originate in the scrotum, and on examination it nearly always is possible to get above the lump. If the lump is confirmed as scrotal, the next question is whether the swelling involves the whole scrotum or whether it is localised to one side or one part of the scrotum. Does the swelling arise from the skin and connective tissue of the scrotum, the coverings of the testicle, i.e. tunica vaginalis, the appendages of the testicle, e.g. epididymis, or the body of the testicle itself? Is the lump cystic or solid? The most important objective in all scrotal lumps is to *exclude testicular cancer*.

Skin
Problems may include sebaceous cysts, warts, chancre and skin cancer, e.g. epithelioma (most common in chimney sweeps and tar workers).

Connective tissue

Idiopathic lymphoedema occurs spontaneously or in response to friction and other triggers. Secondary lymphoedema may result from generalised oedema, e.g. CCF, renal failure. Infections may cause lymphatic obstruction, e.g. *Wuchereria bancrofti* produces the well known elephantiasis of the scrotum. Pelvic cellulitis, ascites and skin infection are other causes.

Tunica vaginalis

This describes a double walled covering of the testis. In health this contains a small amount of fluid which acts as a lubricant for movement of the testis. A large amount of fluid can accumulate to produce a hydrocoele. Hydrocoeles may occur spontaneously or be secondary to underlying disease of the testis, e.g. infection, tumour. Blood may also accumulate in the same way and is known as a haematocoele. In cases of gross infection pus may accumulate to produce a pyocoele.

Testicular appendages

Cysts and swellings occur in the epididymis and spermatic cord, producing lumps that are palpable and separate from the testis, e.g. epididymal cyst, varicocoele.

Testis

Lumps arising from the body of the testis are tumours until proven otherwise.

Hydrocoele

Hydrocoeles are a collection of fluid in the tunica surrounding the testes.

Hydrocoeles may be primary or secondary. Primary hydrocoeles occur spontaneously and there is no underlying cause. They usually occur in men aged over 40. In secondary hydrocoeles, fluid accumulates because of underlying inflammation, infection, trauma or tumour of the testis, and it occurs in younger men.

Primary hydrocoeles may be classified as the following.

- Vaginal hydrocoele, which occurs within the tunica vaginalis and surrounds the testis and does not communicate with the peritoneal cavity.
- Congenital hydrocoele, which is associated with a hernial sac and communicates with the peritoneal cavity.
- Infantile hydrocoele, which extends from the testis to the deep inguinal ring but does not communicate with the peritoneal cavity.
- Hydrocoele of the cord, which occurs anywhere along the spermatic cord, and can occur in women as hydrocoele of the Canal of Nuck.

Objectives

Treatment objectives are to diagnose the hydrocoele, differentiate primary from secondary, treat the hydrocoele and treat the underlying cause.

History

Patients complain of a gradually increasing swelling of the scrotum. In primary hydrocoeles, this is usually painless, although patients may report a dragging sensation. In secondary hydrocoeles, there may be a history of tenderness, inflammation and systemic illness. Ask about genito-urinary infections. In children with congenital hydrocoeles these may fill up during the day when upright and empty at night when supine.

Examination

Examine the scrotum, inguinal region and the testes. Confirm the presence of a scrotal lump and assess the swelling according to the criteria in the introduction to scrotal lumps.

If the testis is not palpable separate from the lump, then a hydrocoele is likely. Does the lump transilluminate? All primary hydrocoeles transilluminate because they contain clear watery fluid. Secondary hydrocoeles may not transilluminate to the same extent because they may contain turbid fluid, pus or blood. A hydrocoele of the cord moves down when traction is applied to the testis. Aspiration of a tense hydrocoele may be necessary to allow palpation of the testis.

Investigations

For primary hydrocoeles, USS may confirm difficult cases. A sample of fluid may be aspirated and sent for cytology and microbiology. The testis is then palpated to confirm a normal shape, contour and smooth surface.

For secondary hydrocoeles, USS is usually performed to confirm the presence of a hydrocoele and to examine the underlying testis. A sample of fluid may be aspirated and sent for cytology and microbiology. If tumour is suspected, ultrasound is mandatory, and so are determinations of serum alpha-foetoprotein (AFP) and human chorionic gonadotropin (beta hCG). If urinary tract infection is suspected, a sample of urine is sent for microbiology.

Treatment

For primary hydrocoeles, aspirate to dryness and review in two to four weeks. If the hydrocoele recurs, a further attempt at aspiration is justified. In the elderly and unfit this can be repeated every two to three months, but in most patients surgery is indicated if the hydrocoele recurs.

In children with a congenital hydrocoele, an inguinal operation is required to deal with the accompanying hernia sac.

For secondary hydrocoele, treatment is primarily of the underlying disorder.

Follow-up

Secondary hydrocoeles should be reviewed at short intervals (one to four weeks) until cancer is excluded. Thereafter, review at regular intervals until evidence shows that the underlying condition is responding to treatment. In primary hydrocoele, review every one to three months and aspirate or arrange for surgery. Complications of aspiration include infection and haematoma.

Post-operative follow-up

In primary hydrocoele, review after four to six weeks to determine the success of the operation and to check wound healing.

Epididymal cyst

Epididymal cysts are similar collections of fluid to hydrocoeles but are separate from the testis. Spermatocoeles are similar to epididymal cysts but consist of turbid fluid that contains spermatozoa. Both may be multiple or multilocular.

Objectives

Treatment objectives are to diagnose the cyst, exclude other causes and treat the cyst.

History

Patients complain of a gradually increasing lump separate from the testes. There is seldom any secondary history, although patients may report an aching or dragging sensation in the testicle, groin or lumbar region.

Examination

Perform a general and abdominal examination. Confirm the presence of a scrotal lump – you can get above it. The lump is smooth, oval and separate from, above and to the lateral side of a normal testis. Epididymal cysts usually transilluminate, and may be multiple and bilateral.

Investigation

None, or ultrasound in difficult cases. Lumps may be aspirated to dryness. Aspiration of clear watery fluid confirms the diagnosis (whitish turbid fluid suggests a spermatocoele). Blood-stained fluid should be sent for cytology and microbiology.

Treatment

Aspirate to dryness in the clinic and review. Epididymal cysts tend to recur after aspiration.

Post-treatment follow-up

Review at one- to three-monthly intervals. If the cyst recurs more than twice, surgery is indicated. Complications of aspiration include haematoma and infection.

Post-operative follow-up

Determine the successful removal of the cyst and wound healing. Generally the scrotum heals very well. Wound infections respond to antibiotics. Successful removal of one cyst does not prevent others from forming in the future.

Haematocoele

Haematoceles are similar to hydrocoeles but *contain blood instead of fluid*.

Haematoceles may result from aspiration of a hydrocoele if the needle causes bleeding within the scrotum. Haematoceles may also complicate surgical procedures of the groin or scrotum, e.g. hydrocoele, scrotal hernia repair. Other causes include trauma, torsion or tumour.

Objectives

Treatment objectives are to diagnose haematocoele, exclude cancer and treat the haematocoele.

History

Determine the onset of the swelling and any precipitating cause, e.g. surgical procedure or trauma. Onset related to trauma or torsion is usually rapid. Tumour causes a more gradual onset. However, sudden onset may occur due to rupture of a small vessel involved in the growth. Patients may ascribe this to an episode of trauma, which may be mild. Testes involved with tumour are more prone to bleeding after trauma.

Examination

Examine the scrotum, inguinal region and testes. A haematocele is usually a tense, firm scrotal lump, similar on examination to a hydrocoele except it does not transilluminate. In addition, there may be ecchymosis of the scrotal skin.

Investigations

Aspiration of blood confirms the diagnosis but does not establish the underlying cause. If tumour is suspected then USS should be performed to define testicular architecture, and measure serum beta-hCG and AFP.

Treatment
If the condition presents acutely, admit for exploration and evacuation of haematoma once tumour has been excluded. In elderly unfit patients, or if the haematocele is chronic, i.e. organised haematoma, a conservative course can be followed with analgesia and a scrotal support.

Post-treatment follow-up
If immediate exploration is not indicated, review at short intervals (one to four weeks) until cancer is excluded. If a conservative course is being followed, review at regular intervals (one to three months) until there is evidence of resolution. Then discharge or give an open appointment.

Post-operative follow-up
Review to confirm the success of the operation and wound healing (at four to six weeks). Complications are similar to those for hydrocoele repair.

Varicocoele
Varicocoele is a malformation of dilated veins surrounding the testis in the scrotum. Varicocoeles may be primary or secondary. The vast majority are primary and are congenital. Their importance is that they may inhibit sperm production because they maintain the testis at a higher temperature than is optimal for spermatogenesis. Secondary varicocoeles are rare but may be caused by obstruction to the testicular vein as it joins the renal vein, by thrombus or tumour extending along the renal vein or by fibrosis caused by excess adrenaline in the blood draining from an adrenal phaeochromocytoma.

Objectives
Treatment objectives are to diagnose the varicocoele, detect secondary causes, treat the varicocoele and treat any underlying cause.

History
Usually young men (teens and early twenties) complain of a generalised swelling in the scrotum that is worse on standing. A patient may also complain of a heaviness or dragging sensation. Varicocoeles may occur in older age groups or in patients with systemic symptoms suggesting kidney tumours or phaeochromocytomas. There may be a history of infertility.

Examination
On standing the scrotum feels full – like a bag of worms. The swelling reduces considerably and may disappear on lying down and on elevation of the scrotum. The testis is normal to palpation.

Investigations
USS of testis and, if indicated, of kidney and adrenal gland. If secondary causes are suspected CT/MRI of kidney and adrenal, and investigation of urinary free catecholamine levels, FBC, urea and electrolytes.

Treatment
Mild cases do not require treatment, especially if they are unilateral. The dragging sensation may be helped by a scrotal support. More severe cases can be treated by ligation of all but one of the veins in the spermatic cord in the groin or laparoscopically by clipping the veins inside the peritoneal cavity.

Post-treatment follow-up

If unilateral and mild, advise and discharge or review once (at four to six weeks) after use of scrotal support to relieve symptoms. If symptoms are persistent or severe, surgery may be indicated.

Post-operative follow-up

Review after four to six weeks to determine the success of the operation (gauged by relief from heavy sensation and resolution of veins) and check wound healing.

Chronic epididymo-orchitis

Epididymitis describes inflammation/infection confined to the spermatic cord and epididymis. Orchitis describes inflammation/infection confined to the testis. Epididymo-orchitis describes infection/inflammation affecting both. It can be acute or chronic. Acute infections are usually investigated and treated as an in-patient procedure and will not be described again here. Chronic infections may be referred to the outpatient clinic due to repeated episodes of inflammation or for investigation of a testicular swelling or hydrocoele.

In children and in men over the age of 35, acute epididymo-orchitis is usually secondary to bacterial infection of the urinary tract, which may have disordered anatomy allowing infection. In younger men the urinary tract is normal and epididymo-orchitis is usually due to sexually transmitted organisms, e.g. *Neisseria gonorrhoea, Chlamydia, Herpes simplex* and *Trichomonas vaginalis.*

In all age groups, epididymitis can be secondary to systemic disease, e.g. TB, *Brucella*, sarcoid and *Cryptococcus*. Other rare causes of testicular infection include the following.

◇ Pyogenic orchitis, which may occur following an episode of generalised sepsis and occasionally destroys the testis.

◇ Viral orchitis, which may occur secondary to influenza and coxsackie virus infection but most commonly is secondary to mumps. It occurs exclusively in post-pubertal patients and starts four to six days after the parotitis to give testicular swelling and a hydrocoele.

◇ Granulomatous orchitis, which may occur following trauma, infection, chemicals or post-vasectomy. The testis becomes enlarged and tender.

Objectives

Objectives are to diagnose epididymitis, exclude tumour or underlying systemic disease, exclude abnormalities of the urinary tract, treat epididymitis and treat any underlying condition.

History

Take a general history for symptoms, which may suggest a systemic cause. Usually, symptoms are confined to the genito-urinary tract, and patients describe recurrent episodes of pain in the epididymis and testis following episodes of dysuria or urethral discharge. This may settle with a course of antibiotics but not completely resolve and it may be a continuing source of symptoms over weeks or months. Ask about sexual encounters to determine the risk of infection and symptoms affecting the patient's sexual partner.

If indicated, ask questions to exclude the rarer causes outlined above.

Examination

Perform a general examination. The scrotum may be erythematous, swollen and tender. A hydrocoele may be present. Try to determine the point of maximal tenderness, i.e.

epididymis or testis or both. The epididymis may feel thickened and hard. The testis may be enlarged, irregular and firm.

Investigations
Investigations include midstream specimen of urine (MSU) or microscopy, and culture and sensitivity (C&S) test of urethral discharge. If cultures are not diagnostic, send blood for immunology for IgG and IgM antibodies to *Chlamydia*. Check U&Es to exclude evidence of renal impairment. In children and elderly men, further investigation of the urinary tract may be indicated to exclude congenital abnormalities or obstruction.

If tumour cannot be excluded, a USS of the testis is indicated, as well as estimations of serum AFP and beta-hCG. If the USS suggests disordered testicular architecture, surgical biopsy/orchidectomy of the testis may be indicated, which may also be necessary for the diagnosis of tuberculosis, sarcoid, malakoplakia and some other conditions.

Treatment
Symptomatic treatment includes analgesia, scrotal support and occasionally drainage of a tense hydrocoele. Children and older men are treated for common urinary pathogens. Chronic epididymo-orchitis in young men may require prolonged treatment with doxycycline, erythromycin or similar drugs. Treatment of secondary conditions is of the underlying condition. Treatment of mumps orchitis is symptomatic.

Post-treatment follow-up
Follow up at short intervals (one to four weeks) until acute infection settles and tumour or serious causes are excluded. Thereafter, follow up at longer intervals (one to three months) to allow time for treatment to work and inflammation to settle. Remember to arrange further investigation of the urinary tract in children and elderly men. Complications of epididymo-orchitis include abscess formation, testicular infarction and obstruction of sperm. Abscess formation is suspected if infection fails to settle and pain and swelling persist. USS may demonstrate pus. Treatment requires incision and drainage or orchidectomy.

Post-operative follow-up
Review with histology and treat the underlying cause appropriately. Complications include wound infection, hydrocoele and scarring.

Testicular tumours
Testicular tumours are the commonest tumours affecting young men. The management of such tumours is specialised, and the general surgical management consists mainly of diagnosis and referral to a urologist and oncologist. It is important to consider the diagnosis in any patient with scrotal pathology, especially since complete cure can be expected if diagnosis is made early enough.

Tumours may arise from all tissue components in the testis, but 90% of tumours are either teratomas (ages 25–30) or seminomas (ages 35–40). Other tumours account for the remaining 10% and include lymphomas (which tend to develop in elderly men), Sertoli cell and Leydig cell tumours.

Carcinoma in situ has been identified with increasing use of testicular biopsy for investigation of infertility. These patients have a 50% risk of developing testicular cancer within five years.

Objectives
Objectives are to diagnose testicular cancer, stage the cancer and treat the cancer.

History

Take a general history. The classical history is of painless enlargement of the testis, but the condition can present mimicking infection, hydrocoele and trauma. The diagnosis should be considered in all scrotal swellings. Weight loss, back pain or shortness of breath may indicate extensive disease. Headaches may indicate brain metastases.

Examination

Perform a general examination. Examine the scrotum and determine the characteristics of the lump or swelling. Examine for distant spread. Examine the supraclavicular fossae for lymph nodes and the chest for bronchial lung metastases, pleural effusions and so on. Examine the abdomen for central lymph node masses and other signs.

Investigations

USS of both testes. Serum estimation of B-hCG and AFP, which is raised in 50–90% of non-seminomatous tumours. These levels may also be raised in seminomas with a teratomatous element.

Definitive diagnosis is by inguinal exploration of testis and testicular biopsy, performed by an experienced urologist. Initial staging is by CXR and by thoracic and abdominal CT scan. Bone and brain scans may be indicated by clinical findings.

Treatment

Treatment is administered by a urologist and oncologist with a special interest. It consists of radiotherapy and chemotherapy, depending on the stage of the tumour.

Post-treatment follow-up

Follow-up is undertaken by the urologist/oncologist.

Index